Terrains and Pathology
in
Acupuncture

Volume One

Correlations with Diathetic Medicine

Yves Requena, M.D.

Paradigm Publications   **Brookline, Massachusetts**
1986

**Terrains and Pathology in Acupuncture, Volume One
Correlations with Diathetic Medicine**
by
Yves Requena, M.D.

Original French Edition
Terrains et Pathologie en Acupunctur
Copyright c 1980 Maloine S.A. Editeur
ISBN 2-224-0613-6

English Edition
Copyright © 1986 Paradigm Publications
ISBN 0-912111-08-9

First English Paperback Edition
Copyright © 1995 Paradigm Publications
ISBN 0-912111-49-6

Library of Congress Number 86-8145

Published by:
Paradigm Publications
44 Linden Street
Brookline, Massachusetts 02146

This book was produced and typeset using software and services
provided by Textware International of Cambridge, Massachusetts.

Translator: Allan Dalcher
Supplemental translations: Paul Zmiewski
Editor: Robert L. Felt
Cover design: Herb Rich III

Introduction
to the
English Edition

Terrains and Pathology in Acupuncture is a welcome addition the the slowly growing collection of mature acupuncture texts available in English. Dr. Requena's approach may at first seem unusual to English speaking practitioners, because he discusses aspects of acupuncture diagnostic and therapeutic logic with which many are unfamiliar. This is not the case in France.

Acupuncture has been an academic arena for French scholars and physicians since Jesuit missionaries returned from China in the seventeenth century with classical texts and clinical reports. Early in this century George Soulie de Morant translated and published the first comprehensive work in French of the major Chinese acupuncture texts. This work has influenced all acupuncture education in the West, and it provoked French and German scientists to study the measurable properties of acupuncture points, meridians and needles. Research, scholarship, debate, translation and decoding, synthesis of diagnostic and therapeutic approaches from classical texts, creation of "pure" as well as "hybrid" schools, re-examination and re-synthesis, have been the French contribution to contemporary Western acupuncture.

What I welcome most about this book is the timely introduction of the concepts of terrain, constitution, and temperament into our literature. That they are presented in a framework blending traditional Chinese acupuncture principles with contemporary psychological and physiological organization should not be surprising, given that Requena is one of the more prolific contributors to the current French "tradition." He studied acupuncture with Dr. Nguyen Van Nghi while attending medical school in Marseilles, after which his scholarly passion led him to rigorously correlate and integrate the medical information of both fields.

Here he takes two of the most common models of symptom organization in acupuncture diagnostics — the six energy levels and the five elements — and combines the first with a psychological inventory test and the second with a system of "catalytic medicine" used to support and prolong the acupuncture therapy. In the first sections of the book he reviews concisely the major tenets of acupuncture and introduces terrain, constitution, and temperament with correlations that are neither forced nor rigid. The latter sections serve as an encyclopaedic tour of the pathology of Shao Yang, Jue Yin and Yang Ming, where he examines traditional acupuncture dynamics in a context of Western-defined physiopathology. It is well

i

indexed, and will serve the practical reader as an excellent reference when pondering patient problems.

I find **Terrains and Pathology** a useful synthesis: for those already comfortable in their understanding and practice of acupuncture it provides a refreshing new point of view; for those just beginning it is a good starting point of orientation for all future study. And there is more to come.

Joseph M. Helms, M.D.
Chairman, Physician Acupuncture Programs
University Extension, UCLA School of Medicine

Berkeley, California, June 1986

Definitions of Terms for the English Edition

Before commencing, it is a good idea to define the term *Terrain* as we have used it and to define other terms frequently used in our discussion that are either nuances of Terrain or that express ways of identifying, improving or balancing a Terrain.

Terrain is "the state of an organism, of an organ, or of a tissue, regarding its resistance to pathogenic agents." If this orthodox definition seems broad, it is nonetheless used in an extremely narrow sense in allopathy and has little consequence for how we treat our patients. When we mean that an individual has a predisposition for diabetes, we say in French that he is "of diabetic terrain." This means nothing more than he or she has a high risk of becoming diabetic, sooner or later, because of their genetic inheritance.

However, a broader definition of the term *Terrain* is commonly used in European medical circles concerned with homeopathy, trace elements and phytotherapy, or herbal medicine. There, the term retains the significance it had in antiquity and in the medicine of the middle ages in Greek, Indian and Egyptian medicine, as well as in alchemy. In this sense, Terrain is the set of an individual's innate predispositions that define his physical as well as psychological reactivity to any type of aggression, considered globally and assuming a close psychosomatic relationship.

Initially, an individual's terrain is determined genetically, but changes throughout life, due to severe climatic changes, drug addictions, infections, vaccinations, surgical operations, traffic accidents, errors of nutrition, excessive sedentarity or excessive physical exercise, or psycho-affective shocks and upsets. In these medical paradigms, the therapist takes into account both a diagnosis of the patient's innate terrain (which may often be subtle and complex) and a meticulous analysis of the specific circumstances that have marked its evolution.

We have retained the term *Terrain* in our translation into English. Our object is to fix in the minds of our readers this broader and more holistic meaning of the term, in the hope of promoting a deeper understanding of the patients we examine and treat.

Constitution is defined as the set of an individual's congenital, somatic and psychological features. One's constitution, then, is his fixed and unchanging genetic heritage. This congenital heritage includes above all the program of a predisposition to certain physical traits, be they morbid or morphological. The vulnerability to infection, for example, is a common trait among those of anergic constitution.

Temperament refers to an individual's innate traits of character, to the psycho-physiological complex that determine behavior. This definition is not far from that of *Terrain*. It applies, above all, to innate psychological behavior as it is determined physiologically.

Terrain Medicines are medical doctrines that consider the individual as a whole, that consider the whole organism, and not only the deficient organ that expresses itself pathologically. *Terrain Medicines* also consider the relationship between people and their environment. They account for climatic, ecological, psychological, telluric and astronomical conditions. In this sense, acupuncture is a real terrain medicine, as is confirmed by the eight rules of diagnosis (Yin—Yang, Inside—Outside, Cold—Heat, Excess—Deficiency) and by the sheng and ke cycle in the five phases. The classic Chinese metaphors of the root and the branch are good illustrations of this way of thinking, as are the correlations between the physiology of the viscera and the seasons, the hours of the day and of the night, the planets, the celestial stems and the terrestrial branches. Acupuncture may be considered one of the most perfect models of a wholistic medicine.

Diathetic or *Catalytic Medicine* is a therapy that uses trace elements prescribed in doses that are infinitesimal but not homeopathic. Even one microgram is still a substantial dose. Here, there is no dilution with dynamization. A trace element's mode of action is catalytic by nature and helps to regularize the enzymatic reactions that occur naturally in the body. This medical doctrine classifies individuals according to their specific morbid predispositions, by way of a meticulous analysis of their morbid or pathological states, into five groups known as *diatheses*, from the Greek diathesis or "predisposition," from which we derive the name *Diathetic Medicine*.

Foreword

The title of this book elicits three questions:

> What is the purpose of introducing the concept of Terrain in a work on acupuncture and how may this be done?

> May we speak of pathology in acupuncture as we do in allopathic medicine?

> Is there a correlation between acupuncture and diathetic medicine? If so, does this correlation deserve to figure in the title of this work and to occupy so much attention in this present study?

To answer these three questions, I think it is useful to present acupuncture and diathetic medicine separately, examining their similarities, and establishing a common ground for the two disciplines.

In discussing acupuncture, I feel it is time to face the more obscure aspects of this medical theory, the more intimate aspects, to come to a better understanding of its nature. Thus, we may more thoroughly comprehend its field of application.

It is no longer advisable for the Western scientific world to ignore the esoteric and metaphysical nature of the origins of acupuncture. Why should we be ashamed of telling the truth, especially when we know that it works? On the contrary, it seems useful to know all the facts and to transpose them into our modern language, to bring them into the light of present day knowledge, instead of hiding behind the simplistic and restricted concept of reflexotherapy, only to save face and court the prejudiced.

Volume One
Table of Contents

Traditional Chinese Medicine and Diathetic Medicine

*E*nergy *flows unceasingly through the Yin and Yang meridians. Energy is immaterial, the body is material; together they form man.*
— *Su Wen*, Chapter 6

Introduction to Acupuncture

The Fundamental Laws

Contrary to the belief shared by many in the Western academic world, acupuncture is not based only on what is known as empirical knowledge. To be convinced of this, we have only to consult the brilliant study by sinologist Marcel Granet, entitled *Chinese Thought*.[1] The development of Chinese medical thought does stem from empiricism, as does any medicine that readjusts its treatment according to experimental findings and experience. It is also based on cosmogenic Taoist theory, the origin of which is almost impossible to trace with any precision, and on Chinese analogical reasoning, with its refined, specific, binary Yin—Yang concept.

This reasoning is fundamental to Chinese civilization and permeates all Chinese speculative thought. The deductions made according to this system form the most fundamental basis of Chinese medicine. It influenced even the earliest practitioners, who classified their findings according to this binary concept, which, intellectually speaking, was probably inherited from Oriental spirituality and from Chinese way of life. In the same way, at a later stage, the same phenomenon occurred in the fields of social and political organization and in military strategy.

In examining the monument of Chinese medical doctrine, it is difficult to separate that of metaphysical or inductive origin from that of analogical, deductive or empirical origin. The basis of this theoretical medical knowledge is found in the earliest known work on acupuncture, the *Nei Jing Su Wen,* which dates from at least 200 BC.[2] A succinct summary of the theoretical elements that stand as laws in Chinese medicine will promote an understanding of this work.

— *First Postulate:* Any living organism, and man in particular, may be considered as an interdependent, intertransforming system.

— *Second Postulate:* Man proceeds from Heaven and from Earth. He is as much a part of one as of the other and incorporates within himself the principles of both. He is, in his organization and in his structure, an identical scale model of the forces and elements found in the universe.[3] As such, he is subject to the same laws and suffers the same variations (seasonal and, specifically, climatic). This second postulate is derived from the Yin—Yang (Heaven—Earth) classification.

Yin-Yang Theory

This is the most famous, and usually the least well understood of all theories. Chinese thought developed a binary classification, whereby everything falls under one of two symbolic categories that represent Heaven and Earth or, respectively, Yang and Yin. The antagonistic and interdependent relationship between Yin and Yang is the universal law of the material world. It is the principle and source of existence of all things. This relationship seems, to the uninformed, a perfect example of empirical classification.

1

Considered Yin phenomena are: the earth, the moon, nighttime, woman, what is cold, heavy or solid, the body, winter and rest. Yang phenomena are: heaven, the sun, daytime, man, what is warm, light or gaseous, the mind, summer and activity. These concepts are original for two reasons: first, they are not deduced from simple empirical speculation. On the contrary, they stem from a Taoist philosophy that invests them with a transcendental meaning and an immanent quality of such extent that each object or phenomenon in the universe consists of two aspects, Yin and Yang. These are at once opposite and complementary. This conceptual paradox defies the foundations of common rationality and the Newtonian paradigm.

From a speculative point of view, Yin—Yang theory predicts the theory of relativity and defies the principle of identity based on mere materialistic observation. In the *Nei Jing Su Wen*[4] we read, ''The appearance, seen from the outside, is no longer appearance.'' Yin—Yang is never a definitive conclusion. Yin contains Yang and can engender Yang. Yin in excess even *becomes* Yang. We must understand that Yin—Yang concepts are not simplistic categories derived from an analogical process, but practical symbols useful in describing the phenomena observed in relativistic terms.

As Marcel Granet points out, Western philosophers have always tried to define these two emblems according to the language of Western doctrines; sometimes as substances, sometimes as forces or energies. We owe the first definition of Yin and Yang to certain Western sinologists among whom Henry Maspero is the leader. In his prewar translations he interpreted Yin and Yang in terms of ''substances.'' He attributed, in the words of Granet, ''to Chinese thought a tendency toward a substantiated duality, and found in the Tao an idea of supreme reality, akin to a divine principle.''[5] This could only lead to misunderstanding.

A second definition is interesting in light of its comparison of Yin—Yang theory with the symbols used in modern physics. Hu Shih, Guiseppe Tucci and D.T. Suzuki agree with such a Yin—Yang representation. Since Yang is represented as a continuous line (—) and Yin as a discontinuous line (– –) they see a prefiguration of undulatory or wave movement (continuous) and of quantum movement (discontinuous). This is not surprising coming as it does from Oriental specialists in energy. On a philosophical level, these relative and complementary symbols allow us to go beyond the body-soul dualism on which our Western religions and philosophies are based. We must also acknowledge the superior insight of the Chinese philosophers and admire the refinement of their speculation.

Yin and Yang were from the beginning used by many theorists, astronomers, practitioners of the arts of divination, musicians and doctors. Based on their use in these fields, we can define two important features of Yin and Yang.

> (1) They are the concrete and antithetical aspect of time and contain the cyclical quality inherent in time.
> (2) They are the concrete and antithetical aspect of space. Here, again, the concept of alternation exists and prevails.

From these two specifics, Chinese thought derived the concept of relativity and the simultaneous classification of spatial and temporal phenomena. It created an original correlation that, in medicine, gave birth to chronobiology long before its time in the West. Thus, the Chinese succeeded in organizing their thought without needing to differentiate between species and types. Marcel Granet writes, "Completely dominated by the concept of efficiency, Chinese thinking moves in a world of symbols made of correspondences and oppositions that we only have to bring into play should we desire to understand or to act." The Chinese had already created the concept of synchronicity that is spoken of by modern day physicists and astrophysicists.

In medicine, Yin-Yang theory led Chinese doctors through the interplay of correspondences and oppositions to a particularly rich idea of man:

(1) Man and the world around him, his environment with concepts of climatic, seasonal and ecological influences;

(2) Man and the world within him, where all the functions thus classified allow for an interplay of multiple correspondences.

This latter thought led the non-anatomist, non-physiologist Chinese to the discovery of correlations that science would only discover some twenty to forty centuries later, and to original relationships that, as far as Western science goes, may not yet have seen the light of day. Recent work in chronobiology has as yet only glimpsed a few of the correlations defined by the Chinese in the *Nei Jing Su Wen*. The simple binary Yin—Yang classification is not, however, the only key to the code. The dual principle may be applied to three, four, five, six or even more variables.

Without going into demonstrations that would take us beyond the purpose of this introduction, the binary classification may be extended to three variables. Thus, man with his feet on the earth and his head in heaven, stands between and proceeds from both. He is, therefore, the geometrical site of Yin and Yang. This explains the divisions of Inferior-Superior, Left-Right and Anterior-Posterior.

- The head pertains to Yang

- The trunk is divided into three levels, each of them Yang, Yin and Yang, and Yin.

- The lower limbs are Yin

- The left is Yang

- The right is Yin

- The front is Yin

- The back is Yang[6]

The topography of acupuncture meridians, their direction and pathways are deduced from the application of this theory to the human body.

The binary classification may be extended to four variables, such as the four seasons — Winter (absolute Yin), Summer (absolute Yang), Spring (Yang in Yin), Fall (Yin in Yang). Spring, the growth of Yang out of Yin, explains expansion and springtime phenomena such as the opening of leaf buds. Autumn, Yin in Yang, describes the decay of Yang and the growth of Yin in aging and decay.

3

These four seasons are also the four directions of the compass, the four ages of life and the four elements — Wood, Fire, Metal, Water — as seen from the center, the neutral point, the fifth element, Earth.

This theory may be further extended to cover five variables, the Five Elements, thus forming a successful system of reference in Chinese thought, owing to the richness of the deductions that the system enables. It governed the emperor's political attitude, the geographical organization of China, the work of the peasants, military strategy, philosophy, arts, sciences, sociology, love, folklore, mysticism and medicine.

The other classifications of four, six, seven, eight, nine and twelve were never as successful as the "Five Elements." These were frequently coupled with the classification by six, as the five elements and the six energies, the foundations of Chinese astronomy, meteorology and calendar. In Chinese medicine, this five element classification is the most prevalent, along with the classification by six. It enabled medical thought of the time to deduce and to explain the relationships among the organs and to explore the depths of human physiology. This will be evident throughout this work. The only other nearly as successful classification was that of sixty-four from the *Yi Jing (I Ching)*. From this classification developed the hexagrams of the *Yi Jing* and an art of divination.[7] This classification was hardly used in medicine where the five elements, or five phases[8] as it was also known, was extensively applied.

The Five Elements

The first laws of physiology and pathology in Chinese medicine were made possible by the development of the postulate of the five elements. We will try to present an overview of this classification. The five elements are: Wood, Fire, Earth, Metal, Water. Each element corresponds to a season: spring, summer, late summer, autumn and winter. Each corresponds to a type of weather: wind, heat, humidity, drought and cold, as well as a flavor: sour, bitter, sweet, piquant (acrid) and salty.

Inside the body, the five elements relate to the liver, the heart, the spleen-pancreas (a coupled organ unique to Chinese theory), the lungs and the kidneys-adrenal gland (another coupled organ). To each of these Yin organs (zang=organ) corresponds a specific Yang bowel (fu=bowel). The five bowels are the gallbladder, the small intestine, the stomach, the large intestine and the urinary bladder. The coupling of organs and bowels creates a relationship known as biao li (outside-inside, or outer-inner lining). Two other specific Chinese functions that do not relate to the viscera, the pericardium (xin bao luo) and the triple burner (san jiao) correspond with the heart and the small intestine to the element Fire. Each organ is also related to a psychic energy, or vegetative soul, its qi. The five qi are: hun, shen, yi, po and zhi.

The list of correspondences is long. To each element corresponds an organ, a bowel, a sense of perception, a tissue, a region of the body, a flavor, a smell, a secretion, a psychic energy and an expression. In the Cosmos an element is related to a specific point of the compass, a planet, a color, a plant, an animal and a metal. In symbolism, the elements correspond to mythical animals, to trigrams,[9] and to numerals. These correspondences are given in the most ancient text, the *Nei Jing Su Wen,* and are shown in Table 1.

4

There are three fundamental laws of human physiology attached to the five elements:

• *The First Law* — A phenomenon classed within a specific element may influence, or be influenced by, another phenomenon that is classed within the same element. The Yin organ and the Yang bowel are coupled and tend to act on each other. The heart, for example, a Yin organ of the element Fire, acts on the Yang bowel of the same element, the small intestine, as it does on the blood vessels.

Table One

Cosmos					
	Water	**Wood**	**Fire**	**Earth**	**Metal**
Hours	Night	Morning	Noon	Afternoon	Evening
Evolution	Stagnate	Birth	Growth	Transform	Decline
Direction	North	East	South	Center	West
Climate	Cold	Wind	Heat	Humidity	Dryness
Season	Winter	Spring	Summer	End of Summer *1	Autumn
Color	Black	Green	Red	Yellow	White
Vegetable	Beans	Wheat	Rice	Corn	Oats
Meat	Pork	Chicken	Lamb	Beef	Horse
Metal	Lead	Tin	Mercury	Copper	Iron
Number	1, 6	3, 8	2, 7	5, 10	4, 9
Symbol	Moon Turtle	Dragon	Sun	Bird	Tiger
Trigram	⚎	⚏	⚌	⚏	⚍

Man					
Organ	Kidney	Liver	Heart *2	Spleen	Lungs
Bowel	Bladder	Gallbladder	Small Int. *3	Stomach	Large Int.
Humor	Fear Distress Delusions of Persecution	Anger Aggression	Joy Mania	Reflection Obsession Difficulties of Ideation	Sadness Depression Self-Control
Shen	Zhi	Hun	Shen	Yi	Po
Flavor	Salty	Sour	Bitter	Sweet	Piquant
Tissue	Bone Marrow Teeth	Muscles Tendons Nails Nerves	Arteries Blood	Fasciae Flesh	Skin
Function	Will	Nerve	Psychism	Nutrition	Energy
Sense	Hearing Ears	Sight Eyes	Taste Tongue	Touch Lips	Smell Nose
Odor	Rancid	Rank	Burnt	Fragrant	Putrid
Excretion	Urine	Tears	Sweat	Saliva	Sputum

*1 August 15   *2 and Master of the Heart   *3 and Triple Warmer

5

• *The Second Law* — There is an exchange of energy among the organs. This exchange is classified according to the five elements; the direction of flow of this energy is shown in Figure 1. This is the "mother-son" law according to which the "mother" is the organ that precedes the "son" to whom she passes her energy. This is also known as the creative cycle.

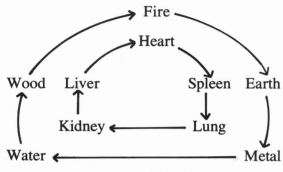

Figure 1

• *The Third Law* — In the state of equilibrium that we know as health, the body's energy is balanced. No single organ or bowel dominates another. This is insured by the system of regulation represented in Figure 2a. This regulatory relationship is known as the "grandfather-grandson" law. However, if an organ begins to retain energy, we say it is in excess. It then "dominates" another organ. For example, if the heart is in excess, it dominates the lungs and this damages them. In western medical terminology, this corresponds to cardiac pulmopathy, a problem in the lung created by an illness in the heart. Or, to give another example, if the kidney (adrenal gland) is in excess, it dominates the heart and the blood vessels. This is the case in pheochromocytoma.

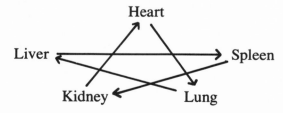

Figure 2a

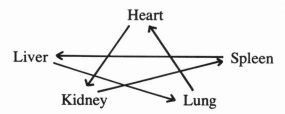

Figure 2b

6

This relationship may also work the other way. If an imbalance in one organ influences the organ that normally dominates it, this is termed impingement (Figure 2b). For example, if the heart impinges the kidney, we have the illness known as cardiac oliguria. If the lung impinges the heart, we have chronic pulmonary cardiopathy.

These three laws governing the five elements enable us to make a wide range of deductions concerning the physiopathology of various disorders, as well as to determine the appropriate therapy. However, the classification by six allows for relationships of almost equal importance.

The Six Energies

If the five phases relate to the five cardinal directions and to five earthly elements, the six energies relate, within the microcosm of man, to the six cosmic energies, or the six periods of the year, each lasting sixty days. Each energy corresponds to a climate in a season. Thus, the six energy cycle represents a year.

These six energies represent the six meridians in man. Each of these meridians is divided in two, making a total of twelve primary channels. Each of these primary channels is linked to the element belonging to the organ it represents. Since there are twelve functions — the five Yin organs, the five Yang bowels, the xin bao luo (pericardium) and san jiao (triple burner) — there is a meridian that corresponds to each. Each function represents a month of the year. All are associated two by two to form the six unit-pair meridians, the six energies. This relationship enables us to determine the period of the year, the month during which the activity of a given function is at its maximum, as well as the period during which activity is at a minimum. In the same way, as every Chinese hour is equal to two of our Western hours, each organ passes through its "hour" of maximum or minimum energy.

In summary, the six cosmic energies have correspondences with the six human energies and form twelve functions. These are classified as six levels of energy — the most superficial is the most Yang, the deepest is the most Yin. This system of levels of energy is a second physiological system relating certain organs to others. It is different from the creative or domination-impingement cycles of the five elements. The six meridians are: Tai Yang, Shao Yang, Yang Ming, Tai Yin, Jue Yin and Shao Yin.

Three Yang	+++	*Tai Yang*, exterior	**Superficial**
	++	*Shao Yang*, intermediate	
	+	*Yang Ming*, interior	
Three Yin	−	*Tai Yin*, exterior	
	− −	*Jue Yin*, intermediate	
	− − −	*Shao Yin*, interior	**Deep**

Figure 3

7

This is another regulatory system that insures the homeostasis of human energy against external aggression and that serves to explain, at least as well as the domination-impingement cycle, the physiopathology of internal imbalances. Modern Western acupuncturists have overstressed the role of domination-impingement among the five elements in their efforts to explain the physiopathology of illness to the detriment of their understanding of the equally important etiological role of the six energies.

Each energy embraces two functions. Each function is represented by a primary channel through which human energy flows in a fixed direction, according to the anastomoses of the meridians. The direction of flow respects two criteria:

(1) The criterion of the energy levels, especially among Yang meridians, that represent the defense barriers against external aggression by the external-internal anastomosis (Yang) of two Yang meridians in a Yang region, the head.

(2) The criterion of the five elements, according to which each Yin organ and its coupled Yang bowel are in an inside-outside (biao-li) relationship.

The energy flow within the meridians begins in the lung meridian, then follows the meridian of the large intestine, the lung's coupled Yang bowel. Both belong to the element Metal and correspond to autumn, drought and the piquant flavor. The stomach follows the large intestine in the energy cycle. Together these two meridians form Yang Ming. Next follows the spleen meridian coupled with the stomach in the element Earth and so forth. Inside the body, there is an internal lung meridian that links up with the kidney meridian and thus respects the direction of flow inherent to the creative or mother-son cycle.

Head

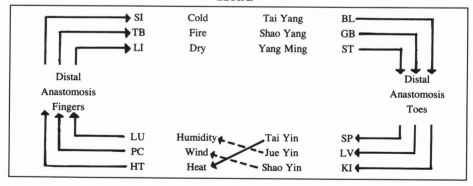

Thorax

Figure 4: Circulation of the twelve principle meridians (chart drawn from the schema of Nguyen Van Nghi). In the cephalic area the anastomosis of the meridians is external, visible, from one Yang meridian to another. At the thorax the anastomosis is internal.

The Twelve Meridians

This classification by twelve is at the origin of Chinese astronomy, meteorology and astrology. There are twelve Chinese hours in a day, twelve months in a year and twelve years in a decaduodenal cycle. Remaining faithful to the postulate "Man proceeds from Heaven and Earth," and to the principle of the implied analogy between the cosmos and man himself, man is divided into twelve organic functions:

- The lung (LU), which assures the respiratory function, but also plays a specific part in the global regulation of body energy.
- The large intestine (LI)
- The stomach (ST)
- The spleen-pancreas (SP). Associated in Chinese thought, the spleen and the pancreas form a single function, wherein is mingled the endocrine and exocrine role of the pancreas, the hematological role of the spleen and an energetic assimilation role unique to Chinese medicine.
- The heart (HT)
- The small intestine (SI)
- The bladder (BL) which includes urethra, ureter, pelvis and renal calyces.
- The kidney (KI) includes the glomerular excretion; the adrenal endocrine (medullar and cortical) function; the baroreceptors responsible for the secretion of renin-angiotensin; the hematological function that must correspond to hematopoietin; and, partially, to the gonads.
- The pericardium (PC) xin bao luo, which we will develop further, corresponds, but not exclusively, to the sympathetic and parasympathetic nervous systems ruling over the heart and more simply to the cardiac plexus.
- The triple burner (TB) which is intimately involved in assimilation and excretion of wastes and in water metabolism.
- The gallbladder (GB)
- The liver (LV)

Each of these organs is responsible for a Yin function (Yin root) and a Yang function (Yang root). Yin concentrates, elaborates and secretes; Yang distributes and moves. Each of these functions is linked to a meridian that assures its energy potential. These are the primary channels (jing mai). In modern texts, particularly in the West, these meridians are named after their corresponding organs. We say, for example, "the liver meridian." Actually, the word in Chinese for liver is gan. Its meridian carries the name of the energy to which it corresponds, that is, zu jue yin. Zu jue yin means choked Yin or small Yin and marks the end of Yin. At the same time, zu jue yin is a intermediary between Tai Yin and Shao Yin. It corresponds to the celestial energy of wind. In other words, if we call zu jue yin simply "the liver meridian," we fail to take into account a great many relationships with zu jue yin energy or with the zu jue yin energy level, as it is sometimes called.

The Concept of Energy in Acupuncture

The Global Concept

In introducing the static and dynamic structures of acupuncture we have shown to what extent the ancient Chinese conception of human physiology is "energetic" and thus much different from our own, which was at first anatomical, then metabolic and biochemical.

In Western medicine, blood and other fluids provide the organs, tissues and cells their fundamental constituents (oxygen, electrolytes, amino acids, glucides, lipids, ions and catalysts) and serve to carry substances formed in certain organs or tissues (hormones, enzymes) to destinations where they influence the functioning of other organs and tissues. The whole system maintains a certain balance thanks to the feedback of various homeostatic regulation factors. In Oriental medical theory, it is energy itself and its circulation through the meridians that governs the activity and the life of an organ.

The meaning of energy in the two systems is therefore different. The Western concept of energy is physical, defined either as a potential or as the result of a chemical or biochemical reaction. In Chinese medicine, energy is a global, syncretistic concept. Every living organism, in particular man, needs energy to live and to maintain its metabolism. Such energy as is taken from the air as well as food is not analyzed in traditional medicine. There is no interest in the breakdown of air into oxygen, nitrogen or carbon dioxide — no more so than in the biochemical mechanisms involved in respiratory exchanges. Energy has a life of its own. Traditional medicine leaves it at that.

The respiratory energy breathed in passes into the lungs and directly into the lung meridian. From there it continues on to the other meridians through their anastomoses, in turn reaching the organs and all the other parts of the body. In the same way, when food arrives in the digestive tract, part of its nutritive energy is absorbed and distributed by the stomach and the spleen-pancreas. The rest continues down the digestive tube to be absorbed by the kidneys or to be eliminated as feces.

What is to be thought of such an energy theory? This nutritive energy theory, for example: if it claims to take into account the same phenomena physiology and biochemistry have described, it is not acceptable. From this point of view it would seem childish, primitive and medically dangerous. If it intends to group the whole of digestion under a sole symbol, it is of little interest in comparison to Western analysis. Western medicine can detect and diagnose pancreatic insufficiency by intubation, testing secretin secretion, and measurement of the fecal fatty acids, nitrogen, amylasuria or blood sugar, and can prescribe pancreatic extracts coherently and scientifically. This highly technical and scientific power cannot be compared to the syncretic, imprecise symbol.

In reality, the Chinese "nutritive energy" is an energy in and of itself, included in the food and absorbed and stored directly. It has nothing to do with "metabolic assimilation." However, some correlations between these two interpretations of energy may exist, and are the subject of a following text.

10

What can we think of this concept of energy? It cannot stem from mere empirical observation as energy is in essence intangible, invisible. It is a theoretical postulate, whose source is metaphysical, or Taoist. The qi, the Taoist breath, corresponds to the energy conceived in other traditions, such as the Greek *pneuma* and the Indian *prana*. Professor J. Filliozat, physician and professor at the College de France, writes:

> The importance of the Prana is revealed in the oldest Sanskrit text. The Prana is not only respiration. It is only one of the basic energies that circulate in the human body and in the entire universe. It gives life to all living things. It is the inner wind, the breath that governs movement. Cosmophysiology, as we must call physiology, is therefore pneumatist, as many Greek philosophers already knew.[10]

The concepts in Chinese and Indian medicine resemble each other to such an extent that Professor Filliozat's statement may be just as well applied in acupuncture to define the qi.

Energy, as it has been defined in acupuncture, circulates inside the body as well as on the surface of the skin, in the organs and through the meridians. Many studies conducted in the most rigorous experimental conditions have shown that along the meridian paths, and notably at the classical acupuncture points, there is a cutaneous resistance that is clearly different from that of the surrounding skin. This was the subject of Niboyet's doctoral thesis and of the research of many of his colleagues, Borsarello, Cantoni and other researchers throughout the world.[11] The Chinese concept of the role of energy in the human body may no longer be considered as metaphysical fiction, but rather as a directly and scientifically measurable parameter. The physiological notion of energy existing in and of itself remains to be seen, as does its direct assimilation and distribution in the abdomen and in the thorax. These concepts should be regarded at least as a plausible reality, or as a global phenomenon situated in a reference system that differs from our own. This difference in the essential paradigm is why, over the years, Eastern and Western physicians have been able to broaden their knowledge of one system, while ignoring the other completely.

It seems incredible that the whole system of energetic physiology, with its laws, its pathology and its correspondence therapy, is to be found in the *Nei Jing Su Wen*. We are asked to believe that when it was written and until the first century of our era, Chinese doctors had never practiced dissection of the human body, unlike the Greeks or the Hindus. According to tradition, the first Chinese dissection took place in the year 16 AD. It was performed at Wang Mang's request on the body of Ing, who was condemned to be tortured to death.[12] The second was in the year 1106. Its results were later made known by Zhang Huang between the years 1527 and 1608.

In light of this knowledge, we must ask two questions: If the Chinese never practiced dissections until the first century, how could they have even suspected the existence of the ten organs and the twelve functions mentioned in the *Nei Jing*? How could they have understood relationships between these functions that science would only rediscover some forty centuries later? Where did their knowledge of meridians come from? Because this concept of energy, as it applies to the cosmos and to man, stems from Taoist metaphysics, so too must the answers to these

11

questions. However, rather than resolved by this knowledge, the problems is only shifted, and we are lead to delve further into Taoist thought.

The Chinese concept of energy is, nonetheless, coherent. It fits into a cosmogeny that explains its origins as well as the transformations that result in physical materialization, giving expression to the laws of transmutation.[13] A. Husson, a French physician who produced a fine Western translation of the *Huang Di Nei Jing Su Wen*, reminds us that in the third forward of the 1955 Chinese edition of the *Huang Di Nei Jing Su Wen*, the *Qiu Zao* or ''creation'' passage describes a four-stage transmutation from the ''invisible'' to the ''visible.''

- Tai Yi: the Universal Quiescence, the original void.
- Tai Chu: the Great Origin, the origin of the breath: Qi.
- Tai Shi: the Great Beginning, the birth and the origin
     of form: Xing.
- Tai Su: the Native State, the appearance of matter: Zhi.

It is only when qi, xing and zhi coexist that illness may
germinate.[14]

Without a thorough comprehension of the concept of energy in Chinese medicine, it is virtually impossible to understand Chinese semiology, pathology and therapeutic principles based on the attempt to eliminate energetic imbalance.

The Body Energies

''Qi is the initial element; it is the celestial emanation that animates the whole universe,'' writes Husson. He also quotes Bridgeman on the difficulty he, as a sinologist, met in the translation of ''qi.'' It sometimes means ''the universal cosmic breath,'' and elsewhere ''man's vital energy,'' or ''the air we breathe'' and often ''the pulse'' or ''essence'' of a viscera.[15] Grains, flavors and odors each have their qi. There is an earthly qi in each element, a qi for Wood, a qi for the Imperial Fire, a qi for the Ministerial Fire,[16] a qi for Earth, for Metal, for Water — all are related to the qi of the five organs. There are six qi for the six meridians: Shao Yang, Yang Ming, Tai Yang, Jue Yin, Tai Yin and Shao Yin. The qi of each viscera is distinct from the qi of the viscera's shen, or psychic emanation: hun for the liver and so forth. (See Table 1.)

In the human body, qi flows through the meridians and its manifestation is the pulse. This qi of the body, the energy of the meridians, goes by the name of zhen qi. However, this zhen qi can take different forms and is then known as rong qi, xue, wei qi, yuan qi, zong qi and jing qi.

Rong qi, ''nourishing energy'' or ying qi, depending on the translation, is the energy that circulates and nourishes tissues and organs. It participates in the elaboration of the organic fluids and of the blood. Apart from this, rong qi follows a precise chronobiology within the nyctohemeral period and is concentrated in one viscera after another for two hours at a time. It also obeys monthly, seasonal, annual, decennial and decaduodenal chronobiology.

Xue, the blood, is considered to be the most concentrated energy. Xue circulates at once in the meridians and in the blood vessels. Thus, a meridian is considered to be a dynamic vector that provokes movement and permits the

12

arteriovenous circulation. There is no clear distinction between blood vessels and meridians. Although they are considered to be distinct, in practice they are so inseparable that we speak of circulation of blood and energy in the meridians in the same breath. There is even a proportional ratio of blood to energy in each of the six meridians.

Tai Yang contains more blood than energy, as does Jue Yin. Shao Yang contains more energy than blood, as do Tai Yin and Shao Yin. Yang Ming contains great quantities of both; it is the meridian sea, out of which the body draws energy and blood. According to certain texts, Yang Ming is associated with, or in rapport with, the main arteries: the aorta, brachial, carotid, iliac and femoral. These considerations are of importance in pathology, when we consider the dissociation of blood and energy circulation within a single meridian, for example, a global downward movement of blood, along with an upward surge of energy.

Wei qi is the "fierce, combative energy from nutrition," says the *Ling Shu*. "It is ferocious, lively, agitated." It circulates in the superficial tissues, the skin, the connective tissues, the muscles and the peritoneum. It radiates to the chest and abdomen. According to the classics, it does not circulate in the meridians and the viscera. In the nyctohemeral cycle, it flows through the face, the trunk and the limbs during the day and at night flows through the viscera. Wei qi does circulate in certain superficial channels, particularly the luo, which are associated with the precapillary anastomoses.

Wei qi is the defensive energy. It protects us from external perverse energies. It opens and shuts the pores, mobilizes and moves rong qi and xue; it is connected to vasomotricity through the luo vessels. It warms up the connective tissues and concentrates in the acupuncture points, the "holes of qi." Wei qi is involved in thermoregulation and represents the whole immune system, from leucocytes to antibodies, histamine, bradykinin and serotonin. In short, it represents all the substances that play multiple roles in our physiology, from vasomotricity, to thermoregulation, to immunity.

Wei qi seems to represent all these aspects, but remains as autonomous as the other energies: it is produced, set into motion and follows its own chronobiology within the nyctohemeral cycle like a precision timepiece. It obeys a seasonal cycle just as rong qi does.

Zong qi, or ancestral energy, is the global product of synthesis of the energies coming from the food we eat (gu qi) and the air we breathe (da qi). It participates directly or indirectly in the production of wei qi, xue, and rong qi. Zong qi is an energy, a sum of elaborated energies. At the same time, it represents an inherited genetic quality that determines our quantitative and qualitative capacity to produce and use all the other energies: wei qi, rong qi, xue, jing. Thus, zong qi is at once the result and the genetic coefficient of energy production. It is also translated, though incorrectly, as essential energy. In a way, it represents our inheritance of terrain and vitality from our parents. The *Ling Shu* also distinguishes zong qi as an autonomous energy: "the essential energy (zong qi) accumulates in the thorax." More precisely, its point of concentration is shanzhong (CV-17), the "master of energy" or hui energy point.

13

The stomach plays a large part in the production of the earthly and respiratory energies and zong qi. It is related to a special meridian, the great luo of the stomach, xu li, which is the "ancestor of the pulse." Coursing through the thorax, xu li passes shanzhong (CV-17) where it causes "pulsations from the tip of the heart to the clothes." Modern Chinese authors remind us that the force of the pulse of zong qi is considerable. It passes through xinmu, or juque (CV-14), the mu point of the heart, and through the lung to reach the throat.[17] Lower down, this force heads toward the abdomen, through qichong (ST-30), on the femoral artery, also called qijie, and on down to the foot. It is written in the *Ling Shu*, "Downwards it enters qijie; upwards it ascends to the respiratory system."[18] In other words, zong qi also represents the dynamic force of the cardiac and respiratory pumps. It is the hemodynamic function of the respiratory and circulatory systems, and also a vector of energy within the meridians, since it is impossible to dissociate the circulation of blood and energy.

Yuan qi, or original energy, represents a potential of life, an energy potential given to an individual at conception.[19] Yuan qi dwells in the kidneys and in the "exterior kidneys" or testicles.[20] The kidneys are related to the adrenal glands in Chinese physiology and to the precursors of the sexual hormones. We must keep the kidney-adrenal gland connection in mind throughout our studies of Chinese medicine. In Chapter 8 of the *Nan Jing,* it is written that "the original energy is the spring {the source} of the twelve meridians." As the modern Shanghai authors say, "The gonads are the motors of the human body's activity."[21] Thus, the physical function of the meridians and zhen qi (the meridian energy) is inseparable from the yuan qi stored in the kidneys and the gonads. Yuan qi is, then, the spring of the twelve meridians, their source.

The eight "miscellaneous channels" connect yuan qi to the body as a whole. Chong mai in particular connects the energy of the kidneys with the primary channels. This is why we may read in the texts that chong mai is the "sea" of the twelve primary channels:

> {This meridian} begins in the genitals, ascends toward the upper part of the body; its energy flows outside the body and disperses on the chest. It flows within the meridians as well, passes into the arteries, which we may feel beating beside the navel.[22]

Yuan qi, the "inherited energy,"is also linked to the unfathomable program — the design of the Tao, the primary energy, or tai yi — of which yuan qi is the initial spark. This sea of all energies, yuan qi, constitutes capital fixed at birth that diminishes during an individual's life. When yuan qi runs out, one meets death. This is something like the fixed capital of the gametes of our sexual endocrine physiology, which diminishes with genital activity. It is also similar to the prostaglandins.[23] The Taoist sexual ascetic techniques, which are similar to most other religions or mystical codes, are closely related to the economy of yuan qi, which is why, in Taoism, they are known as techniques of longevity, or "immortality."

Just as shanzhong (CV-17) is known as the "dwelling" of zong qi, rong qi dwells in zhongwan (CV-12), wei qi dwells in xiawan (CV-10) and yuan qi dwells in the kidneys and the gonads. More precisely, the location is the space between the two kidneys, at the point mingmen (GV-4), known as the "door of light, door of destiny." In the gonads, the location of yuan qi is in huiyin (CV-1), the

14

"meeting of the Yin," and changqiang (GV-1), "always strong." These are the pelvic origin points of the two miscellaneous channels ren mai and du mai that form the dividing lines between Yin and Yang, right and left, back and front, respectively. Between the symphysis pubis and the navel are two other important points, guanyuan (CV-4) and qihai (CV-6) on the ren mai. The ren mai is the sea of all the Yin meridians and du mai is the sea of all the Yang meridians. Also known as the "voluntary course of energy," this meridian, which obviously relates to the cerebrospinal axis, plays an important role in Indian and Taoist ascetic techniques.

Jing qi, the "essential energy,"in the sense of quintessence, is also known as the acquired essential energy, jing. Translation presents a problem; it is synonymous with germs, grain, semen and sperm. Each organ nourished by rong qi and wei qi synthesizes its own jing, which is stored in the kidneys and is mobilized on demand. Chinese medicine also distinguishes an inherited jing, distinct from acquired jing, but which induces the activity of acquired jing. Acquired jing and inherited jing are nevertheless physiologically referenced as one. The concept of jing qi calls to mind the visceral endocrine activity, which depends on the adrenal glands, the kidneys and the gonads. Here again, a relationship with the prostaglandins, or with both the notion of DNA and RNA messages and HLA immunosystems, are tempting assumptions. Jing qi dwells in the kidney, in the broader Chinese sense of the term. It may be mobilized on request within the preferential circuit of the eight miscellaneous channels, and thus interpenetrate the twelve primary channels. These miscellaneous channels energize[24] the five curious bowels, which are distinct from the ten viscera and the twelve functions of the primary channel network. These five curious bowels are: the marrow (spinal and bone marrows), the arteries, the gallbladder, the uterus and the brain.[25] The concept of endocrinology forms an incomplete picture of jing qi, unless we incorporate within endocrinology the concepts of neurology and neuroendocrinology. Both zong qi and jing qi are known as "essential" energies, whereas yuan qi is called the "original" energy. Since zong qi is also called the "ancestral" energy, we should retain the adjective "essential" especially for jing qi.

In summary, the energy that circulates within the meridians (zhen qi) is composed of rong qi, the nourishing energy; wei qi, the defensive energy; xue, the blood; zong qi, the ancestral energy; yuan qi, the original energy; and jing qi, the essential energy. Each of these energies implies a preferential circuit, is produced differently, and obeys a precise chronobiology, specific to the hour, day, month, season and year.

The Other Meridians

The Eight Miscellaneous Channels (Jing Qi)

These eight channels are the preferential flow paths of the energy of which we have just spoken, jing qi, which energizes the curious bowels.[26] They are coupled two by two as follows:

du mai — yang qiao mai
chong mai — yin wei mai

yin qiao mai — ren mai

dai mai — yang wei mai

These meridians, too, obey a precise chronobiology. One opens every Chinese hour, the equivalent of two of our astronomical hours. It is essential to proper treatment to consult the universal calendar of openings.[27] A specific point, the special opening point, or meridian key point, should be needled at the moment of its opening. Each miscellaneous channel's opening point is located on a primary channel. Besides playing a role as a route, or canal, to energize the curious organs with jing qi, the miscellaneous channels, with the exception of the dai mai, are also shunts situated on the primary channels. This enables communication between upper and lower parts of the body.

Not surprisingly, the Yang miscellaneous channels shunt onto Yang primary channels and have Yang key points. The yin miscellaneous channels shunt onto Yin primary channels and have Yin key points. When the energy in the primary channel is excessive and its circulation disrupted, the excessive energy can be diverted into the miscellaneous channel and the flow of energy in the primary channel is reestablished. This is true regardless of whether the source of the excess is internal or external.

According to the ancient texts, the miscellaneous channels are the great rivers. When there is a heavy storm, the small rivers overflow and the large rivers fill with the excess. For example, when the zu shao yang energy is excessive, an excess of emotional energy in the meridian, the symptomology will be anger, insomnia and even hypertension. The point to needle is fengchi (GB-20). This point is located in the posterior aspect of the neck, below the occipital bone. It is related to yang wei mai and can divert the excessive Yang energy out of the upper extremity and into the miscellaneous channel allowing the energy to descend, relieving the blockage that might otherwise have occurred. Modern Shanghai authors poetically write that fengchi (GB-20) enables us to hide the Yang in yang wei mai.

The pneumatic role of the lung, the organ known as the "master of energy," which is so important in activating the circulation of rong qi in the primary channels, is also involved in the circulation of jing qi in both the principle and miscellaneous channels. The lung is effectively the crossroads of the twelve primary channels and the coupled miscellaneous channels du mai and ren mai.[28] In other words, du mai and ren mai are the "oceans" in which the primary channels converge (Yang in the back; Yin in the front), through which flows rong qi, propelled by the lungs, which are themselves propelled by zong qi. However, in these two miscellaneous channels, as well as in the other six, jing qi also flows, propelled by yuan qi. Yuan qi acts as a motor for the primary channels also. Thus, we realize the existence of intimate interpenetrations of energy and of multiple relationships between the two networks.

16

Energy Circulation

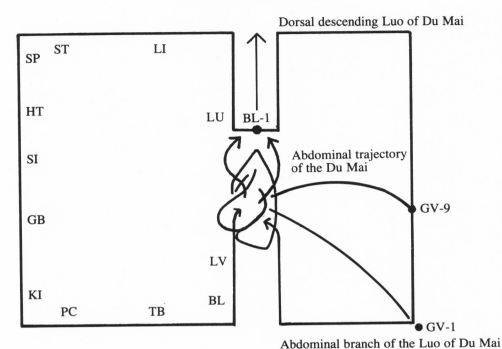

Figure 5: The intermediary role of the lungs between the larger circulation of the principle meridians and the smaller circulation of the curious meridians, du mai and ren mai.

The Secondary Channels

Our study of the Chinese energy system would be incomplete if we were to neglect the 48 secondary channels (luo mai) which are linked to the twelve primary channels (jing mai), to form a single, all-encompassing energy network (jing luo). To each primary channel are linked four secondary channels. The whole forms what we may call a meridian unit. This unit is composed of one primary channel (jing mai), associated with a tendinomuscular channel (jing jin); a distinct channel (jing bie); and two luo channels, the transverse and the longitudinal luo.

The tendinomuscular channel (jing jin) is more superficial than the primary channel to which it is linked. Its energy nourishes the skin, the muscles, the tendons and the nerves in the territory that it reaches. The tendinomuscular channel (TM) of the liver governs the big toe, the dorsum of the foot, the inner part of the calf, the inner and posterior parts of the thigh, the external genitalia and the abdomen beneath the navel. A disorder of this TM may result in superficial pain (neuralgia, tendinitis) or even joint pain.

The distinct channel (jing bie) provides a shortcut, a shunt, for the energy that goes from the surface to the organ related to the meridian unit. It shunts the primary channel and is involved in those illnesses that affect the organs and superficial tissues simultaneously.

17

The transverse luo channel (luo mai) is a link between the meridian unit of a Yin organ and that of the Yang bowel with which it is coupled through the distal anastomosis (fingers or toes). The transverse luo of the liver, for example, enters the primary channel of the gallbladder and is, in effect, a precapillary energy shunt. Another luo coming from the gallbladder meridian enters the liver, thus establishing a connection in both directions.

The longitudinal luo channel (luo mai) goes deep and connects the organ and the surface directly.[29] A disorder of the liver luo channel may result in a genital pathology such as pruritis or external genital eczema.

Therapeutic Use of the Jing Luo System

There are those in the Western world who have tried to present Chinese medicine as a blind, stab-in-the-dark, empirical method, by which we needle here and there trying to obtain one result or another. The more we become familiar with Chinese medicine, the more we realize that this is the opposite of the truth. We are dealing with a complex and coherently elaborated theory with detailed parameters of the circulation of energy along the meridians, their internal and external anastomosis, different levels of energy and relationships between different types of energy within different parts of the body. It is statistically unthinkable that such a system was elaborated by way of trial and error needling of hypothetical acupuncture points. Not only would our Chinese ancestors have needed to discover, according to their various afflictions, the 365 points on each side of the body, but also the "recipe" for treating each point. They would have needed to invent the whole theory to explain the incredible success of their random needling.

It is true that one law of acupuncture, as set forth in the *Nei Jing*, states that any painful spot on the surface of the body may be considered an acupuncture point and may be needled. This reflexotherapy technique is certainly somewhat empirical. It extends only to pain and does not constitute an etiological treatment. On the other hand, volumes and volumes of Chinese texts describe in detail illnesses caused by energy imbalance and present a coherent semiology of the various aggressions suffered by the meridians. Each of these descriptions is supported by a body of consistent therapeutic laws. To illustrate the coherency of Chinese semiology, as well as the consistency of its therapeutic framework, let us examine the case of aggressions against the liver meridian, or zu jue yin, to use its real name.

Aggression Against the Primary Channel (Jing Mai) and Against the Liver (Gan)

When a disorder is internal and affects the liver, tradition[30] directs us to needle the rong and shu points (LV-2 and LV-3) of the liver meridian. This is true for cases of organic disturbance from an advanced stage of energy imbalance caused by internal or external aggression against the liver energy. In the first stage of the disorder — the functional stage, before there is lesion of the organ — we are dealing with an imbalance of the energy among the five elements. If this is the case, damage is limited to the principal channels and we may reestablish the energy balance and bring the condition under control by treating several points.

The therapeutic attitude is not, however, codified. We must first establish the program of the imbalance according to the symptoms, if we are to be able to reestablish equilibrium. We may want to needle ququan (LV-8), the tonifying point of zu jue yin, to increase the energy in the meridian, or we may want to do the opposite, needling the dispersion point, xingjian (LV-2). We may want to harmonize the energy, by needling the luo points, thus shunting energy towards the gallbladder. The extensive traditional symptomology describes the symptoms according to the origin of aggression, external or internal, and according to its gravity, functional or organic.

Another technique, known as the shu-mu technique, brings into play points that are related to the medullary neurovegetative reflexes, which have been known to the Chinese since the origins of acupuncture. The shu point of the liver is located over the medullary level D9, D10. It is paramedian at the level of the sympathetic chain, on the urinary bladder meridian zu tai yang. The acupuncturist may choose between these two techniques, between balancing the meridians or using this medullary technique, or may use both simultaneously.

Aggression Against the Distinct Meridian (Jing Bie)

The symptomology of the jing bie, or distinct meridians, is described by some authors (such as Nguyen Van Nghi) as intermittent. Symptoms appear, go away and then come back again and are usually unilateral. The organ and the superficial region that the meridian crosses are affected simultaneously. The symptomology of the distinct meridian of the liver is different from that of the primary channel and consists of acute genital pains that are sudden and brutal. We can also mention certain forms of infectious urethritis and certain opthalmic migraines, caused by the penetration of the perverse energy into the ascending internal pathway of the distinct meridian that leads to the eye. Once we have diagnosed the affection, its treatment is specific. According to the "technique of opposites," we needle LV-3 and LV-8 on the affected side and LV-1 on the opposite side, or only LV-1 on the opposite side.

This technique is effective for treating primitive facial neuralgia caused by disorders of the stomach and large intestine distinct meridians, whose pathways cross the corresponding facial areas. It may originate in the distinct meridians of the liver and the gallbladder. This technique is capable of good results in disorders where mere reflexotherapy may temporarily relieve, but never cure.

Aggression Against the Tendinomuscular Meridian (Jing Jin)

According to the Chinese, the tendinomuscular meridians are vulnerable to aggression of an external, climatic or traumatic nature. When the TM of the liver is affected, the symptomology is as follows: Pain in the big toe, extending to the internal malleolus; pain in the tibial tuberosity and in the inner knee; pain and spasm in the medial thigh.

Any external damage along the path of the TM meridian, such as a sprain or a twisted muscle, may be the cause of a disorder in this meridian. This is often the case with muscular pain. The spectacular relief provided by acupuncture treatment of traumatology (sprains, strains) is a good example of TM meridian treatment. The jing and shu points are usually needled in such circumstances.

19

In ancient texts dealing with the TM of the liver, we read:

> The Yin of the genitals is disturbed and becomes useless. This is why, in cases of repeated intercourse, when the Yin is wounded, the Yang becomes impotent and erection of the penis becomes impossible.

This explains the penial vasomotor phenomenon of priapism, regardless of its etiology. Infra-umbilical pain and hernia are also mentioned.

Aggression Against the Luo Meridian (Luo Mai)

The luo meridian of the liver suffers only rarely from aggression. If the energy is excessive, scrotum and penis dilate: hydrocele. Treatment consists of needling ligou (LV-5). When the energy is deficient, we find acute and severe pruritis of the scrotum and of the labia majoris for which we must needle taichong (LV-3).

Simultaneous Aggressions Against the Primary Channel (Jing Mai) and the Miscellaneous Channel (Jing Qi)

Simultaneous energy imbalances may occur in primary and miscellaneous liver channels, as is sometimes observed in pregnancy and delivery accidents (chong mai and primary liver channels) or in hernias (ren mai and primary liver channels). In such cases of simultaneous imbalance the semiology and pathology may be different from cases involving either of the two meridians separately. A close study of the traditional texts is essential to understanding this difference.

Each meridian imbalance is associated with a distinct semiology and pathology. In light of this statement, it is interesting to note that we have considered stimulating the point taichong (LV-3) in three of the different pathologies described as examples. The first concerned an aggression against the primary channel of the liver; the second, an imbalance in its TM meridian; the third, a case of deficiency in the luo meridian. However, in each instance, this point has been employed in association with other points, according to an appropriate therapeutic strategy that takes into consideration the specific rules of each meridian.

The frequent use of this point is because taichong (LV-3) is a specific point on the liver meridian, the shu point. Shu points, as a class, possess special energetic properties. The Chinese texts speak of specific indications for taichong, the "supreme assault." It is located in the depression distal to the junction of the first and second metatarsal bones. It is needled in cases of genital infection and pain, metritis, dysuria and uterine bleeding. These indications correspond to the symptomology of the various liver meridians. Treating them solely on the reputation of the one point presents two major risks. First, we might not understand the therapeutic mechanism we are setting into action and thus treat blindly, possibly aggravating the disorder we are trying to cure. Secondly, we might perform an incomplete treatment, which will be partially or totally ineffective because we are ignorant of the strategy involved.

Taichong (LV-3) has the specific reputation of relieving opthalmic headaches. When we needle this point and stimulate the needle, manually or electrically, we obtain almost immediate relief of the migraine. Nonetheless, when we remove the needle, all the pain comes back in a few minutes if the treatment has not reduced the energy imbalance, which was the origin of the migraine. This example enables us to grasp Chinese reasoning about energy.

As we have seen, out of seven disorders, only one has anything to do with the organ as such and could be termed an organic illness. This is why the Chinese do not speak of the "liver meridian," but give to the meridian the name of the specific energetic quality it represents. Our comprehension of energetic disorders is furthered by the realization that the liver meridian is known as zu jue yin, rather than gan jing. We speak of a Jue Yin level disorder so long as the illness is only energetic. If the imbalance persists beyond this reversible stage, the illness may attack and eventually provoke lesions of the organ — gan, the liver. Only at this stage are we dealing with what may be termed an organic illness. Based on this example, we can make the following statements:

- An autonomous energy flows through the body, taking on specific, conventional aspects to account for activities of specific sectors.

- This energy obeys laws of balance and or interaction between the various functions by which it is engendered, or to which it is destined.

- Some external and internal factors can temporarily disrupt this energy circulation and be the source of disorders that themselves provoke compensatory reactions within the body.

- If the compensatory mechanisms are overwhelmed, there ensues a definitive imbalance that leads to organic lesions.

The fundamental stage of an illness which precedes organic lesions, the stage at which the illness is present as a functional disorder, was perfectly understood and assimilated by Eastern medical practitioners thousands of years ago. This understanding was not limited to energy mechanisms, but specially included semiological projections. Thus, Chinese medicine represents a key for unlocking the mysteries of functional disorders that, for the most part, have stymied our too substantialistic, too organically oriented Western therapeutic logic. This is essential to our study of the correlations between acupuncture and catalytic medicine.

Etiologies in Chinese Medicine

The exhaustive list of the causes of illness, according to acupuncture theory, is as follows: cosmic perverse energies, irregular perverse energies, emotional disturbances, malnutrition, fatigue, sexual overindulgence, traumatisms, germs, parasites, intoxications and genetic factors.[31] Of this list, three classic etiologies stand out: cosmic perverse energies, emotional disturbances and malnutrition. All the others are self-evident and most often explained by cosmic, emotional or nutritional factors.

21

Etiology One: The Cosmic Perverse Energies

The six cosmic energies that govern meteorology and the cycle of the seasons (in chronological order: wind, heat, humidity, fire, dryness, cold), and any external energy that becomes excessive and attacks the body, may be considered to be perverse, as it is harmful to our health. The six cosmic energies are: Jue Yin, Shao Yin, Tai Yin, Shao Yang, Yang Ming and Tai Yang. These coincide with the six paired meridians and follow one after the other throughout the course of the year. Man tolerates and adapts to these changes — "Man responds to Heaven and to the Earth."

However, this state of harmonious balance may be disrupted under two circumstances. Of the first, human circumstance, it is written in the *Su Wen*, "If a man suffers the attacks of perverse energy, it is because his essential energy is already weakened." The causes of this weakening are multiple: emotional upsets, poor nutrition, sexual overindulgence, overwork, traumas and genetic factors. The second, cosmic circumstance, is displaced cosmic energy (cold weather during the summer, for example) that breaches the body's defense barriers and penetrates into the body, resulting in weakness.

Chinese meteorologists invented a calendar according to which each year was assigned two numbers that correspond to two types of weather. Their calculation according to the laws of domination or submission (impingement) of the six energies, allow the determination each year of the actual succession of the energies, as well as the variations of what would be normally predictable.[32] Such a calendar enabled them to foresee meteorological (and medical) disorders that would threaten those in other than excellent physical condition.

When we speak of xie, perverse energy, we mean any external aggression — climatic, bacterial or viral, isolated or endemic. Afflictions are codified in terms of perverse energy enabling us to extend our energetic reasoning. Thus *cold*, which is Yin, will be a perverse energy that, by attacking one of the meridians and eventually an organ, will precipitate a clinical condition that is Yin in nature.

The organism's defense system is represented by the superficial cutaneous energy, wei qi. There are three possible methods of aggression:

> The perverse energy penetrates the secondary channels, in particular the most superficial, the tendinomuscular meridian, and from there gains the primary channel and the organ itself.
>
> The perverse energy penetrates the most superficial energy, wei qi, and finds a pathway deep into the body: wei qi, rong qi, xue.
>
> The perverse energy may penetrate the primary channels, where as a rule it comes against the strongest of the defense barriers, the most Yang: first Tai Yang, then Shao Yang, then Yang Ming, etc.

Each of these three scenarios of aggression corresponds to a specific mechanism and calls for different therapeutic sanctions. Thus, any external affliction, when seen in the light of the Chinese energy code, allows us to pinpoint the mechanism of penetration of the perverse energy into the meridian-organ complex and to establish an appropriate treatment. For example, when the perverse energy is in the tendinomuscular meridian, perverse energy plus tendinomuscular energy yields primary channel energy. The normal balance of the triple burner and pericardium is disrupted. The tendinomuscular meridian is in excess and the primary channel is consequently deficient.

Clinically, the state of excess manifests itself by Yang symptoms: inflammation, pain, redness and swelling. The treatment required is tonification of the primary channel to expel the perverse energy. This reasoning may be applied to a sprain, as well as an insect bite, since both invasions will yield to the same energetic defense.

When the perverse energy is not chased out naturally, by acupuncture, or by any other therapeutic treatment, it passes from the tendinomuscular buffer meridian directly into the primary channel. At this point the primary channel is in a state of excess, whereas the tendinomuscular meridian is deficient. The tendinomuscular symptoms are thus Yin by nature, the pain is dull and is felt during rest and at night. Lumbago, which has become chronic, for example, could be thus described. Medication may possibly relieve the pain without affecting the physiopathological process. The treatment of tendinomuscular deficiency is dispersion of energy in the primary channel.

The curious perverse energies cause infective, toxic endemoepidemic diseases. They were studied meticulously from the fourth to the sixth centuries BC: "They enter the respiratory tract and pass into the stomach and the intestines." These are the "cold" and the "latent heat" diseases. Here "latent" is the concept of incubation. Adverse climatic conditions, or poor nourishment or hygiene facilitate penetration of the organism.

The Chinese accord to the words "cold" and "hot" a far more extensive and systematized meaning than that of our popular language, as in our expression "to catch a cold." The Chinese dialectic is a code. For example, an insect bite or a spider bite produces symptoms of calor, tumor, dolor and rubor (inflammation, swelling, pain and redness) which tell us that the bite is an excess of Yang of external origin. Perverse heat energy has penetrated into the TM meridian. From this codification stems the appropriate treatment. Perverse heat energy is not merely a mystical symbol used to mask ignorance of the actual aggressive agent — the venom, its chemical composition and the allergic reactions it produces. It is a coherent dialectical system that uses symbols to efficiently relate cosmic conditions and treatment to the energy system of the human body. The use of this code in no way contradicts Western reasoning and analysis; it is certainly complementary. We may say that Cosmic energy represents, in pathology, the level of Heaven.

Etiology Two: The Emotional Energies

Self-awareness is what sets man apart from the other animals. Speculative thinking represents a revolution within evolution. Man's fundamental axis is Shao Yin, which is composed of two organs, the kidney and the heart. The kidney, dwelling of yuan qi, stores jing qi, the essence. The heart is the royal palace, the sovereign, in which zong qi and shen[33] are stored. The kidney and the heart serve to balance each other and are kept in balance through the interplay of the five elements. Together the two represent man's quota of energy and the relationship of

23

this energy with conscious thought, with the brain. They form the psychosomatic axis.

The stresses of modern life weaken jing qi and disturb shen. Emotional instability, too, weakens shen and thus jing. This explains the mental and sexual hygienic principles of Taoism that are treated in Chapter One of the *Nei Jing Su Wen* and are of fundamental importance. This Shao Yin axis, fundamental to Chinese medicine, helps us to understand conscious thought dysfunction, as well as behavioral problems. To this axis is associated a system of psychosomatic relationships, whose code is a part of the theory of the five elements. Each shen corresponds to a specific organ and is manifested through a particular emotion. Joy corresponds to the heart, anger to the liver, sadness to the lung, reflection to the spleen and fear to the kidney.

This code enables us to explain the neurovegetative phenomena of the emotions. We may make the following deductions: an excess of emotion is harmful to the corresponding organ; a problem of an organ will find echo in its corresponding emotion. Thus, sadness is harmful to the lungs, but problems in the lungs make the patient sad. In Chinese medicine, a mood or behavioral disturbance is not merely a psychiatric symptom, but an imbalance of energy among the five organs and six bowels, and some very specific energy disorders in the corresponding meridians. Hypomania, for example, is an imbalance in the longitudinal luo channel of the stomach. The opposite is also true: innate or acquired behavioral phenomena can perturb the energy of the corresponding Yin organ or bowel. This perturbation is perfectly codified. An excessive emotional energy will usually cause an excess, even a blockage, of the circulation of energy in the corresponding meridian. This is why in treatment we may have to disperse the energy in the meridian and also unblock it to reestablish a normal circulation of energy.

In summary, the emotional energies represent a second etiology of illness, at the level of Man. They explain psychosomatic illnesses and serve as a code for the understanding of their mechanisms in Chinese energetic physiology. Chinese medicine is thus, by definition, a psychosomatic medicine.

Etiology Three: The Nutritive Energy

The Chinese have insisted on the part nutrition plays in the cause of disease. Nutrition represents a third etiology: since food comes from the ground, its origin is the Earth. Of the three origins, Heaven (perverse energies), Man (emotional energies) and Earth (nutritive energies), the latter is the most material, the most Yin. Of the three etiologies, the third is the most likely to affect the organ directly, by etiogenic process, without passing through a meridian. From the food absorbed, the spleen synthesizes five flavors, each of which corresponds to a Yin organ and a Yang bowel. The sweet flavor corresponds to the spleen, piquant to the lung, salty to the kidney, sour to the liver and bitter to the heart. Food of a particular flavor that is absorbed in normal quantities is beneficial to the ''form'' of the organ, the matter of the organ, as opposed to its energetic level. Food of any flavor that is absorbed in excessive quantities is harmful to the corresponding organ. Sweets in excess, for example, injure the spleen (diabetes). The Chinese pharmacopoeia is based on these relationships.

The flavors that are Yin go to the Yang organs, just as the Yang flavors go to the Yin órgans. The more a food has a Yin flavor, the more Yang energy it contains. Salt, the most Yang flavor, for example, contains the most Yin energy (most concentrated in matter and emanating the least energy). It is linked with the kidney, the most Yin organ. It corresponds to the Yin in the Yin. Drugs that belong to the Yin in the Yin encourage evacuation, such as purgatives. Evacuation here means elimination of matter. This remarkable classification was introduced by Nguyen Van Nghi, based on experiments with animals in which the corresponding herbs of the Chinese pharmacopoeia were studied.[34] When a flavor is in excess and is recognized as pathogenic, there are two therapeutic strategies. The first is to treat the disorder with food of the flavor that dominates the flavor that is in excess. This strategy treats according to the law of domination-impingement. The second strategy uses acupuncture and will be developed further on in the text. To conclude our discussion of the three etiologies we may say that external factors (Heaven) act on energetic equilibrium, the most immaterial aspect of man, the most Yang. The internal, emotional factors (Man) act on the equilibrium among the five elements, the intermediate aspect. The factor of nutrition (Earth) acts directly on the organs, which represent the most material aspect of man, the most Yin (xing). This schematic rule is by no means absolute, but it illustrates the rule that in Chinese medicine no organ is treated as a single entity. Every organ enters into multiple relationships with the human energy system. This rule will serve as a guideline for our study of acupuncture specialty by specialty.

Therapeutic Considerations — Acupuncture Points

Shu-Antique Points

In our discussion of the five elements, six energies and the various meridians, we have gradually established a clear overview of the essential therapeutic principles. We must now introduce the shu antique points. On each meridian there are five important acupuncture points: ting, rong, yu, jing and he,[35] each of which corresponds to an element, and thus to a Yin organ, a Yang bowel, a cosmic energy, an emotional energy and a flavor, as shown in Table 1. Thus, for the Yin organs (zang) — the heart, the lungs, the kidneys, the liver and the spleen — the rong point is Fire, joy and heat. Rong can be needled when an organ is injured by cold. We shall, for example, treat a disease of cold in the kidneys by needling the rong (heat) point of the kidney principle meridian, known as rangu (KI-2). Rong also represents the bitter flavor. When an excessively spicy (piquant) flavor dominates the liver (metal triumphs over wood), we may needle the rong point of the liver meridian, xingjian (LV-2), which dominates the piquant flavor, destroying the excess.

We determine the point of tonification on each meridian according to the logic of these shu antique points. The point of tonification is the point corresponding to the phase that precedes the phase of the organ we intend to tonify. Here we are using the creative cycle and specifically the mother-son law. For example, if we want to tonify the heart, which is correlated to the element Fire, we must treat the point on the heart meridian that represents the element Wood, since Wood is the mother of Fire. Thus, we stimulate the ting point, shaochong (HT-9), the most distal point on the meridian.

To disperse the energy in a meridian, we apply the same logic in reverse. To disperse the heart meridian (again, Fire), we stimulate the point which corresponds to the element Earth, the shu point, since Fire creates Earth. Both of these techniques have been proven scientifically.[36] Once again we are tempted to insist that these tonification and dispersion points were not determined randomly, but determined by the five element doctrine.

Other Fundamental Points of the Meridians

• The luo point is the point of origin of the luo mai (transverse and longitudinal) meridians. It is to be needled for imbalance in these meridians, to open the energetic ''precapillary anastomoses.''

• The yuan point is the opening point of the energetic ''post-capillary sphincter'' and is to be needled in association with the luo point when we wish to allow the passage of energy from one meridian to its coupled meridian. According to the *Nan Jing,* it is the point at which yuan energy is distributed in the meridian. It also plays an important part in the penetration of perverse energy into the meridian.

• The xi point is the point of the meridian for disobstruction, jue (obstruction, obstacle). It is classically indicated in emergencies. The xi point of the lung, kongzui (LU-6), for example, is to be needled in cases of respiratory distress or severe hemoptysis.

• The arterial point is the point where we can feel the pulse in an artery passing over the meridian path, and according to which we can determine the excess or deficiency of the blood and of the energy of the meridian and its organ. This point is to be needled with extreme prudence.

• The heavenly window points are generally located in the cephalic region or in the neck. These points act as safety valves and are able close off the flow of energy whenever there is a rush of energy towards the upper part of the body. These do not exist on all meridians. When an excess of energy stagnates in the cephalic region, these points are able to oppose the descending energy and thus disturb the circulation in the meridian. For this reason, the point is also called an arterial point. One of these points, renying (ST-9), correlates to the carotid glomera, and is indicated for arterial hypertension. Indeed, an excess of energy in the cephalic region corresponds to hypertensive hot rushes and may provoke cerebrovascular accidents.

Remote Energy Points

• The beishu and mu points[37] are where the energy of the viscera is concentrated. For each function there is a dorsal beishu point (sympathetic chain) and a thoracic or abdominal mu point (plexus), thus there are twelve beishu points and twelve mu points. Besides these, there is a beishu point for the diaphragm and one for the du mai, without an anterior correspondence. There are also two posterior and anterior points where the yuan energy and the jing energy emerge. These points act on the dorsal and ventral emergences of the du mai and ren mai axes.

These miscellaneous meridians are related to neurological functions and circulate jing qi. When we stimulate the beishu and mu points we are acting on the jing of the disturbed function in an effort to regularize its relationships with the jing of the body in accord with the Yin—Yang principles. On the other hand, when we stimulate the meridian points, we regulate the rong qi. This is a somewhat schematic distinction and is still only theoretical.

- The he points have a specific action on the bowels. These are:

Point	Number	Relation
zusanli	ST-36	he point of the stomach
shangjuxu	ST-37	he point of the large intestine
xiajuxu	ST-39	he point of the small intestine
yanglingquan	GB-34	he point of the gallbladder
weiyang	BL-39	he point of sanjiao triple warmer
weizhong	BL-40	he point of the bladder.

- The hui points[38] have a specific action on the tissues:

Point	Number	Relation
dazhu	BL-11	hui point of the bones
yanglingquan	GB-34	hui point of the muscles
geshu	BL-17	hui point of the blood
taiyuan	LU-9	hui point of the arteries
shanzhong	CV-17	hui point of energy
jugu	LI-16	hui point of the marrows
zhangmen	LV-13	hui point of the organs
zhongwan	CV-12	hui point of the bowels.

- The curious meridian key points will be frequently referred to in this study:

Point	Number	Relation
houxi	SI-3	opens du mai
shenmai	BL-62	opens yang qiao mai
zhaohai	KI-6	opens yin qiao mai
lieque	LU-7	opens ren mai
zulinqi	GB-41	opens dai mai
waiguan	TB-5	opens yang wei mai
gongsun	SP-4	opens chong mai
neiguan	PC-6	opens yin wei mai

Other Points on the Meridians

Altogether, there are 360 cardinal points, each with a precise indication. They conform to the physiology of the meridian on which they are situated and to its organ, or correspond to the properties of the organ in relationship to the production or circulation of a body energy, or to the vulnerability to penetration of perverse energy.

Conclusions

Throughout this brief overview of acupuncture, I have insisted on the philosophy, or system of thought, which is the basis of Chinese medicine. I have tried to demonstrate the internal coherency of this philosophy and to show that it is far more than mere reflexotherapy, which is how, until recently, Chinese medicine has been viewed.

To reduce acupuncture to the level of reflexotherapy is to take the risk of being less accurate, less effective, less etiological. Although such an attitude may be born out by research, both scientific experimentation and clinical experience tend to make us doubtful and wary. Experimentation poses the difficult problems of protocol, especially if the object of this experimentation is to unify or standardize acupuncture. It also ignores completely the placebo effect. Clinically, such an attitude would be like conferring a drug formulary on a layman, so that he or she might practice medicine.

The demonstration of the internal coherency of acupuncture theory has been foremost among my intentions, as has the revelation of the psychosomatic nature of Chinese medicine. Indeed, in Chinese traditional medicine, psyche and soma are inseparable. In this sense, our discussion will serve as a good introduction to catalytic medicine and its correlations with acupuncture. In practice, the acupuncturist as well as the catalytic practitioner is faced with a patient who presents a number of disparate symptoms that classical semiology is unable to explain or to interrelate. This forces the conclusion that the origin of the problem is emotional and requires accepting all the imprecision and sense of failure that such a conclusion entails.

With this supplementary code of pathogeny, the therapist may understand and may treat his patient. The acupuncturist does not disregard the emotional origin of some functional disorders, but his approach is different. He thinks in terms of energy, not of psychopharmacopoeia, and of harmony between body and mind, restoring order to the system that was imbalanced. We must also say that Chinese medicine is not limited to acupuncture. The word doesn't even exist in the Chinese language. The ideogram we translate as ''acupuncture'' means ''needles and fire.'' This reveals the importance attributed to moxa, which is used to cauterize the acupuncture points directly or indirectly. Chinese medicine also involves massage and energetic gymnastics (taijiquan). On the pharmacological and hygienic plane, Chinese medicine involves precise dietary and pharmacological prescriptions, which follow the classification of the five flavors and correspond to therapeutic properties that were codified before and during the Hui dynasty.

The number five and the five elements, with all the physiological, organic and psychological correspondences that the theory entails, open our eyes to the possibility of a link with the five diatheses and the five catalysts with which Menetrier has classified symptoms, pathology and behavior, and which we will now introduce.

28

Notes

[1] Marcel Granet (22). According to Granet, Chinese medicine is related on one hand to the schools of sorcery and numerology from which comes the doctrine of divination and the magical arts, and on the other hand to the Taoist philosophy, from which stems the "doctrine of immortality."

[2] According to Soulie de Morant, the *Nei Jing* was written during the 18th century BC. He notes the mention of stone needles in the *Nei Jing*. This would imply that the origin of acupuncture is neolithic. According to Huard and Wong, the *Nei Jing* was written much later, 206 B.C.-220 A.D. These authors explain in detail all the alterations made to the text up until its latest version in the 15th century.

[3] This represents an assumption, probably of metaphysical origin, that Taoism shares with Greek, Indian and Hebrew metaphysics.

[4] Chamfrault (7). His translation of the *Hoang Ti Nei Jing Su Wen* will be frequently quoted in the present work, and unless otherwise specified it is this, the Chamfrault translation, which we reference.

[5] Maspero (43).

[6] Nguyen Van Nghi (67).

[7] Wilhelm and Perrot (117).

[8] In Chinese medicine, the five elements are better expressed as five phases. This term expresses the concepts of motion and change in time that is inherent in these five categories. Nonetheless, both terms are commonly used.

[9] This proves the correlation between Chinese medicine and the school of the *Yi Jing*.

[10] J. Filliozat (20), p. 448.

[11] This discovery has since been completed with Rumanian, French and American works on thermovision and the electrobiography of Dumitrescu. (See Laugt, A., "L'electrobiographie, These pour le doctorat en medecine," Grenoble, 1978.)

[12] Maspero (43).

[13] *The I Ching, Book of Changes,* is the work that deals with changes and their consequences through symbolic hexagrams. Each level of the hexagram is composed of a continuous line (—) that is Yang, or a discontinuous line (– –) that is Yin. This correlates acupuncture and the *I Ching* and supports the view of Yin and Yang as forces rather than substances.

[14] Husson (28), p. 22.

[15] Bridgeman, quoted by Husson (28), p. 22.

[16] The Imperial Fire relates to the heart viscera and small intestine, the Ministerial Fire to the pericardium and the triple burner.

[17] Roustan (98), p. 28.

[18] *Ibid.* This obviously suggests the large arteries over the Yang Ming that are related to the stomach and thus to the xu li.

[19] Like zong qi, this potential partly depends on the genetic inheritance. However, it relates as well to the "anterior heaven," in other words, the immaterial or not yet materialized, Tao, the principle of the universe.

[20] Roustan (98), p. 28.

[21] *Ibid.*

[22] *Su Wen,* Chapter 60; *Ling Shu,* Chapter 65.

[23] The amount of gametes diminishes even without sexual activity because of the periodic maturation of the gametes in both sexes. This is obvious in ovulation; our current knowledge of the prostaglandins is insufficient, and figures here as an hypothesis. In a philosophical and non-biological way, we must understand yuan qi as destiny, which determines the length of our life. When our capital of yuan is finished, death results, whether from disease, age or simply "accident."

[24] We can offer this neologism in acupuncture, meaning to vascularize or innervate, in order to transport energy through the meridian to the target.

[25] *Su Wen* (8), Chapter 11, p. 54.

[26] Chamfrault and Van Nghi (10). See also, Nguyen Van Nghi (67), p. 204-231.

[27] Nguyen Van Nghi (62), pp. 125-164.

[28] Requena (78), pp. 337-348.

[29] See *Ling Shu* (8), Chapter 10, 11, pp. 374-380; Nguyen Van Nghi (67); Nguyen Van Nghi (65).

[30] According to the *Su Wen* and the *Ling Shu.*

[31] Nguyen Van Nghi's list, according to the relatively new treatise *Trung Y Hoc* from Hanoi.

[32] *Su Wen* (8), Chapters 65, 67, 68, 69, 70, 71. See also: Nguyen Van Nghi (67), pp. 43-70.

[33] The shen is the product of the five visceral qi, or the five psychic essences of the five organs.

[34] Nguyen Van Nghi (67), pp. 43-70.

[35] In the pinyin transliteration system, the ting and jing points are both spelled *jing*. We shall retain the former convention of referring to them as ting and jing respectively, in order to distinguish between them.

[36] We can mention among many other works those of the Rumanian Stoicescu *et.al.* (108), and of Mussat (52) on the radioscopic manifestations of the points.

[37] For the sake of clarity, the yu (iu) points of the back will be called beishu. The yu points, the third points of the meridians, will be called the shu points.

[38] Nguyen Van Nghi (67), pp. 406-407. These are traditional antique Middle Age points that were classified according to the *Huang Di Nei Jing Su Wen*.

Introduction to Diathetic Medicine

Life as we know it depends on a perpetual exchange between the environment and the constituents of organic matter, thanks to the pulmonary and cutaneous respiratory systems, the intake of food and the excretion of wastes. These exchanges take place at a rhythm that we are only beginning to be able to calculate, in any case, much more rapidly than we might have supposed.

— M. Polonovski

Diathetic Medicine

Acupuncture is a medicine where treatment consists of the physical stimulation of special cutaneous sites, by way of needles, massage and moxibustion. It is a manipulation of energy. In diathetic, or "catalytic" medicine, treatment consists of the prescription of trace elements. This too is a manipulation of energy. The aims of these two medical theories are so close that from the beginning the pioneers of diathetic medicine have tried to relate their practice to acupuncture.[1]

In diathetic medicine the concept of energy is expressed more scientifically with a less symbolic code. The matter — energy duality, fundamental to Chinese thought, finds clear expression in the study of biological phenomena. It is astonishing to find, through an elementary analysis of living matter, that 99.9% of its constituents are plastic elements (oxygen, carbon, nitrogen) and that only .1% is made up of atoms indispensable to the functions of life: the trace elements. This amazing disproportion led Gabriel Bertrand to write, at the beginning of the twentieth century, "the organism appears to be like an oligarchy where vast amounts of passive elements are governed by very few catalytic elements."

Gabriel Bertrand's discovery was only the continuation of the work of Berzelius, who more than a century earlier had noticed a similar chemical phenomenon in plants:

> The mere contact of some substances with others can provoke a set of chemical reactions. Combinations may dissolve or give form to mixtures without the apparent participation of the substance that caused the reaction.

From this fundamental chemical and biochemical discovery stems the concept of catalysis. Of the hundred elements classified by Mendeleeff, only about thirty seem to possess this peculiar catalytic quality. These are still known as the transitory or catalytic elements. These elements are active, even when present only in trace amounts, hence their name: *trace elements*.

In treatment, minute quantities of these trace elements can act on and modify a given metabolism. Many experiments have confirmed this original hypothesis as well as the concept of critical active concentration. The infinitesimal active threshold is a law of trace element theory. For example, when there is no manganese at all in the culture medium, certain mold cultures, the *Sterigmatocystis nigra,* will not grow. A concentration of 10^{-10}g allows the development but not the appearance of the reproductive organs. At 10^{-9}g manganese concentration, the first yellow conidia appear and at 10^{-8}g the black, reproductive conidia grow. Around 10^{-7}g there is a maximum growth and any further concentration inhibits growth. Similar phenomena are observable in animals.

If one adds manganese traces to a deficient diet, the lifespan of rats increases by 12%. A total deficiency of manganese always leads to testis degeneration. Under similar circumstances, chickens present bony formations called "perosis." A manganese violet histochemical reaction on bone sections shows a high manganese bone concentration, which is even higher in the areas of bone formation. We can relate this fact to the phosphate catalytic property attributed to manganese by Roche and Courtois. However, between the laboratory results and practical medicine, there is a gap that is difficult to fill. We must praise Jacques Menetrier whose patient and meticulous research, beginning as early as 1932, filled that gap.

Historical Background

In his first published work, 22 years after he began his research, Menetrier himself stressed:

> Since 1932, we have dedicated our work to the study of the trace elements and to empirical experimentation in this domain, following the lines of research established by Gabriel Bertrand and by his school, and according to the methods of J.U. Sutter.[2]

By 1942, Menetrier had recorded more than 10,000 worldwide biological experiments with catalysts. He was the first person to think of the medical applications possible and to methodically investigate the clinical effects. As he wrote at the time, the new discoveries in the realms of physiology, endocrinology, neurology, physiochemistry and morphopsychology allowed medical science to take a closer look at the "human factor" in illness and to reconsider the old problem of terrain, so dear to the ancients since the days of Hippocrates.

During the same period many other authors were working on the same problems: Abrami, Achard, Biot, Carrel, Delor, Laignel-Lavastine, Reilly, Leriche, Jacquelin, Besancon, Nicolle, Roger, Mauriac, Lumiere, Vernes and Vernet (in association with Corman's work on morphopsychology). Also, we can include the first ideas of Freud on the subconscious, the first lessons of atomic physics by L. de Broglie and V. Henri, and Gabriel Bertrand's equally important work in organic chemistry.

Toward the end of 1943, at Menetrier's initiative, a biological research center was established and dedicated to the methodical and experimental study of the trace elements. The first step of this study was the polyvalent examination of patients, comparison between different diagnoses and the search for therapeutic indications for the trace elements. Meanwhile, therapeutic testing was begun with great care, centering on arthritis and tuberculosis. Menetrier himself admitted that

34

the initial research was empirical. Nonetheless, the results of his research lead him to a number of conclusions, as early as 1954:

> There is no doubt of the existence of diatheses, or terrains, which unite many different symptoms.
>
> These diatheses constitute etiological entities. The proof of this is shown by the multisymptomatic action of an isolated element or group of elements.
>
> Taken regularly in similar quantities these elements alter the clinical picture and can solve a problem either temporarily or permanently. This is specific to a diathesis, not to a symptom.
>
> This therapeutic effect enables us to more precisely define the limits of a terrain and to link this terrain to apparently aberrant or contradictory symptoms. It is the basis of a new clinical attitude and of a better understanding of organic receptivity.
>
> The action of the trace elements is basically regulative, equilibrative and adaptive as well as experimentally psychophysiological.
>
> Trace elements act on physiological as well as psychological symptoms that have the same value for the prescription.
>
> The active dose of a trace element is a dose of about one-millionth of a gram. The activity of the trace element is therefore clearly qualitative, not quantitative.[3]

Other French and foreign researchers collaborated with Menetrier. In time, methodical research and empirical studies led to the creation of what we have come to call in French the "medicine of the functions," or "diathetic medicine." Its basic principles have remained unchanged, as have the five diatheses published by Menetrier in 1954, to which only a few details have been added over the years. Diathetic medicine has appealed to more and more physicians since its introduction and is flourishing in many countries. Numerous experiments are carried out in hospitals and laboratories and the number of practitioners is increasing steadily. This "medicine of the functions," with its abundant medical references, is now a reliable non-allopathic medicine. Veterinary doctors have become interested in the experimental study of the trace elements and have proven that their action goes beyond the placebo effect.

The Diathesis

A diathesis is a morbid state somewhere between health and illness. It may be considered a state of malfunction and of deregulation of the physiological functions, psychosomatic as well as organic, or as an intermediate stage in the evolution of a functional disorder into an organic lesion. These definitions are analogous to the Chinese concept of the function that corresponds to a meridian, which is linked to a specific viscera. In theory, a functional deregulation in the meridian may eventually lead to organic troubles in the related viscera.

35

The biologist H.P. Klotz asked:

> Is the difference between functional and organic a matter of nature, or simply of degree? The analysis of this deregulation is biochemical. We look for the initial disorder and the site of the enzymatic blockage. When the blockage is known, it can be treated and the problems solved.

From this point of view, any metabolic disorder, signaled by symptoms, a specific syndrome or by a specific behavior, may be related to a trace element that is responsible for the deregulation. An author who published an introduction to the method gives the following poetic example:

> Like a river that travels from barrier to barrier, from the mountains to the sea, life progresses from one reaction to another, oriented by the law of the masses and aided by the enzymes, from the unmetabolized to the metabolized molecule.

> What if a barrier is closed? An enzyme missing?

> The river leaves its bed, floods fields and meadows; the metabolism is detoured from its normal course and digs new channels, whose consequence will be illness, either through lack of vital substance or because of the presence of a new toxic substance. Open the barrier; bring the enzymes to life — the flow of energy returns to its bed. The gravity of the flooding depends on whether or not the disrupted metabolic chain was an essential one, whether the disruption lasted a short or long time and whether the detour was destructive or not.[4]

This comparison is somewhat prophetic and may be extended to acupuncture if we replace the river with the meridian and consider a group, a network of channels, rather than a biological chain. It is in this way that a diathesis is defined in terms of a specific catalytic trace element. According to Bert, Vallee and Hoch, a metal that is present in the biological matter is included in different compounds and plays very different roles.

As most of these compounds and the part they play in biological reactions are not yet defined, and as only the sum of their metallic atoms can be measured, the biological interpretation of their analysis is, to say the least, problematic.[5]

Thus, only through clinical experience and observation may we be sure of the mechanisms involved, and in this sense, we must be grateful to Menetrier for his systematic classification of metals according to diathesis.

A diathesis can thus encompass many chronic, ill-defined disorders that are difficult to categorize as classical pathological syndromes. Its diagnosis demands a meticulous study of the patient's symptoms and behavior. It is not accomplished the other way around, by an analysis of the classical syndromes relating them to a single diathesis. It would be difficult to relate a clinical picture to a single diathesis. It is well known that personal characteristics vary from one to another and depend on the individual constitution. Let us not forget the words of Sir William Osler, who wrote:

It is certainly necessary to know what illness the specific patient has contracted, but is it not more important to know what patients contract specific illness?

The ability to grasp an order amongst the disorder, unity among the many, is the results of clinical experience. It is this experience that enabled Menetrier to write a description of the five diatheses.

The Five Diatheses

• The arthritic or allergic diathesis corresponds to the trace element manganese.

• The hyposthenic diathesis corresponds to the trace elements manganese-copper.

• The dystonic diathesis corresponds to the trace elements manganese-cobalt.

• The anergic diathesis corresponds to the trace elements copper-gold-silver.

• The diathesis of maladaptation corresponds to the trace elements zinc-copper and zinc-nickel-cobalt.

The reader will find descriptions of physical, psychological or intellectual behavior, of syndromes and of symptoms defining each of these diatheses in specialized literature.[6]

Each of these diatheses will be reviewed in detail and related to acupuncture. The secondary metallic ions — cobalt, copper, nickel, zinc, iodine, sulphur, phosphorus-antimony-arsenic, fluoride, bromine, silicon, aluminium, magnesium, potassium, lithium, barium, strontium, bismuth, iron, boron, rhenium, selenium and so on, take us from the present subject and are detailed in other literature.

The Examination of the Patient

Dudan wrote:

> To avoid a symptomatic and only temporarily effective treatment, we have to determine the diathetic origin that is actively present through an attentive and discriminating examination. The therapist will thus discover the weaknesses of the individual terrain, whose importance may no longer be ignored.

This statement expresses the originality of the method. A diathesis is first recognized during questioning and is then confirmed by way of physical examination. According to the pioneers of diathetic medicine, the interview must include questions covering at least three generations: "Diseases of the ancestry of the parents, previous personal diseases, diseases of the siblings and diseases of the children."

37

Such an interview will bring to the surface much useful information about the family, its genetics and the patient's own individuality. In the interview, the physician gets to know his patient's inherited terrain, his personally acquired pathology, his weak points, his ability to resist diseases and his intolerances or incompatibilities. The physician can group these various elements into behavior groups. The study of the family helps to uncover more or less predominant functional problems and actual morbid states that tend to be more lesional. The vital destiny of an individual is related to the sources and stage of his disorder. The morbid state, with the comprehension and firm support of the doctor, may often be favorably influenced, even permanently.[7]

These statements remind us of those of the Chinese ancients, whose preoccupations were equally preventive and for whom the doctor-patient relationship was inspired by the desire for a deep comprehension of the patient as a whole: ''The patient is the trunk, the doctor his branches: if there is incompatibility between branch and trunk (biao ben bu de),[8] the perverse energy cannot be subjugated.''[9]

Correlations between Diathetic Medicine and Acupuncture

I must repeat that I am not the first to attempt this comparison. It is interesting to note that the only physicians and researchers who have shown an interest in establishing a correspondence between the two systems, based on energy manipulation, have been those who were specializing in diathetic medicine. Menetrier suggested, then confirmed, the existence of relationships between the two systems. He also proved their complementarity and added, ''Acupuncture seems to be catalytic in its effects.''[10] Without limiting acupuncture to this definition, I agree wholly with Menetrier, who began in 1954 to study acupuncture points electronically, notably concerning their electrical resistance in correlation with the diathetic states. In 1967, Menetrier wrote:

> Whatever our understanding of the Yin—Yang principle, of the five elements and of the circulation of energy, we can verify two facts: Acupuncture is a medicine thousands of years old that is based on the principle of exchange and regulation, and there are known electrical phenomena at the acupuncture points that are altered during treatment with needles. One day (probably through electronic research) the physical mysteries of acupuncture will be unlocked, and diathetic medicine will be enriched by new ways of knowing and new ways of acting. We do not mean by this to discredit the existence of irrational or metaphysical phenomena.[11]

Faced with the difficult problem of plotting electrical resistance in the acupuncture points over time, the attitude of the first trace element experimenters, which was based on clinical experience and on therapeutic application, is valuable. This attitude, which was, and is still clinical, may be easier to adopt in the present study, as there are only two proposals to compare. Clinical pictures and behavior

38

are already well-defined in both medical systems. The comparison of the two systems was just waiting for an acupuncturist to come along.

Can this effort bring any irrational phenomena to the surface? We believe not. We believe, instead, that there are some phenomena that remain unexplained. Can this come to involve certain metaphysical concepts? I am sure of it. This brings up the questions: Why? How? These must answered with circumspection and with the legitimate curiosity of scientific pragmatism. This may shed light on the identity and the nature of facts, whereas a prejudiced, defiant attitude can only perpetuate the darkness and blind ignorance that has been, until recently, the rule in Western medical circles.

To facilitate this comparison, it is necessary to introduce the diagnostic concepts of Chinese medicine as well as the concepts of *constitution* and *temperament*. These ideas are essential to Chinese diagnostics. It is the remodeling of these concepts to create a new classification in Chinese pathology that justifies the title of this book, *Terrains and Pathology in Acupuncture*. Any order, any cohesion that becomes apparent in clinical practice is worthy of consideration. Just as the description of these diatheses does not betray classical pathology, a focus on constitution and temperament in no way betrays the oriental tradition. The general framework of diatheses is contained in the purest traditional texts. We will demonstrate this point throughout the course of this work.

Notes

[1] Menetrier (44).

[2] *Ibid.*, p. 26.

[3] *Ibid.*, p. 30.

[4] Laboratoire Labcatal (33).

[5] We are far from knowing all the 10,000 enzymes that we believe to exist.

[6] Menetrier (46).

[7] Laboratoire Labcatal (33), p. 54.

[8] ''The patient (ben) is the fundamental element; the secondary is the physician (biao), a common agreement is the factor of cure,'' notes Husson on the biao ben bu de.

[9] *Su Wen* (28), Chapter 13, p. 109.

[10] Menetrier (44), p. 98.

[11] Menetrier (45), p. 47.

Examination of the Patient

*Before we begin needling, we must know precisely what role the mind plays.
Life is engendered in the meeting of the earth's energy with that of heaven.
Life conserves the essence of this combination. The essence is composed of
two elements, one of which comes from the cosmos {the air} while the other
comes from food {the earth}. These two elements engender the shen {the
spirit} and the po {the secondary soul} which comes and goes with the
essence.*

— *Ling Shu, Chapter 8*

The Eight Rules of Diagnosis

The rules of traditional Chinese diagnosis are common to most forms of medicine and share the attitude of semiological investigation: interrogation, inspection,
palpation. These rules are expressed in Chinese in the following way:[1]

— look
— listen and smell
— question
— touch

These are the four elements of diagnosis. The object of this examination
differs from that of Western medicine as Chinese diagnosis pertains to energy balance, rather than anatomopathology. Thus, symptoms are codified in a very different language. Also, the acupuncturist looks at different things, feels and pal-
pates different parts of the body and asks questions that are very specific, yet different from those asked by a Western doctor. At the end of his examination, the
acupuncturist selects, classifies and compares the results of his examination. Just
as the diagnosis is expressed in terms of energetic balance the laws of energy
govern his comparison and his reflection. We are referring to what is known in
Chinese medicine as the eight principles.[2]

The expectation of this diagnostic inquiry is well expressed in the *Trung Y
Hoc:*

> To observe and to assess the illness is to apply the basic theories of
> Yin—Yang, of the five phases, of the organs and the bowels, of the
> primary channels and the secondary channels, of rong and wei ener-
> gies and of the qi {energy} and of the xue {blood}.[3]

This is, of course, what is suggested by the discussion of energetic physiology in
the first chapter. This diversified approach is intellectually structured according to
the Yin—Yang dialectic. This dialectic gives birth to the eight principles, which
are:

Yin—Yang
Interior—Exterior
Cold—Heat
Deficiency—Excess

These eight rules represent the fundamental aspects of diagnostic reasoning in acupuncture. Nguyen Van Nghi has studied these rules in detail[4] and many other authors have examined these principles and their dialectical extensions.[5] It is always the Yin—Yang duality that presides over the other six principles: the phenomena of heat, exterior phenomena and excesses are by nature Yang, while interior, cold and deficiency are by nature Yin.

In each category, there are several different signs that may be discovered through interrogation and examination. We may thus determine if an illness is Yin or Yang, interior or exterior, cold or hot, or caused by a deficiency or an excess of energy. For example, in an illness caused by heat,[6] the symptoms are sudden and high fever, anxiety, dislike of heat, thirst, a red face, constipation, oliguria, reddish dark urine, a rough, yellow-coated tongue and a rapid pulse. Diseases caused by the cold, on the other hand, are characterized by moderate temperature, lack of thirst, pallor, diarrhea, polyuria, a white tongue and a slow pulse. More complicated Chinese pictures are possible when cold and hot are mixed or symptoms of false cold and false heat coexist.[7]

The terms interior and exterior, as they are used in diagnosis, pertain to the location of the illness within the body:

> When perverse energy invades the surface and is localized in the main meridians and the secondary channels, the illness is of the exterior. On the other hand, when the perverse energy gains the organs or the bowels, by way of the main meridians, the illness is internal, that is, of the interior.[8]

Diseases caused by emotional factors, fatigue and nutrition are interior.

Since the Yin—Yang discrimination presides over the eight rules, symptoms have to be interpreted and associated to define an illness. An illness may be, for example, interior, cold, and due to either excess or deficiency. However, these associations agree with the logic expected of the Yin—Yang principle. For example, an illness of heat (Yang) will be particularly felt on the surface of the body (exterior, Yang). There will be symptoms in the upper portion of the body (Yang) rather than the lower, hot skin and cheeks, headache, anxiety (all of which are signs of the excessive ascent of Yang), dry throat, thirst, an excess of energy, acceleration of the pulse and beating arteries. When cold invades the body, the disturbance is interior (Yin). One will feel "frozen to the bones." The lower (Yin) portion of the body is affected; the feet and the trunk will be cold. The movement of perverse humid energy is that of cold, as dryness is the same as heat.

Wind can penetrate anywhere: in the upper and lower extremities, into the skin, the connective tissues, the bones and the viscera, both inside and out. Wind is capable of provoking innumerable illnesses. Once again, things become more complicated when wind combines with cold, heat or humidity. These countless clinical pictures include the whole range of human pathology, which explains why there are numbers of Western medical volumes dedicated to their description and enormous medical encyclopedias, as well as the ever increasing mass of medical documents. In Chinese medicine we need only index the symptoms and to classify each according to the eight principles of diagnosis to determine the global nature of the disease. Then, one may diagnose the abnormal circulation of energy within the meridians.

The language of Chinese medicine, by definition, enables the acupuncturist to decode symptoms and adopt a treatment under any circumstances, even if the patient presents an illness with an unknown Western etiology, such as multiple sclerosis; or a disease that is not recognized as a pathological entity, as was the case with Barlow's disease only twenty years ago; or other unnamed diseases.

The Four Elements of Diagnosis

The eight principles allow selection and classification of clinical symptoms according to the four elements of diagnosis.

Look

We must first examine the overall condition of the patient. We examine the face and specifically the complexion, regarding its color and the localization of certain pigmentations.[9] We look at the eyes, the color of the conjunctiva and of the sclera, faults of visual convergence, the presence or absence of tears, the presence of capillaries and the brightness of the patient's eyes. We also look at the nose. We check whether the nose is dry, humid or cold and whether it is blocked. We pay attention to the color of the tip of the nose.[10] We also look at the lips: whether their color is red, black, blue, or pale; if they are swollen, dry or contracted; or whether there is any deviation.

In the mouth, we assess the condition of the teeth: their brightness, their degree of humidity and the condition of the tongue. The analysis of the tongue should be extremely precise. As in all the other sensory organs, all twelve functions are effectively represented in the tongue. The examination of its coating, its color, its thickness and the difference between one part of the tongue and another, is an important element of Chinese diagnosis.[11] We also look at the fingernails, at the fingers and at the hands to see if they are thick, smooth or rough. We look at the limbs in the same light to see if they are contracted, emaciated or powerless. A particularly interesting area, worthy of close inspection, is the inner side of the forearm, the "one-meter pond."

Listen and Smell

The tone of the patient's voice, the sound of his breathing, the aspect of his cough or of his hiccup, to which we must listen attentively, are also important diagnostic tools.[12] In healthy people, as it is written in the *Trung Y Hoc,* "energy does not smell." It is in this text that we find detailed descriptions and interpretations of the many body odors.

Questioning

In the *Trung Y Hoc* we read, "To question the patient about the past and present signs of his disease is one of the four methods of diagnosis."[13] In acupuncture, as in diathetic medicine, this interrogation of the patient is an essential element of the diagnosis. The patient's emotional make-up is just as interesting as his physical constitution and the role of "mental" activity is equally important. In Chapter 13 of the *Su Wen,* we read:

> The Emperor Huang Di asked of Qi Bo, "You have already spoken
> of the fundamental rules {of diagnosis}. You have said that the
> essential thing is to pay attention to the complexion and the pulse. I
> understand this. But are there not other important points?"
>
> "Yes," answered Qi Bo, "the clinical examination must include
> another fundamental point."
>
> "And what is that?"
>
> "It is the interrogation."
>
> "And how does one interrogate a patient?"
>
> "We must choose a quiet and secluded place and make our patient
> feel at ease. In particular we must have the patience to gather all the
> information about the history of the illness and to have the patient
> describe in detail all their symptoms. We have also to appreciate the
> state of our patient's mental energy, whose presence is a good sign
> and whose absence is a bad one."[14]

As already mentioned, the orientation of this inquiry follows the eight rules. Analyzing the symptoms at the onset and during an illness helps to differentiate deep and superficial symptoms, Yang and Yin, hot and cold, excess and deficiency. The ancient texts describe and classify the different aspects of perspiration, headaches, pains, paresthesia, stools and urines, appetite, thirst, the appeal of one flavor or another, the presence or absence of deafness, of tinnitus, of visual disturbances and of dysmenorrhea according to the eight rules of diagnosis. In short, all the functional symptoms that can be gathered during a systematic interview similar to our Western interview, yet classified according to the eight principles, instead of apparatus by apparatus, as in Western diagnosis.

The intellectual approach that leads to the diagnosis of a particular energy imbalance is vividly apparent during the interview. This is especially the case when a Western physician leads the questioning. By the questions we ask, we effectively "feel-out" the ambivalence of the enquiry. The indications given us by the patient fall, instinctively and logically, into two different and specific groups. The Chinese classification of the signs and symptoms according to the eight rules need not be learned by rote. For example, through the Yin—Yang dialectic we may logically distinguish between the cold or warm aspects of a diarrhea, between an illness that is interior or exterior, between a deficiency or an excess of energy.[15] In acupuncture, as in Western medicine, semiological particularities, symptoms and syndromes are related to specific functions or viscera. This link may not be invented, but must be learned, just like the correlations learned in any training.

Obviously, the correlation code is the same in any medical system. An anuria is a disorder of the urinary function. Thus, a Western medical background can without doubt help when we practice Chinese medicine. However, if in Western medicine a symptom or a sign is related to an anatomophysiological function, the same sign or symptom in Chinese medicine corresponds not only to that function, or viscera, but also to its corresponding energetic entity. The liver function, for example, includes not only the liver meridian, the zu jue yin with all the specificity of this meridian energy, but also the genitalia, the lower urinary tract, the face, the eyes, the nose and the lips. In other words, even though we all agree that the disease is located in the bladder, a retention of urine causing an anuria may be a blockage of the energy in the liver meridian. Thus, certain points of the liver meridian will require stimulus. Note also that a liver problem may cause disorders that are classified as otorhinolaryngologic or opthalmic diseases, such as allergic rhinitis, conjunctivitis or keratitis.

Another example that we have already discussed is diarrhea. We may discover diarrheas of kidney origin (zu shao yin), as in certain cases of melena or ulcerative colitis. In other words, while the Chinese semiology cannot be said to be contradictory to our own, its code is more complex and contains sizable differences that can lead to misunderstandings and errors of energetic diagnosis, if we are not extremely careful in interpretation. This code cannot be improvised. It must be learned, and in this learning, classical medical knowledge may be a handicap. The main problem lies in the presentation of the material. The classical texts of Chinese pathology were compiled according to a logical model that is different from Western pathology. In our search for meaning, to understand the semiology of the most obvious as well as the most subtle of signs, we must hunt through labyrinths of chapters dealing with pulses, fevers, seasonal variations, topographic descriptions of the meridians and of their symptoms. We must comb other more general chapters dealing with the emotional aspects, the mental aspects, Yin—Yang theory, excess and deficiency, or look again to those chapters that examine the global imbalance of rong qi or of wei qi, the blood, or the global ascending or descending energy, the blockage of energy such as jue, or the abnormal counter-clockwise circulation of the energy within the meridians.

In short, Chinese semiology and pathology are like a puzzle and the symptoms, to be understood in the Chinese sense, must not be removed from the physiology nor from the specific disturbances of this physiology that are the Chinese energetic physiopathology.[16] Some of its mechanisms are obscure in certain texts and clear in others. Often one must read several texts to compare and contrast their contents to understand their real importance. For example, the *Da Cheng,* a text from the middle ages, notes a specific symptomology for each acupuncture point. This helps us understand some symptoms and to relate these to a physiology that agrees with the physiological properties of the point, as with the example of taichong (LV-3).

This fundamental aspect of Chinese medicine has been improperly studied and neglected by most Western acupuncturists for far too long, probably because of the difficulty we find in the synthesis of these texts and our cultural medical conditioning that leads the Western physician to adjust his diagnosis exclusively according to the semiology he has been taught in medical school.

Finally, the taking of the Chinese pulses, a fundamental element of diagnosis in acupuncture, increases the difficulty faced by the Western physician, as it is highly subjective, difficult to interpret and goes against our habits and our objective, Cartesian reflexes.

Palpation

Of the four elements of diagnosis, the greatest difference between Western and Chinese medical systems is found in the methods of palpation and pulse taking. The object of Western palpation is to explore the deep viscera: the spleen, the liver, the stomach and the colon. The same technique is used in the palpation of the natural orifices and cavities. We exaggerate only a little in saying that this is a material exploration that conforms with the anatomopathological spirit of Western medicine. In Chinese medicine, palpation is an exploration of that which is superficial: the skin, the subcutaneous tissues and the pulsations of the arteries. This exploration of the surface is, according to the Yin—Yang dialectic, an investigation of the immaterial and energetic. This is equally within the spirit of Chinese medicine.

• **Examination of the integument**

To the experienced eye, the aspect of the skin along the pathway of a meridian reveals any morbid perturbations in that specific meridian network. Clues of an energy imbalance may be visible as changes of skin color, changes in temperature or changes in thickness. A cellulitic infiltration in the concerned territory and the presence of reflex dermalgia are meaningful symptoms. The Chinese doctor looks for and feels the fine capillary beds on the skin. He looks for balance, excess or deficiency of the venous system or of the arterial pulses throughout the vascular territory. An original technique of diagnosis in Chinese medicine is the taking of the pulses at both wrists over the radial artery.

• **Taking of the radial pulse**

In the most ancient texts, such as the *Nei Jing Su Wen,* pulse taking is described and its results are commented on. The index, middle and ring fingers of both hands are applied on both wrists of the patient: the middle fingers are placed over the radial arteries, which are felt over the radial styloid, with index and ring fingers on either side. Thus, three positions are fixed on both sides: the *inch,* the *bar* and the *foot,* a total of six positions over the two radial arteries. These correspond to the lung meridian points: taiyuan (LU-9), jingqu (LU-8) and lieque (LU-7). The difference in pressure over these arteries distinguishes the deep and superficial pulses. There are a total of twelve tactile impressions, or twelve positions related to the twelve functions of the twelve main meridians. These twelve positions, according to some modern Western acupuncturists are, respectively:

Pulse:	The left wrist foot positions
Superficial:	Kidney
Deep:	Bladder
Pulse:	The left wrist bar positions
Superficial:	Liver
Deep:	Gallbladder
Pulse:	The left wrist inch positions
Superficial:	Heart
Deep:	Small Intestine
Pulse:	The right wrist foot positions
Superficial:	Pericardium
Deep:	Triple Burner

Pulse: The right wrist bar positions
Superficial: Spleen
Deep: Stomach

Pulse: The right wrist inch positions
Superficial: Lung
Deep: Large Intestine

The differences of the pulse qualities indicate the energetic excess or deficiency of any function in comparison with other functions. However, the taking of radial pulses needs much discussion.

As has been noted by Nguyen Van Nghi, the twelve functions felt in the pulses were not mentioned in Chinese medical texts until the 14th century AD.[17] In the earlier texts of the *Su Wen* only the pulses of the organs are considered, excepting a single bowel, the stomach. Even more important is the knowledge that at the left and right inch positions are felt the Yang kidney and the Yin kidney respectively, from the time of the *Nei Jing* to the epoch of the *Yi Zong* (1792). Elsewhere, Faubert describes five ancient and modern classifications and supports the complete inversion of the *Nan Jing* system: bowels reflected in the superficial pulse, organs in the deep pulse. This theory was accepted by J. Lavier and by J. Worsley, but with the substitution of Yin and Yang kidneys on the left wrist and the triple burner on the right.[18]

These irregularities demonstrate the extreme complexity of this topic, as well as the obvious divergence between authors and schools. Even if we were to agree unanimously on a schema, the information is confusing and difficult. The information we must gather to make a diagnosis according to the eight principles is not only quantitative, but also qualitative. With incredible subtlety, the traditional Chinese doctor must be able to recognize illnesses of cold, of heat, of the interior or of the exterior, which have invaded a given function, solely by the qualitative aspect of the corresponding pulse. Depending on the case, an aspect of the global radial pulse may determine the diagnosis. Thus, to be an expert in pulse diagnosis, an acupuncturist must be able to recognize twenty-eight different pulse qualities. These are: floating, deep, slow, rapid, gliding, rough, empty, full, long, short, excess, small, hurried, retarded, hollow, bowstring, intermittent, hard, soft, weak, dispersed, fine, hidden, moving, excited, thready, changing or quick.[19]

Each of these pulse qualities is defined by a metaphor. The hollow pulse, for example, is "like the smashed stalk of an onion, with a gap in the middle." This pulse is symptomatic of hemorrhage. The full pulse arrives "in great waves, like on the sea." The information gathered during the taking of the radial pulses is not limited to this information alone. In Chapter 49 of the *Ling Shu,* entitled "General Advice," we read that in addition to the specific information concerning each function, there is another, more global technique.

By feeling the pulses of both wrists simultaneously, it is immediately possible to determine which global pulse, the left or the right, is dominant. This relative excess of one pulse over the other is then appreciated by degrees. The right global pulse is known as qi hao and reflects the Yin; the left pulse is known as ren ying and reflects the Yang. If the left pulse is twice as ample as the right, Shao Yang is affected. If it is three times as ample, Tai Yang is affected. Four times as ample, and it is Yang Ming to which we must attend. If the right pulse is twice as ample as the left pulse, Jue Yin is affected. Three times as ample indicates Shao Yin, four times indicates Tai Yin.[20] Thus, the diagnosis is not only based on the five movements and the twelve meridians, but also on the six energies and the six unit meridians. Each complements the other. In addition to this comparison of right and left pulses, it is also possible to compare radial and peripheral pulses. For example, the intensity of the pulse in qi hao may be compared with that of a pulse taken on the carotid artery, at the point renying (ST-9).

• Examination of the peripheral pulses

To complete our discussion of the role of pulse taking in Chinese medicine, we must examine the peripheral pulses. Qi Bo, the ancient Chinese physician, lists these thus:

> "The ultimate numbers of the Heaven and the Earth begin with one and end with nine. Heaven is one, Earth is two, Man is three, and three times three is nine which corresponds to the number of 'peripheral regions' (ue). Man is composed of three parts that each have three possible observation posts: to decide the chances of survival, to control illnesses, to harmonize and finally to eliminate perverse energies."

> The Yellow Emperor asked, "What is meant by the three regions?"

> Qi Bo replied, "Upper, middle and lower, these three regions of the body each have three observation posts: heaven, earth and man. To do a good job, it is necessary to offer good instructions. In the upper region, the post of Heaven refers to the two frontal arteries, whence passes the qi of Shao Yang of the limb, the biliary vesicle.[21] The post of Earth in the upper region refers to the arteries of the two cheeks; the Man of the upper region refers to the arteries in front of the ears {ermen, TB-21}.

> The Heaven of the middle region refers to the Tai Yin of the hand {jingqu, LU-8}; the Earth of the middle region refers to the Yang Ming of the hand {hegu, LI-4}; the Man of the middle region refers to the Shao Yin of the hand {shenmen, HT-7}.

> The Heaven of the lower region refers to the Jue Yin of the foot, {wuli, LV-10}; the Earth of the lower region refers to the Shao Yin of the foot {taixi, KI-3}; the Man of the lower region refers to the Tai Yin of the foot {jimen, SP-11}.

> Therefore, the Heaven of the lower region is symptomatic of the liver, the Earth is symptomatic of the kidneys, and the Man is symptomatic of the energy of the spleen and stomach."[22]

Qi Bo's explanation generates two observations. First, most of the Western textbooks on acupuncture make little mention of these peripheral pulses. Second, the radial pulse is usually considered only in its quantitative aspect. In the description of where and how to take the pulse, many disagreements exist in China as well as in the West. Thus, Chinese pulse diagnosis never ceases to be a cause of argument for the layman and among acupuncturists. To the layman, it seems impossible to assess the health of the various bodily functions simply by feeling the radial pulse. Among acupuncturists, besides the internal disagreements about this diagnostic tool, some have rejected the concept of pulse diagnosis outright and do not accord it any credibility. Often their arguments bear weight. They refer to Qi Bo himself, who states, ''The morning is the best time to take the pulse, as the Yin energy is sleeping, and the Yang energy has not yet risen.''[23] Before the patient breaks his fast, the slightest perturbation is clearly perceptible. These practitioners argue that it is almost impossible, without a wide margin of error, to take the pulse at any other time of day. Let us imagine our first afternoon appointment, at around 2 p.m., with a patient who has just had lunch and probably a cup of coffee as well.

Other acupuncturists think that without radial pulse diagnosis, there can be no good acupuncture. To soothe this argument, the least we can say is that pulse diagnosis is the most subjective aspect of Chinese medicine. It depends on the acupuncturist's values; it varies with the time of day, the seasons, the temperature; and it is not a scientific and objective means of diagnosis. Nevertheless, it occupies an important position in the traditional texts of acupuncture and the information gathered during its study must not be neglected. It might eventually help to correct an error of diagnosis. Thus, it is true that what constitutes the strength of a medical art may also be its weakness.

Any modern scientific approach that tries to assess the variations of the pulse over the radial artery objectively, according to position and depth, deserves to be considered. Such a study may be able to clarify the ancient and traditional statements. Some Western authors, many of them French, have begun studies of pulse diagnosis and to date have shown fragmentary results.[24] Their approach to pulse diagnosis seems to be the most logical and most Cartesian.[25] In the meantime, it seems useful to moderate certain exaggerations found in the ancient texts themselves. In the *Ling Shu,* for example, it is written:

> The complexion, the pulse, the symptoms, form a whole like a voice and its echo, like the roots and leaves of a tree; one cannot imagine the one without the other. The complexion, the pulse and the symptoms must accord {A Yang pulse with Yin symptoms has a poor prognosis.}[26]

Thus, the ancient text returns to clinical observation. All things being equal, pulse diagnosis is only one of the three points of the diagnostic triangle: pulse, symptoms and complexion. In the present state of our limited mastery of pulse techniques, it seems primarily important to perfect our methods of clinical observation. In this perspective, the physical, constitutional and emotional aspects of a patient's condition have an importance that we fail to see at first glance through our didactic analysis of the eight principles and the four elements of diagnosis. However, we find in the classical texts that there is ample and explicit material to enable us to define various constitutions or temperaments and that a psychological approach is thus perfectly plausible, as we would expect of a medical paradigm defined as essentially psychosomatic.

Constitution and Psychosomatic Factors

In our effort to establish a diagnosis according to the traditional Chinese methods, we are interested in any element that may help us to understand patients and their suffering. Thus, the ancient remarks pointing out the interaction between social factors and physiology are relevant to our times:

> To practice medicine is to come to the aid of the people. In this matter there are five mistakes. . .

> Before examining the illness, one must inquire if the patient has not been socially outcast, for if such is the case, rather than any external perverse invasion, this might engender an illness within called tuo ying {prolapse of nutritive energy}. If the patient has become financially ruined, this is the shi jing {loss of essence}, immobilizing the qi among the viscera, and by their overlapping, provoking an illness.

> At the time of examination, one can find nothing in the organs, no somatologic alteration; the diagnosis is undecided. The emaciation progresses each day. The qi is empty, the essence is gone. If the illness is severe, the qi is gone, there are shivers with occasional convulsive terrors. Severe illness burns up the wei qi on the exterior and undermines the rong qi in the interior. It is a severe shortcoming for a doctor to know nothing of the emotional states of an illness. Such is the first failure.[27]

Qi Bo had previously enlightened the Emperor about the importance of the physical constitution and vigor of the patient in these terms:

> Normally the body is in the same state of fullness or of emptiness as is the breath; the opposite would be pathological. Normally, the breath abounds when the nutrition is perfect; the breath is empty when nutrition is deficient; the opposite would be pathological. Normally the blood is deficient or in excess at the same time as the vessels; the opposite would be pathological.[28]

This distinction between the normal and the abnormal is important to an understanding of the differences between the physical appearance of a patient and the results of our examination. Such a distinction may be made only by reference to what is expected and what is expected involves the assumption of good nutrition, a healthy emotional life and a solid constitution. Notice that in his observation of the patient, Huang Di makes the subtle distinction between energy, qi (or breath) and blood. The two are intimately linked.

Blood and Energy in the Body

Blood and energy are the two Yin—Yang poles that define the physiology of an individual; blood circulates through the blood vessels, energy through the meridians. Through the correct use of acupuncture points we may act upon one or the other, bringing each into balance.

This aspect of physiology and its therapeutic implications, even though clearly explained in the *Ling Shu,* are often neglected. In Chapter 49, Huang Di asked of his physician:

"Can one understand how a person might have more or less of blood or of energy?"

Qi Bo replied, "Those who are large and fat have more of energy. Those who are muscled, fleshy, have more of blood. Those who are small and fat have less of energy. One must keep these factors in mind when one needles an illness."[29]

Therefore, we should not be surprised to find the following in the chapter from the *Su Wen* titled "The normal and the abnormal — needling according to the stoutness of the constitution":

Huang Di asked, "Does one needle for any illness in the same way?"

Qi Bo replied, "No, when there is a patient with a robust constitution, one must needle deeply and let the needle stay in place a long time. When the patient is very fat, one must needle deeply, leaving the needle inserted for a long time, needling many times in succession. It would be necessary to needle less deeply for a thin patient and leave the needle in place less time. When the patient is of a strong constitution, but with weak muscles and soft flesh, one must needle deeply, leave the needle in place for a long time and needle many times in succession. If he is of a strong constitution, with tough muscles and firm flesh, one must needle less deeply and leave the needles in for less time."[30]

In the *Su Wen,* Qi Bo states:

Before regulating the energy, one must always, no matter what the illness, quell the blood stagnation until the blood and the energy are balanced.[31]

This global constitutional aspect that is visible at first glance may be either confirmed or modified by morphophysiological observations that reflect the relative aspects of blood and energy.

Primary among these morphological observations is the facial complexion. This is part of the first element of diagnosis, looking. We must be able to compare constitution and complexion and to appreciate the variance to make a precise diagnosis. We read in the *Ling Shu,* in the chapter entitled "Conditions of the Energy and of the Blood According to Certain Physical Signs":

A reddish yellow complexion indicates normal Yang heat.[32] If the complexion is greenish and whitish, there is a lack of Yang heat. If it is blackish, there is more blood than energy.[33]

Certain secondary morphological signs support the physical aspect of the complexion. In the same chapter we read:

A hairy and full face in man means strong blood and strong energy.

An emaciated face, on the contrary, means a deficiency of blood and of energy.[34]

To Huang Di's question, "Can we assess the condition of the blood and of the energy on the basis of the physical signs?" the physician Pac Ko answers:

In the upper part of the body, if in the stomach, zu yang ming, blood and energy are strong, the beard is soft and profuse and is shorter. If energy and blood are deficient, there is no beard and many wrinkles.

In the lower part of the body, a deficiency of blood and energy leads to the absence of hair, and there is often an imbalance of wei.[35]

Notice in this last sentence the correlation between constitution and morbidity, or vulnerability to illness, which is the central interest of this work. Note too, that the constitution, which determines the complexion, may also influence the pulse. As Qi Bo says:

Constitution is variable — some people have more energy than others. The pulse varies too, it may be shorter or longer.[36]

To complete our study of the concepts of blood and energy in Chinese medicine and to understand the following chapters, it is essential to note that the proportional variability of blood and energy is dependent on the physiology of the meridians. Indeed, each meridian may be defined according to its quantity of blood and energy. Pac Ko wrote:

Tai Yang has always more blood than energy.
Shao Yang has always more energy than blood.
Yang Ming has much blood and energy.
Tai Yin has always more energy than blood.
Shao Yin has much blood and little energy.
Jue Yin has always more blood than energy.

Influences of the Viscera on Physical Characteristics

Another concept that supports a constitutional theory is that of the influence exerted by a preponderance of energy in a specific organ on an individual's physical features. Judging from the title of the chapter devoted to this concept in the *Nei Jing Ling Shu,* itself the most ancient text known, this is surely among the earliest observations that created the Chinese tradition: "The teachings of the old masters."

To assess the condition of the energy within the five viscera, we have only to look at the facial complexion. We can also assess the energy of the five viscera in the patient's constitution. If his shoulders are broad, it means his lungs are strong; if his scapular girth is large, his heart is strong; the strength of his liver depends on how big his eyes are, and so on.[37]

The organs and the bowels are all thus analyzed. These comments may be incorporated into corresponding discussions of the various constitutions.

One detail must be stressed. Inspection of the complexion is just as important as examination of the physical particularities in any assessment of constitution. This is important because the complexion is an element of diagnosis that must not only be considered as a momentarily pathological phenomenon, but also as a natural variation related to an individual's specific constitution. Thus, a red complexion, whose pathological interpretation is an excess of heat (Yang) in the upper part of the body, may also indicate a constitutional aspect. It may be either the plethoric, reddish complexion of the sanguine patient (a Yang constitution), or the erythrosic complexion of a timid, dystonic patient (a Yin constitution). Both complexions, however, identically signify an excess of Yang in the head, but the clinical interpretation differs. The former will lead the physician to fear a vascular accident, while the latter signifies an emotional disturbance with an excess of energy related to the heart or the pericardium.

All these subtle considerations are usually perceived by the acupuncturist during his diagnostic program, even if he does not verbalize the procedure. We frequently speak of intuition, or "the knack," in defining this natural ability. This is often nothing more than systematic analysis, which could easily be described if we were to take the trouble to do so. In any medical system that recognizes the importance of terrain, it is easy to relate constitution and morbidity. In Chinese medicine, direct observation of the patient already allows classification within Yin and Yang categories according to the patient's behavior. The signs of Yin or Yang energy that are indexed using the eight rules of diagnosis apply as well to morbidity as to behavior. In the *Ling Shu,* the physician Qi Bo himself gives an example to Huang Di:

> Those who have an excess of Yang have faster minds and faster energy. They are people who speak rapidly, who are prompt and are often ill because there is an excess of energy of the heart and of the lung. Their energy is always in excess and accelerated. That is why it is mobilized at the first opportunity.[38]

The Vietnamese treatise on Chinese medicine, the *Trung Y Hoc,* relates the Yin—Yang manifestations according to the second of the eight principles, and describes Yin and Yang patient groups:

> *Yang Group:* the patient turns his face outwards, towards the light, he looks for company, sleeps on his back with his limbs outstretched, he feels light in the body, he is anxious and talkative, he likes coolness, his breathing is strong, his pulse is accelerated and superficial, his body is hot.

> *Yin Group:* the patient turns his face inwards, towards the wall, towards darkness, he enjoys being alone, he sleeps on his belly, with his limbs coiled, he is quiet, not talkative, his breathing is weak, he likes the heat, is not thirsty and his urine is clear, his pulse is deep and slow and his body is cold.[39]

Extending these descriptions of Yin and Yang groups to the functional characteristics linked to Yin or Yang constitutions, there are abundant relationships between the viscera, the energetic functions and the psyche. This concept, which is

53

included in the traditional Chinese medical texts, introduces the direct meeting of psyche and soma, inherent to the Chinese vision of constitution.

Psychosomatic Relationships in Acupuncture

In the *Ling Shu,* we find descriptions of the volume, the position and the constitution of the various organs, together with their relationship to specific behaviors and moods. In Chapter 67, "The Viscera," the ancient doctor specified:

> When the heart is small and firm, the perverse energy cannot attack it. But anxieties and fear damage the heart. If the heart is big it can resist anxieties but the perverse energy can attack it easily. If the heart is in a higher position than normal, one lacks memory; if it is in a lower position, one catches colds easily and is fearful.[40]

These statements, which may appear to be merely empirical, are understandable when we realize that in energetic theory, the heart is the dwelling of the shen, or the psyche, which is sometimes translated as the "mental energy." There are five shen, in other words, one shen per organ. These shen are qi, the psychic emanations of the organs.

The word shen has also been translated as "vegetative soul." In fact, the physiological activity of each organ finds its immaterial, psychic expression in a human attitude, a behavior or a mental activity that is proper to each organ. This is why, reciprocally, the observation of a patient's behavior allows the physician to assess the activity of the organ to which the behavior corresponds. Remember that the word *humor* has a double meaning. On one hand it means *organic* fluid, on the other, it means mood, which according to the *Webster's New World Dictionary,* varies according to the body fluids. This point of view can be found in any ancient medical doctrine, be it Greek, Indian, Chinese or Arabic.

In acupuncture, the five psychic humors are the emanations of the five organs: anger, joy, reflection, sadness and fear. (See Table I.) A sudden or prolonged, constitutional or circumstantial excess of a humor may lead to an imbalance of the internal energy of the organ, or of the meridian. This is the functional stage of an illness and may lead to more serious damage of the visceral matter, the organic stage. This is an emotional etiology.

The *Nei Jing Su Wen* describes at length and on several occasions the unfavorable emotional or physical circumstances, their target organs and the illnesses caused. Here are two representative passages:

> Grief damages the energy of the heart; severe cold weather can directly damage the energy of the lungs; anger can directly damage the liver; intercourse in a state of drunkenness, or the feng {wind} during a strong perspiration, can directly damage the spleen; an excess of fatigue or of debauchery can directly damage the energy of the kidneys.[41]

> Anger reverses the flow of the qi, and the qi escapes through coughing and vomiting. There is hematemesis and diarrhea (sun xie). Joy softens the qi, enlarges the feelings, helps the circulation of the rong and wei, and the qi is comportable.[42]

54

Sadness narrows the heart and enlarges the lungs, which infringe on the superior burner; the rong wei cannot radiate; there is an excess of internal heat that dissolves the qi. Fear spoils the essence[43] and blocks the superior burner; the qi turns back in the opposite direction, expands the inferior burner and does not circulate.

Fear shakes the heart, unbalances the mind, makes the thoughts wander and disorganizes the qi. Overwork makes us gasp and perspire. It creates an internal and external void, it wastes the qi. Thinking delays the heart, concentrates the mind, and immobilizes the correct qi, in a knot.

For a better understanding of this psychosomatic relationship we might also link together all the factors included within a given element and assume the existence of correlated constitutions. For example, if we consider the element Wood (Table I), which corresponds to the liver (organ) and to the gallbladder (bowel), the corresponding humor is anger and its qi is the hun. The hun is analogous to the patient's internal movement, what pushes him toward exteriorization and action in the outside world. The English sinologist, Needham, considers it to be the qi of neuromuscular activity. Its expression is acclaim.

An important chapter of the *Ling Shu*, entitled "The Role of the Psyche," analyzes the correlations between the organ, its corresponding emotion and its morbidity. Of the liver we read in this chapter:

When there is deficiency of energy in the liver, one becomes anxious and scared; when the energy is in excess, one becomes irritable, one is always angry.[44]

We can read in the *Su Wen* that the ability to make decisions depends on the correct functioning of the gallbladder. When grouped together, all these scattered factors gradually enable us to construct psychosomatic profiles, one element after another. This does not constitute a new and dissident approach. All the information comes from the texts. Also, Chinese tradition classified this information according to five types that correspond to the five elements. A complete chapter of the *Ling Shu* is dedicated to this classification and is titled, "Typology According to the Five Reigns or Five Elements." The first question that Huang Di asks about the concept of constitution is explicit:

"Tell me about the relationships between a man's physical constitution and his energy."

The physician Pac Ko replied, "The wood type has a greenish complexion; his trunk is long, his shoulders are broad, his hands and feet are small and he is a hard worker."[45]

Notice the similarity between the Wood types and Hippocrates' bilious constitution, or the muscular constitution in contemporary classification by Sigaud. In this typology, one can interplay all the possible correlations within an element and in the biao-li arrangement of organs with bowels, or if we prefer, with their meridians. But all the correlations in Chinese physiology are not summarized in the five elements. The six energies have a similar position and many aspects of pathology and behavior, many more than are usually considered, are explained by man's six celestial energies, the six unit meridians (Figure 4). Here is an example given by Qi Bo:

> There are people who are always sleepy. This is because their stomachs and intestines are overdeveloped, their tissues are very thick and heavy, and the defensive energy flows through these tissues slowly, remaining longer in the Yin than in the Yang.[46]

These viscera correspond to a unit meridian, the Yang Ming, of shou yang ming (large intestine) and zu yang ming (stomach).

The *Ling Shu* also mentions a typology based on the unit meridians. This typology is described in Chapter 72, "Relationships Between Man and the Cosmos." This classification allows us to situate the different variations of blood and energy relative to each unit meridian and thus to integrate the more physiological aspects of these respective amplitudes.

For example, a Tai Yang person is one where Tai Yang is the dominant meridian in his physiology, which will therefore contain more blood than energy. Thus, his attitude, personality and morbidity will be influenced by the characteristic features of the two segments of the Tai Yang, the small intestine meridian (shou tai yang) and the bladder meridian (zu tai yang).

It is also interesting to note how the ancient texts considered the psychological examination of the patient. The conditions of the interrogation are specific: questions on one side and perception of the mental energy on the other. Qi Bo says:

> If we want to examine our patient according to the principles of diagnosis, we have to observe the degree of emotivity, the general condition and the sensitivity of the skin to know the nature of our patient.[47]

Qi Bo's most fundamental observation, however, concerns the first point on the urinary bladder meridian, jingming (BL-1). It is located on the superior edge of the internal canthus of the eye and means "insight," "brightness of the glance (or eye)" and "reflection of the vital essence."[48] The ancient doctor necessarily conjoins this subtle observation of the patient's eye with the taking of the pulse. In Chapter 17 of the *Su Wen,* which defines the basic principles of this practice, we read:

> The taking of the pulse and the inspection of jingming inform upon the excess and deficiency in the stores {viscera}, on the vigor or the weakness of the receptacles {bowels}, and on the fullness or decline of the body constitution. Through the confrontation of this information we can determine the chances of survival.[49]

Later in the same chapter, he states:

> Jingming is what we use to look at things, to identify their color and measures. To see white as black, good as bad, is a deficiency of the jing that is stored in the five viscera.[50]

In other words, what we see in jingming, the brightness of an individual's eye, is his level of consciousness, his way of looking at the world around him. Jingming, as its name indicates, is nothing less than the emanation of the jing, the essence of the five organs. Thus, the level of consciousness cannot be separated from the organic physiology.

The sinologist Granet states it clearly, but with a more general meaning, when he writes, "The more or less harmonious mixture of elements that belong to wood, fire, earth, metal and water characterize an individual's xing."[51] He goes on to say, "The xing, the manner of being, corresponds to a certain aptitude to exist, to a quota of life, to a specific temperament."[52]

Jing, the essential energy, and shen, the mental energy, are intimately linked, as we can see from Qi Bo's statement regarding the changes of consciousness that precede a coma:

> The head is on the side of clairvoyance (jingming). When the head falls and the look is drowned, the essential shen is on the verge of collapse.[53]

Qi Bo explains clearly in the chapter, "The Concentration of the Energy of the Meridians in the Eyes," in the *Ling Shu:*

> The site of concentration of the "essential energy" of the five viscera is the eyes. In the eyes all the meridians meet and link with the brain, and from the brain go to the back of the neck.[54]

Thus, when we assess the brightness of the eyes, we assess the essence of the meridians that converge at and proceed from the eyes. Recall an anatomical detail of importance: all the meridians link with the eyes through their secondary, or distinct, channel. Each channel (jing bie) passes through the heart, the dwelling of the shen. Qi Bo concludes in the last chapter:

> The eyes are the outer door of the heart, and thus of the soul.[55]

Automatic or intuitive perception, which is often instinctive, plays an important part in the elaboration of a diagnosis when we speak of a patient's general attitude, of the way he looks. This is also true in interpersonal relationships at every moment of our lives. But if we try to verbalize what we feel, or simply to increase our awareness of what we perceive (most of the time in subconscious impressions), we realize to what extent the information we receive is multiple and heavy with meaning. This aspect of diagnosis, the focus on the psyche of the patient through the psyche of the physician, was not neglected in traditional Chinese medicine. The ancients valued it over the purely technical elements that nonetheless make the greater part of the texts.

As an epilogue to our discussion of "matter and spirit," we have Qi Bo's answer to the Emperor's question:

> "You have often talked about form (xing) and spirit (shen). What is xing? And what is shen?"

> Qi Bo replied, "In the study of the pulse and of the meridians, to objectify what one cannot touch, or what one cannot understand at once, is what we call xing (revealed by the senses).

Shen refers to illumination, the opening of the spirit, premonition, the active comprehension of the inexplicable, that which one alone sees while the others watch. That which shines in the obscurity as when the wind drives away the clouds, is called shen.''[56]

Conclusions

After this discussion of the classical aspects of Chinese psychosomatic medicine, we are led to envisage an original attitude of classification. It is certainly legitimate and desirable to value the traditional notions of constitutions and temperaments as special frameworks upon which we may base a new classification — the psychophysiological profile of an individual. Around this center revolve his morphological features, whose importance is relative, and his vulnerabilities, to which correspond the major syndromes of the meridians, as well as the energy imbalances of the blood, of wei qi, of jing qi and all the functional qi related to perturbations in these meridians.

We may thus consider acupuncture a ''terrain medicine.'' This facilitates its comparison with other, similar medical systems. Such a classification makes possible a new synthesis of semiological and pathological aspects that otherwise are scattered throughout the ancient and modern texts. The coherency and efficacy of this synthesis facilitates diagnosis as well as treatment. In the context of these psychophysiological profiles, which are none other than the Chinese constitutions or temperaments, it is necessary to study specific syndromes and illnesses within a Western anatomopathological framework, apparatus by apparatus. This is true since it is senseless to ignore the clinical, paraclinical and biological factors that modern medical diagnosis and research have developed for the definition and classification of syndromes.

It seems wiser to interpret these Western syndromes in Chinese terms, thus establishing a correlation with traditional energy theory, rather than the other way around. If we recodify our Western symptoms, syndromes and illnesses according to energy terminology, we discover with no little surprise that within a single Chinese energy imbalance, we may group two or more of our syndromes. The association of various energy imbalances is made coherent meridian by meridian, or better still, element by element, or energy by energy. We thus confirm the clinical association of syndromes to diatheses or terrains that are empirically elaborated. Just as important is the realization that these associations of diverse affections are made in accord with a semiological analogy.

A good example of this are certain cases of neurovegetative dystonia, or of epilepsy, spasmophilia and tetany that are so similar to one another that their differential diagnosis presents a problem. It is equally difficult to diagnose an association of tetany and epilepsy. In Chinese medicine, these affections are grouped as a common disorder, which is represented as an imbalance of energy in the liver meridian (wood), or more precisely an imbalance of Jue Yin. As a second example, consider an imbalance occurring in the stomach meridian. An imbalance of Yang Ming may be at the origin of a hiatal hernia, of an acute pulmonary edema, of a perforated ulcer, of a heart attack or of a stroke.

What principle of coherency in Chinese medicine groups the various illnesses that Western medicine has separated and classified as neurology, endocrinology, psychiatry or gastroenterology? Is not the existence of the meridians themselves and of the energy that flows through them readily differentiated as: wei qi, rong qi, jing qi, yuan qi, xue? Beyond obedience to the principle of unity in our use of more or less identical therapeutic sanctions against disorders that affect such different systems, there is the question of our comprehension of how and why this therapeutic unity is effective. As far as our basic diagnosis is concerned, we must understand our patient "energetically." In daily practice we find that the more we are able to come to a precise definition of a specific energetic imbalance, the more effective we become as practitioners. This often has an all-or-nothing dimension.

If we wish to go to the heart of acupuncture, it seems just as important to be able to handle the symbols by which acupuncture has been codified and transmitted and to allow them their full expression. Only then may we appreciate the clinical and physiological developments of this medical paradigm — the general sense of the Chinese concepts in their meeting with the modern language of physiology and biology. Our classification of six temperaments takes on an additional dimension when we become aware of the strict correspondence by five or by six with the classification of the trace elements developed by the practitioners of catalytic, or diathetic medicine. Thus, the preoccupations of a metaphysical medical theory, developed several thousands of years ago, find echo today in the empirical observations and experimental demonstrations of the school of diathetic medicine. It is at the meeting point of these two schools of thought where we must begin.

Notes

[1] Nguyen Van Nghi (67), pp. 327-373.

[2] *Ibid.*, pp. 326-373.

[3] *Ibid. Trung Y Hoc* is a Vietnamese text frequently quoted in Nguyen Van Nghi's work. We do not, at present, have any complete French or English translation of this work.

[4] *Ibid.*

[5] We must mention the particularly fruitful research done in this field by J.M. Kespi.

[6] External heat or noxious hot energy (bacteria, germs, are classified as heat since their penetration within the body provokes clinical symptoms of heat); the same reasoning applies to the other energies.

[7] Nguyen Van Nghi (67), pp. 331-333.

[8] *Ibid.*

[9] *Ibid.*, pp. 339-340.

[10] *Ibid.*, pp. 327-373.

[11] *Ibid.*, p. 348.

[12] *Ibid.*

[13] *Ibid.*

[14] *Su Wen* (59), Chapter 13, pp. 140-141.

[15] Kespi (32).

[16] Word introduced in the title of his book by Nguyen Van Nghi.

[17] Nguyen Van Nghi (67), p. 360.

[18] Faubert (19).

[19] Nguyen Van Nghi (67), pp. 354-373.

[20] *Ling Shu* (8), Chapter 49, pp. 475-476.

[21] From here one observes the heaven (Yang) of the heavenly region (Yang), which is to say, for man, the Tai Yang.

[22] *Su Wen* (28), Chapter 20, p. 134.

[23] *Su Wen* (8), Chapter 17, p. 68.

[24] Cantoni, Borsarello and the ASSMAF, and Bricot in Marseille.

[25] Verdoux (115).

[26] *Ling Shu* (8), Chapter 4, p. 323.

[27] *Su Wen* (28), Chapter 77, p. 363.

[28] *Ibid.*, Chapter 53, p. 220.

[29] *Ling Shu* (8), Chapter 49, p. 500.

[30] *Ibid.*, Chapter 38, p. 452.

[31] *Su Wen* (66), Chapter 20, p. 331. Of this stagnation, Zhang Zhi Cong says, ''The presence of perverse energy is an obstacle to the circulation of the blood and causes pain. To ease this pain, we have to needle the local ahshi points before regulating according to the tonifying or dispersing method.'' Mentioned by Nguyen Van Nghi (66), p. 331.

[32] Yellow=earth=stomach; red=fire. This can easily be understood by the physiology of the stomach.

[33] *Ling Shu* (8), Chapter 65, pp. 512-513.

[34] *Ibid.*

[35] *Ibid.*

[36] *Ibid.*, Chapter 5, p. 337.

[37] *Ibid.*, Chapter 29, pp. 436-437.

[38] *Ibid.*, Chapter 67, p. 519.

[39] Nguyen Van Nghi (67), p. 330.

[40] *Ling Shu* (8), Chapter 67, p. 472.

[41] *Ibid.*, Chapter 39, pp. 517-518.

[42] This represents the most favorable condition, but the word ''joy'' has to be more precisely defined. (See Shao Yin.)

[43] Jing qi; see the passage on social transfer and financial ruin.

[44] *Ling Shu* (8), Chapter 8, p. 348.

[45] *Ibid.*, Chapter 64, p. 511.

[46] *Ibid.*, Chapter 80, p. 557.

[47] *Su Wen* (28), Chapter 21, p. 139.

[48] *Ibid.*, Chapter 17, p. 115.

[49] *Ibid.*

[50] *Ibid.*

[51] Granet (22), p. 330.

[52] Note that the Chinese ideogram transliterated as xing is different from the one that gives jing, but their meanings are very close to each other. Ultimately we can consider jingming like a mirror image of the xing.

[53] *Su Wen* (28), Chapter 17, p. 116.

[54] *Ling Shu* (8), Chapter 80, p. 556.

[55] *Ibid.*

[56] *Su Wen* (28), Chapter 26, p. 154.

Conformation
of the Five Diatheses
and the Five Elements

The five reigns, or five movements — Wood, Fire, Earth, Metal and Water —
encompass all the phenomena of nature. This is a symbolism that applies
equally to man.

— *Nei Jing Su Wen, Chapter 64*

Introduction

It is immediately apparent that there are correlations between the five diatheses, as they are defined by Menetrier, and the five elements that are the basis of the physiology in traditional Chinese medicine. Indeed, when descriptions of physical, intellectual and psychological behavior, as well as the actual syndromes presented by patients, are classified by the various diatheses, everything between the five diatheses and the five elements seems to coincide. This is presented in schematic fashion in Figure 6.

If we refer to the table of correspondences of the five elements (Table I) and confirm it with the five diatheses, we can see that the allergic diathesis corresponds to the element Wood; to the optimistic or aggressive temperament (Wood-anger); to allergies of the respiratory system (rhinitis, seasonal asthma) linked to the liver (Wood-liver); and to migraines, linked to the gallbladder (Wood-gallbladder). These correlations are confirmed by Chinese pathology.[1]

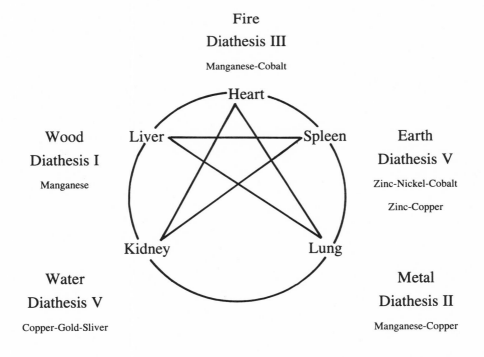

Figure 6: Correspondences of the Five Diatheses and the Five Elements

The hyposthenic, corresponding to Metal, is related to the temperament of sadness (Metal-sadness); to pulmonary disorders, such as tuberculosis and chronic bronchitis (the Metal organ is the lung); to chronic colitis as well as to other disorders of the colon (the Metal-bowel is the large intestine).

The dystonic, corresponding to the element Fire, is related to signs of anxiety, emotivity and anguish. We know the role played by the heart (Fire) as the ruler of the psyche in this pathology. The dystonic is also related to vascular, arterial and venous disorders ("the heart rules the arteries") and to coronary diseases and arteriopathy. The anergic, corresponding to the element Water, is depressive and suicidal, feels overcome and has a distaste for life (Water-fear).[2] There is a table of correspondences,[3] established according to the most fundamental texts of traditional Chinese medicine, that is provided for reference to the detail of these correspondences.

Diathesis I and the Element Wood

Diathesis I: *Allergic or Arthritic Diathesis*

Associated Trace Element: *Manganese*

Element: *Wood*

Organ: *Liver*

Bowel: *Gallbladder*

A Study of the Physical, Intellectual and Psychological Behavior

The psychological characteristics of the patient classified as belonging to the allergic diathesis (Diathesis I) are optimism, activity, dynamism and enterprising behavior.[4] "He needs activity and inactivity brings on multiple disorders and a feeling of intoxication. . .eventually {he is} restless, nervous, unsteady and frequently emotive."[5] He is, therefore, an active, enterprising individual. On the borderline of pathology, according to Menetrier, he can "present a veritable aggressivity." We can compare these characteristics with the knowledge we gained through the reading of the traditional Chinese texts. We know that the element Wood corresponds to the liver and the gallbladder and that its emotional expression is anger.[6] We read in Chapter 64 of the *Nei Jing*:

> The five reigns or movements — Wood, Fire, Earth, Metal and Water — encompass all the natural phenomena. Its symbolism can also apply to man: Wood types have a green complexion, are tall with broad shoulders, small hands and feet, and they are hard workers.[7]

There is, thus, a visible correspondence between the temperament of Diathesis I and the Wood constitution as described by the Chinese. The liver, moreover, is the dwelling place of the soul, though not just any soul, but of the hun, one of the five vegetative souls, according to the translations of Nguyen Viet Hong.[8] It is also translated as the dwelling place of the rational soul (Hubotter), or the spiritual soul (Veith). According to Ban Gu, as quoted by Needham, the hun "corresponds to the continuous propagation; it is the small Yang; it presides over the instincts, all the things that lead man outwards."[9] According to Needham, the hun is the qi of neuromuscular activity.[10]

This last interpretation links not only Wood types with Diathesis I, but also the constitution termed *muscular* by Sigaud and *bilious* by Hippocrates, as was mentioned in the introduction. We can easily understand one of the characteristic features proposed by Menetrier on this Diathesis: the allergic "seems to badly tolerate rest, which inhibits him." The physical behavior of these individuals includes two particular characteristics that the practitioners of diathetic medicine term "morning fatigue" and "diurnal unrest." Morning fatigue, which makes it difficult for the patient to get up and get going in the morning, may be explained analogically by the fact that Wood is the element that corresponds to spring and to the morning. An imbalance in Wood energy will therefore lead to difficulties with the initiation of movement in the corresponding period. On the other hand, as soon as activity has initiated the muscular activity of the liver and the gallbladder, the individual warms up. He can even get too excited and experience the typical diurnal unrest with its evening euphoria. With a greater degree of imbalance we find that he has difficulty in getting to sleep. This is also described by Menetrier and corresponds in acupuncture to the etiology of insomnia from an excess of Fire in the liver and in the gallbladder.[11] In Chinese physiology:

> The gallbladder is the judge who decides and condemns, who makes all the decisions; the liver is the general who elaborates the plans.[12]

A temporary blockage of these functions can justify morning fatigue and delay the initiation of movement. Aside from the gross physical features, we find in Diathesis I the eventual presence of nervous tics that may be explained in terms of neuromuscular activity. They may also be explained as an internal energy imbalance in the liver.[13]

The Syndromes

The syndromes that are included in Menetrier's Diathesis I — the allergic or arthritic diathesis — may be compared with the physiological and pathological correspondences of acupuncture. These include: migraine, digestive disorders, allergies, arthralgia, neuralgia, cardiovascular syndromes, genital syndromes, endocrine disorders and disorders of the phanera (hair and nails).

Migraines

The real migraines, the post puberty hemicrania of the adult individual, that occur most frequently in women and electively in the premenstruum and at the time of ovulation, are directly related to a disturbance of the gallbladder and liver. The pathway of the gallbladder meridian explains the radiation and the consistency of the pain, associated with fronto-orbital cephalalgia. Among acupuncturists, this corresponds to a liver disturbance, more or less associated with the gallbladder, but occasionally of the liver only.

Digestive Disorders

According to Menetrier, digestive disorders in Diathesis I are hepatic, with morning sickness, difficult digestion and bilious vomiting. The analogy between the gallbladder, the liver and Wood is obvious: bitter taste in the mouth and biliary vomiting, swelling of the ribs (or flatulence) are all, according to Chinese practice, signs of liver and gallbladder malfunction. With these syndromes, Menetrier associates intestinal problems such as colonopathy of the right side. This is in perfect correspondence with the Chinese etiology defined as excess of gallbladder.[14] Menetrier also mentions a possible pathological outcome to this diathesis, "the renal and biliary lithiasis."[15] This pathology corresponds to the gallbladder; however the renal pathology does not correspond exactly and seems

68

to be illogically associated with Diathesis I. Acupuncture might be the key to explaining this paradox in introducing the idea of mixed diatheses.

Allergies

The allergies — childhood eczema, asthma, hives, rhinitis, cutaneous and mucosal allergies — are in relationship with the seasons. They are of climatic or geographical origin and can be found in the allergic diathesis. We refer here to contact eczema or photosensitization, not infectious eczema. These symptoms are precisely related to a liver meridian pathology. In acupuncture theory, rhinitis, asthma and allergic sinusitis are linked to an upsurge of the energy of the liver to the pharynx through its internal pathway. This excessive ascent of energy takes place most frequently in the spring, at which time the liver energy (Wood energy) is at its maximum. We generally treat these disorders by using the calming points of the liver meridian.[16]

Arthralgia

The arthralgia from which Diathesis I takes part of its name may be acute and severe, without accompanying joint deformity and, at a later stage, joint rigidity. Typically, the pain is erratic and sometimes of a muscular type. Clinically, it is an acute inflammatory bone and neuromuscular disease without rigidity or deformity. As far as the muscular pain goes, the correspondence with the element Wood and its related viscera (liver, gallbladder) is obvious. As for the inflammatory bone disease, this coincides with an imbalance in the main gallbladder meridian. In the *Ling Shu* it is written of the gallbladder main meridian:

> In bone diseases, we must needle the points of this meridian. Wherever this meridian passes, there are pains in the articulations.[17]

This is the reason behind Nguyen Van Nghi's clinical gallbladder picture, "any bone disease."[18] We shall notice that, in acupuncture, the allergic component relates mainly to the liver meridian and the arthritic to the gallbladder. At a later stage such a distinction can be important.

Neuralgia

Neuralgias, for example certain sciaticas described in Diathesis I, are by nature "primitive." In acupuncture we know of a type of sciatica located on the gallbladder meridian's external pathway. The intercostal neuralgia precisely follows the pathway of the main and tendinomuscular gallbladder meridians. To these neuralgias we may add certain facial or temporal neuralgias, and frontal and occipital headaches, which are located on that same meridian pathway.

Cardiovascular Syndromes

In Diathesis I we find palpitations, acute and erratic precordialgia, tachycardia from stress, primitive hypertension (usually severe with headache, visual labyrinthic and auditive disturbances) or hypotensions. Palpitations and acute and erratic precordialgia relate to the liver's energy that may surge forth at the chest and disturb the cardiac and respiratory energies.[19] In acupuncture, functional hypertension is a classic example of such a disorder. Acupuncture recognizes that the excess of liver energy with an excess of heat in the gallbladder is among the

69

possible causes of hypertension, the treatment of which consists of the needling of fengchi (GB-20). This point "calms the heat of the head." Associated headache, visual and labyrinthic disorders should not be a surprise. The gallbladder meridian in its lateral and posterior pathway travels through the ear before connecting with the triple burner in the point known as ermen (TB-21). Primitive hypotension is due to an insufficiency of the liver energy (q.v. Pathology of the Temperaments).

Genital Syndromes

Hypermenorrhea is also related to a disorder of the liver energy. In the *Nei Jing* and in all the Shanghai medical texts, we find dysmenorrhea as part of the clinical picture of liver malfunction. Modern Shanghai authors call it the "dark liver."[20] The uterine fibroma represents a main symptom of Diathesis I. Since the liver energy plays a great part in the physiology of the blood as it is directly related to chong mai, it is the miscellaneous channel that governs blood and gives "pelvic swelling" in women.[21]

Endocrine Disorders

Hyperthyroidism is part of Diathesis I. The role of the liver in this endocrine disorder is mentioned in the classic acupuncture texts.[22]

Disorders of the Phanera

Disorders of the fingernails, hair and teeth are included in Diathesis I. The fingernails belong to the element Wood: "The liver governs the muscles and the fingernails,"[23] and therefore only fingernail problems fit into both systems. We cannot however set aside the teeth. Dental arthritis indicates a disturbance of the energy of the gallbladder, and is one of the foremost symptoms associated with Diathesis I. Nor may we rule out the hair, as we may see in a study of Jue Yin.

Family History

One striking element of the diathetic practitioner's approach to his patient is the refinement of his examination. To determine the patient's specific diathesis, nothing is left to chance, not even the family history. The concept of genetically transmitted disorders was not unknown to the *Nei Jing Su Wen,* but it was not considered to be a diagnostic tool. The *Trung Y Hoc* from Hanoi lists genetics among the nine causes of disease, but here again, no specific diagnostic method is described. The interrogation of a Diathesis I patient includes a careful study of family history. The practitioner will often discover that his patient's parents had suffered from similar disorders and in particular from allergies that the patient may also transmit to his children.[24] According to Menetrier, "The arthritic inheritance is frequently obvious" and, "The more aggressive the symptoms are, the more heredity bears the burden."[25]

This is certainly food for thought for all acupuncturists. This should inspire our efforts to focus on preventive medicine and to outrace such determinism. One disorder considered by Sal to be often hereditary is arterial hypertension.[26] Classic Chinese doctors call stroke "the wind that goes straight to its target" and consider the liver to be responsible for the disorder.[27]

Conclusions

Virtually all the physical, intellectual, psychological and pathological aspects found in Diathesis I correspond to the element Wood and are directly related to the liver and the gallbladder. Just as we speak of the arthritic-allergic diathesis in diathetic medicine, we may speak of a Wood diathesis in acupuncture. This is the Wood constitution. In these patients we frequently find some personal history of allergy (sun, insect or food allergies) or of arthritis. The same people will later suffer from one or several of the clinical symptoms we have mentioned in the context of this diathesis.

Diathesis II and the Element Metal

Diathesis II: *Hyposthenic Diathesis*
Associated Trace Elements: *Manganese and Copper*
Element: *Metal*
Organ: *Lung*
Bowel: *Large Intestine*

A Study of the Physical, Intellectual and Psychological Behavior

Asthenia in the evening is the landmark of this diathesis. In Chinese medicine, it is said that the lung is the master of energy. It is understandable that hyposthenic patients whose lung function is weak are easily tired out. They use little energy, have long rests and periods of sleep. They are slow and inactive. They know how to organize, says Menetrier, their periods of rest and relaxation.[28] Their complexion is pale and white. In acupuncture, Metal relates to the color white. Their intellectual and psychological behavior is defined in this way: chronic inability to apply their concentration to anything and to stick with an idea; absentminded at school or at work; chronically inattentive; easily intellectually fatigued, pessimistic, sad; calm and measured, "they would rather think than get carried away."[29]

This sudden fatigue, lack of energy, slowness and palor fit into both systems. According to the *Su Wen,* "The lung is the master of energy."[30] In Chinese medicine, the vegetative or animal soul, po, dwells in the lung.[31] Nguyen Van Nghi translates the po as the vital fluid and assigns its pneumatic quality to this energy, a quality that, we recall, may be found in Greek and Indian medicines. Ban Gu, according to Needham, relates the po to the continuous pressure, the small Yin. It governs feelings and all the external stimuli man feels inwardly.[32] According to Needham it is the qi of the neurosensorial activity. All these references describe the hyposthenic patient as psychologically tied to the influence of the world around them. They are more passive than active and are centered around the affective and intellectual effects neurosensorial messages have upon them. With inhibition or a rupture, the hyposthenia can turn into schizophrenia (hebephrenia with catatonia and abulia). These subjects fit into Hippocrates' lymphatic temperament, as we shall see in the lymphatic disorders of the reticulo-endothelial (lymphadenites) and pulmonary systems (tuberculosis). In the *Nei Jing,* the Metal temperament is described as follows:

> Their complexions are white, their heads small, their shoulders narrow, their feet and hands small.[33] They are simple, meticulous and wise; they make good judges.[34]

72

This view finds echo among the diathetic practitioners:

> The older the hyposthenic becomes, the more habitually sparing of
> his activity he becomes. With time, he develops into a wise man who
> knows the difference between agitation and activity.[35]

A Study of the Syndromes

Here again, there are obvious similarities. These individuals are "pulmonary," they present colic and respiratory pathology relative to the bowel and the organ of the element Metal.

Clinical Respiratory Syndromes

Patients classified in Diathesis II suffer from rhinitis, pharyngitis, laryngitis, tracheitis or bronchitis.[36] In acupuncture this whole respiratory sphere is dependent on the lung meridian. The sinusitis and otitis complained of by these patients depend on the large intestine (shou yang ming) as we can see according to the shou yang ming meridian pathway and to the acupuncture treatments we generally reserve for these cases.

The pathology of the ear is not obvious, but Chinese doctors describe infectious otitis among the disorders of the large intestine's distinct meridian: "loss of hearing, deafness of external origin."[37] These symptoms frequently occur in childhood, but may also be part of an adult pathology. Some more specific, severe infectious diseases, such as any form of tuberculosis — pulmonary, intestinal, genital — as well as primary infections are included in this diathesis. Laennec used to say, "Tuberculosis is the disease of sad passions." Here we find the Chinese correlation between the lungs and sadness. Pleuritis and lymphadenitis are also part of this diathesis and confirm once again a correspondence with the lymphatic temperament. In the hyposthenic diathesis we find another pulmonary syndrome, asthma. Not the allergic asthma, but the asthma that complicates "chronic bronchitis" and is related to upper respiratory tract infections. In acupuncture, this is "lung" asthma, or asthma from a deficiency of lung energy.

Colonic Syndromes

Chronic enterocolitis, colitis (left and transverse), sigmoiditis and rectocolitis are all part of the colonic pathology. There is no need to point out the pathology of the large intestine. Notice that Wood (liver, gallbladder) and Fire (small intestine) colonic disorders usually affect the right colon. When these disorders are related to Metal, they are usually located on the transverse and sigmoid colon or throughout the colon. Roughly and with many exceptions, there are some territories where the bowels impinge upon the colon, as may be noticed in colonopathy of splenic origin, which is usually right-sided.

Cutaneous Syndromes

Among the typical features of the hyposthenic diathesis are the clinical cutaneous syndromes, such as certain eczemas usually associated with other hyposthenic symptoms and acne. These symptoms are understandable, given the relationship

Metal-lung-colon-skin. The acupuncturist's tendency to think of a Metal imbalance whenever he is faced with a cutaneous disorder is justified in this case. Other clinical syndromes, such as hypothyroidism with sensitivity to cold, certain forms of dysmenorrhea with hypomenorrhea (due to hypofolliculinemia) and cryptorchidism, which do not easily fit into this context, require further information to describe effectively.

Family History

Among the most serious antecedents we frequently find tuberculosis, and even more frequently we find hyposthenic symptoms. The hyposthenic diathesis is the most easily transmitted. As Picard[38] frequently mentions, there are some whole families who would benefit from a manganese-copper treatment.

Conclusions

The hyposthenic diathesis corresponds to the element Metal in acupuncture with an obvious correlation: Metal-autumn-white-sadness-lung-colon-skin. The correspondence extends throughout the realms of physiology and psychology. It is incredible that Menetrier could have empirically grouped within a single diathesis some areas that at first glance are alien to each other: the lung, the colon and the skin. In acupuncture these are related to the element Metal, implicating a specific behavior, complexion and frame of mind. The Metal diathesis in acupuncture is easily recognizable. Indeed, we regularly find that the patient who, as a child, suffered from rhinopharyngitis, sinusitis or eczema, is a victim today of asthma, of chronic left colitis, emphysema or chronic eczema.

Diathesis III and the Element Fire

Diathesis III: *Dystonic Diathesis*
Associated Trace Elements: *Manganese-Cobalt*
Element: *Fire*
Organ of the Imperial Fire: *Heart*
Bowel of the Imperial Fire: *Small Intestine*
Organ of the Fire Minister: *Pericardium*
Bowel of the Fire Minister: *Triple Burner*

A Study of the Physical, Intellectual and Psychological Behavior

When the dystonic patient suffers from asthenia, exercise fails to alleviate the condition as it does for a Wood type asthenia. His fatigue is global and cyclical, gradually increasing during the day and reaching a peak toward the end of the afternoon. The patient feels weak and heavy especially in the lower limbs.[39] This syndrome reminds us of the cyclical behavior and pathology of the pericardium: global fatigue followed by a hypertonic phase corresponding to alternating periods of joy and depression.[40]

This diathesis is often seen as secondary, indicating aging of the fundamental energy. The patient suddenly feels he is getting old. This is a turning point in his life, as previously he was "jolly and optimistic," according to Menetrier.[41] Intellectually the patient suffers from loss of memory — initially the loss of recent memory, which gradually becomes total. Anxiety, nervousness, emotivity and excessive worry are the psychological symptoms of Diathesis III. They are identical to the pathology of the heart and pericardium meridians, considered to be an etiology of the depressive states, expressed as an excess of Fire.[42] The memory impairments are secondary to the imbalance of the heart luo channels, as we have shown in our study of the heart.[43]

We can compare this with the general description of subjects presenting a Fire constitution as detailed in the *Nei Jing:*

> Fire types have a red complexion, a small head, a pointed chin, and rounded back, shoulders, hips and belly. Their hands and feet are small; they walk fast, are agile and active and very energetic. They plan ahead but are very sensitive, and don't often keep their promises. They don't generally live to be very old.[44]

Patients of Diathesis III fear not being able to cope, according to Sal.[45] They tend to exaggerate their worries. Their anxiety brings on impressions of heart constriction and tightness in the throat. They are subject to unreasonable panic and spasmodic tears with no apparent reason. The syndromes exhibited by the

75

Diathesis III patient reveal his neurovegetative dystonia, which is related to the hysterical aspect of his personality. Syndromes, psychology — everything agrees with the pathology of the pericardium meridian: alternating phases of hysterical laughter and the opposite, sighing, whimpering and crying. A very thorough study of the qi primordial energies of the body has been done by Nguyen Viet Hong, concerning the shen that dwells in the heart as specified in the *Su Wen*.[46] This shen was defined as the "vital spirit"[47] or mental energy by Nguyen Van Nghi and as the "transforming power of fire" by Ban Gu. "It is the great Yang that puts order into the mixed confusion of the psychosomatic unity of the organism." According to Needham, the shen is the qi that governs instinct and emotions and is at the origin of the metabolism.[48]

We can understand why a shen imbalance may lead to an emotional disturbance, "the mixed confusion," and why that disturbance moves towards the change of life: andropause or menopause. Almost all subjects feel suddenly older, a sign of the weakening of the shen, whereas those of the dystonic constitution feel their emotions scattered and spent. The great Yang is unable to put order into the mixed confusion. This is the meaning of the Chinese expression of "emotional qi of the heart," which has been translated incorrectly as "joy."[49] Joy is also the capacity to be moved emotionally and goes well with the corresponding qi of the heart. It is in this sense that joy is spoken of in the *Su Wen*, in a phrase on eugenics and longevity: "Nowadays, we think only of satisfying the heart."[50] Nguyen Van Nghi comments, "To fulfill the heart is to hurt the shen. Heart and joy are related. An excess of joy damages the heart."[51] It is now possible to understand why the Chinese considered Fire individuals likely to have shorter lives than others.

A Study of the Syndromes

As with the previous diatheses, the correspondences between each of the diathetic characteristics and the traditional descriptions of Fire is complete.

Neurovegetative Dystonia

Neurovegetative dystonia is the syndrome that dominates the Diathesis III repertoire. It affects all the plexuses: the pelvic; the cardiac plexus with precordialgia, constriction; the digestive plexus with colitic spasms; the mediastinal plexus with some distension. To this picture Menetrier adds numbness and formication in the hands and forearm. This corresponds to the pathways and pathology of the primary or tendinomuscular pericardium channels.[52]

Cardiovascular Symptoms

The typical symptoms of Diathesis III are hypertension, arterial diseases, venous pathology mainly located in the lower limbs with weakness, fatigue and malleolar edema at the end of the day,[53] intermittent arteriopathic claudication, angina with main artery diseases. According to the *Nei Jing*[54] the pericardium rules over the arteries. Nguyen Van Nghi sums up the pericardium pathology by including "All the venous and arterial disorders."[55]

76

Digestive Disorders

The clinical duodenal ulcer picture, with its periodic epigastric pains relieved by food and recurring a few hours after meals, is a part of Diathesis III.[56] It can be related to the small intestine, the bowel coupled with the heart in Fire and which has a duodenal territory. Small intestine hypermotility can affect the right colon as can the gallbladder in Diathesis II. Thus, Fire dominates Metal[57] and causes organ and bowel problems.

Renal Excretory Disorders

Oliguria, uremia and renal elimination disorders in general are to be included in this diathesis. The correspondence with Fire, which rules over the qi of metabolism, involves above all the triple burner (the bowel of the Fire Minister). The kidney is a part of the triple burner. More specifically, the Yang kidney is even referred to as the "Fire Minister" in certain texts. The evolution from benign arthralgia to arthrosis is a sign that, toward the middle of his life, the subject is moving into Diathesis III, the diathesis that covers the beginnings of arteriosclerosis. Urticaria, eczema, lichens, angioneurotic edema, hemorrhoids and headaches — all these symptoms plainly correspond to the specific physiopathologies of the bowels or the organs linked to the Fire element that corresponds to the diathesis in question.

Conclusions

The dystonic diathesis corresponds to the element Fire in acupuncture. This is true in the psychological, intellectual and physical profiles as well as the syndromes and illnesses associated with each system. The number and complexity of the Fire organs and bowels — heart, small intestine, pericardium, triple burner — must lead the practitioner to cautious reasoning based on deep functional and physiological knowledge. This is why it is difficult to establish a meticulous correspondence for the first two diatheses. The dystonic diathesis covers somewhat less material than does Fire in acupuncture. To go deeper into the relationships between the two medical systems, it is necessary to introduce the six temperaments, four or even five of which overlap the element Fire.

Diathesis IV and the Element Water

Diathesis IV: *Anergic Diathesis*

Associated Trace Elements: *Copper-Gold-Silver*

Element: *Water*

Organ: *Kidney*

Bowel: *Bladder*

Water corresponds to the kidney-bladder complex. It is related to the north, to winter, to cold, to darkness, fear and will power, to salt, to the ears and to the bones and marrow. This fourth diathesis covers severe infections, advanced functional disorders that give way to lesions and malignant and severe tissue degeneration. Diathesis IV is occasionally said to be of constitutional origin; however, more generally it indicates a veritable pathological evolution. For this reason it is vital to recognize this moment in sufficient time when the functional disorder becomes a lesion. Proper therapy applied at this time may avoid or delay degeneration.

A Study of the Physical, Intellectual and Psychological Behavior

The onset of fatigue may be either gradual and insidious or rapid and brutal, characterized by a general loss of vitality, by a sensation of exhaustion. The intellectual disturbances of the anergic subject are defined as being obsessional and leading to memory loss. Psychologically they lose interest in neighbors, friends, family and professional life; they want to be left alone. They lack will power and feel that life is meaningless and absurd. They become indifferent to death, and contemplate, or even attempt, suicide.[58] This behavior corresponds, in acupuncture, to the element Water (kidney, bladder). Water is the element of fear and its pathology in Chinese medicine is related to the adrenal gland, to cortisol and to adrenaline. Cortisol links Water to the pathology of infectious disease. Adrenaline is the flight or fight hormone according to classical physiology.[59] Water individuals are described in the *Ling Shu* as follows:

> Water types have a blackish complexion. They have a big head, narrow shoulders, fat stomachs. They like movement, and their spine is longer than normal. Often they are dishonest.[60]

Passing weakness, exhaustion or even constitutional failure lead the Water subject to this anergic state. A frequent cause of depression, according to the Chinese, is a renal deficiency:

> A lack of Water cannot balance the heart Fire that, uncontrolled, ascends to the head and causes anxiety, anguish, depression, insomnia.[61]

The jing dwells in the kidney and corresponds on an emotional level to the zhi, the will to live.[62]

A disorder of the will — a disease or an exhaustion of Water — leads to a distaste for life, to abulia, loneliness or suicide. We see this in the elderly who let themselves die, the old elephant who leaves the herd to wander off and die alone. The given quantity of jing, determined genetically, decreases during the course of life until the aging process leads to death.[63] This expenditure of jing comes about in cycles that are numerically determined. The number seven governs women's cycles. The number eight governs the cycles of men.[64] We can read, for example:

> When men are 56 years old {7x8} the liver energy is depleted[65] and their testicles deteriorate, muscles and tendons weaken, the heavenly gui[66] vanishes, the jing decreases, the kidney functions weaken,[67] and the body is heavy and tired.[68]

The element Water is related to the winter; the trigram Kan ☵ is the trigram of immobility, of death. It is not difficult to grasp that the life cycle, having been through the warning decrease of the shen (Fire-heart) passes into the decay and exhaustion of the jing that dwells in the kidney (Water).

This is the inevitable evolution towards old age which corresponds to the anergic diathesis and towards the degeneration of the tissues which brings on death. This evolution can, however, be suddenly accelerated or prematurely oriented towards an anergic stage. It is easy to understand why Menetrier considers that the diagnosis of this diathesis is a "question of life or death,"[69] and why he urges physicians to prescribe copper-gold-silver trace elements to avoid such an outcome.

A Study of the Syndromes

The list of severe, acute and degenerative diseases included in the anergic diathesis should be no surprise.

Rheumatological Pathology

Arthritis and various rheumatisms — rheumatoid disease, spondyloarthritis, the Gougerot-Sjogren syndrome — are typical of this diathesis. All these afflictions pertain to renal imbalance, and thus to the jing, the cortisol metabolism that governs bones and marrow.

Intestinal Pathology

Ulcerative rectocolitis, a sign of deficiency in the Yang kidneys,[70] and Crohn's disease may be related to the descriptions of the kidney meridian imbalance described in the *Nei Jing Su Wen* as dysentery and melena.[71]

79

Infectious Syndromes

In Diathesis IV we find infected eczema, nasal allergies with sinusitis, severe or complicated suppurative otitis, sinusitis, parodontitis and tonsillitis, severe and recurrent coccal (mainly staphlyococcal) pulmonary or dermatologic infections (such as acne, boils or anthrax), osteomyelitis,[72] acute and severe meningitis, pulmonary, bony, lymphadenitic and visceral tuberculosis, erratic recurrent cystitis and fevers of unknown origin. All these syndromes indicate renal insufficiency, the loss of and the inability to mobilize the jing energy (Yang-kidney-adrenal gland-medulla). The inability to synthesize jing, cortisol and wei is present, along with defensive energy from cortisol secretion to the whole range of macrophage and lympho-histiocytic immunity mechanisms.[73]

The insertion of Shao Yin occurs at the point of concentration of the kidney energy, lianquan (CV-23). This point is located above the Adam's apple in the depression at the upper border of the hyoid bone. Thus, it is in the thymus zone. The thymus-adrenal gland-bone marrow junction falls under the territorial jurisdiction of the kidney. It is easy to understand how severe infections can occur when the kidney is insufficient. This is also a pathology of perverse energy in the distinct renal meridian that passes through the heart: "acute cardiac pain, fullness in the chest and ribs, pain and swelling of the throat, trouble swallowing and spitting."[74] If we relate this description to the diathesis of a patient who has a red, sore throat (red-Fire-perverse heat) and more specifically with rheumatic fever (a constant complaint among anergic patients), we can understand the relationship between streptococcus, the tonsils, the heart and the kidneys. The treatment in acupuncture is no mystery: stimulation of kidney and heart (Shao Yin) meridians.[75]

Degenerative Syndromes

Leukemia, Hodgkin's disease, neoplasms and general senility with death by natural causes are included in this diathetic state.

Severe Neurological Syndromes

The degenerative medullar and cerebral diseases, such as multiple sclerosis, syringomyelia, amyotrophic lateral sclerosis and Parkinson's disease fit into this category. These disorders justify our concept of exhaustion of the jing from old age or by constitutional predisposition, aggravated by factors of pollution. Mental pollution, such as that caused by a death in the family resulting in a depressive reaction or by too much work or worry, as well as physical pollution resulting in the chelation of ions through food, insecticides, food additives, and drugs (medullar aplasia, for example, produced by noramidopyrine),[76] can all contribute to aggravation of the insufficiencies of age or constitution.

Menetrier is correct to write, "The anergic diathesis involves most of the causes of imbalance and of artificial aging of living creatures and is a disease of civilization."[77] This disease is as old as man and his psychological greediness; his sensorial dependency on stimuli and his reactions to them are to blame. The Emperor Huang Di asked:

80

> I have heard that the ancient men lived until the age of one hundred years. Nowadays a man is already exhausted at the age of fifty. Who is responsible, man or the circumstances?

The doctor Qi Bo spoke of the jing and told the Emperor that man is obsessed with satisfying his heart, which is to say that he is obsessed with sensory and affective gratification. There are good reasons to look deeper into the pertinent answer of the good doctor.

Conclusions

The anergic diathesis does indeed correspond to Water. Water governs the kidneys, adrenal glands and the bladder physically, intellectually, psychologically, pathologically and even philosophically. The acupuncturist who is cognizant of this correspondence is in a position to be of help to the diathetic practitioner in his efforts to prevent or to correct this diathesis. Our concern goes beyond therapy, however, to eugenics. We may invite our patients to modify their behavior, according to the principles of "long life," the physical and spiritual practices of conservation developed by the Taoists.

We will occasionally meet patients who are constitutionally anergic, or, more precisely, of the Water constitution. In their family history or in their childhood we will find serious infectious episodes, recurrent sore throats, otitis, boils and septicema. Often we find that these patients remain vulnerable to infection throughout their lives.

To paraphrase Menetrier, in a general way, any patient with a chronic condition needs copper-gold-silver. As a correlate, in Chinese medicine every chronic disease signifies a kidney yang deficiency, or a deficiency of the kidney qi. For such chronic conditions we would need to apply moxas often and for a long time to mingmen (GV-4) and xuanshu (GV-5).

Diathesis V and the Element Earth

Diathesis V: *Misadaptation Diathesis*
Associated Trace Elements: *Zinc-Copper and Zinc-Nickel-Cobalt*
Element: *Earth*
Organ: *Spleen-Pancreas*
Bowel: *Stomach*

According to the classical authors, the misadaptation diathesis is not, strictly speaking, a diathesis, as it is not a true morbid disposition.[78] Sal stresses:

> It may complicate one of the other four diatheses, or it may, because of various stress factors, become the vector that causes an otherwise apparently healthy person to evolve towards one pathological diathesis or another.[79]

This syndrome of misadaptation, explain Menetrier and Sal, the loss of the ability to adjust, is "frequently due to a malfunction of the cortico-hypothalamo-pituitary axis," which results in either a pancreatico-pituitary imbalance, an adreno-pituitary imbalance or a gonado-pituitary imbalance.

This statement calls for several comments. First, the element Earth is by definition the center. In other words, it is associated with a state of balance, rather than with a morbid state. Second, the spleen and the stomach, which are related to the middle burner, occupy a central metabolic position. From the raw nutrient materials, the spleen and the stomach synthesize and distribute rong and wei energies as well as blood and other organic fluids. Third, the spleen and the stomach correspond to the yi. This is thought, reflection, or the activity of the cerebral cortex which is particularly well developed in human beings, who are the summit of phylogeny. The cerebral cortex coordinates peripheral information and controls the more primitive subjacent formations, the bulb and diencephalon, with the hypothalamus and the pituitary gland.

The spleen and the stomach are the dwelling of the yi, the cognitive and reflective aspect of mental activity. In the *Su Wen* we find the statement, "The psychic function of the spleen is reflection and worry."[80] In acupuncture, one cause of imbalance in the spleen is too much worrying. "An excess of worry," goes the saying, "harms the spleen."[81] In Chinese medicine, the spleen and the stomach control and regulate the hypothalamo-pituitary axis. Neurophysiologists, constantly on the lookout for new substances among the endocrine secretions, have recently discovered with some surprise a gastric hormone, gastrin, right in the middle of the cerebral tissue. This news interested many acupuncturists who consider the cortico-hypothalamo-pituitary axis to be the yi in its psychosomatic function.

Pancreatic malfunction of pituitary origin is ruled by the yi organic feedback mechanisms. Again, too many worries may damage the spleen. Adrenal gland malfunction of pituitary origin, on the other hand, is caused by pancreato-splenic

82

hyperactivity, in acupuncture an excess of the spleen which affects the kidney (adrenal gland). Traditionally, Earth dominates Water. If we assume that the gonad, wherein dwells the jing, is under the dependence of the kidneys, gonadal malfunction of pituitary origin is caused in the same way. However the liver may also be involved. The liver is the organ that synthesizes the precursor of cortisol and of the sexual hormones. The liver is affected as Earth destroys Wood. In acupuncture, stress and overactivity are not the only causes of splenic misadaptation. Perverse humidity and an excessive intake of sweets are apt to aggravate and harm a spleen that is constitutionally weak, or has become so due to bad living habits. This may be an insight into the etiology of diabetes.

A Study of the Physical, Intellectual and Psychological Behavior

The asthenia associated with Diathesis V is short-lived. It arrives as hypoglycemia with sudden fatigue before meals accompanied by acute hunger pains.[82] Intellectually, the patient feels temporarily vacant and depressed.[83] If things get worse, we see a cyclothymic attitude: temporary depression and abulia[84] that give way to intellectual and emotional elation. This cyclothymia is not psychotic. Menetrier explains this by saying that ''there is no actual pathology''[85] in this syndrome which remains at a functional stage. A real psychotic syndrome accompanied by real organic damage would not respond to zinc-copper or zinc-nickel-cobalt treatment, because of the powerful action of the metallic zinc-copper ion. This ion might, instead of helping the patient, accelerate the degenerative or proliferative process.[86]

The cyclical nature of this asthenia may be explained by the nutritive function accorded to the spleen in acupuncture. Food is absorbed, metabolized and sent into circulation by the spleen and the stomach. The spleen is the first served, as is the stomach. Thus, as soon as there is intake of nourishment, the insufficiency of functional energy in the spleen and stomach is diminished. The patient feels better. The pancreatic glycemic regulatory mechanisms provide an explanation for hypoglycemic attack that is relieved by eating. The impression described in Diathesis V of being empty-headed and out of contact with one's own intellectual capacities is also found in Chinese semiology in cases of deficiency in the spleen:[87] ''heavy-headed,'' ''floating sensation in body and head.'' From a psychological point of view, the depressive episodes signal an excess of worries which is harmful to the spleen. As Nguyen Van Nghi says, ''The symptoms of aerogastria and aerocolia are typical in cases of splenic aggression and among predisposed subjects are prodromic symptoms to depression.''[88]

Menetrier reminds us that it was Selye who discovered ''the relation between adrenal malfunction of pituitary origin and the loss of the ability to adjust to stress.''[89] For the ancient Chinese this relationship was explained by the domination of the spleen over the kidney; of the yi upon zhi; of thought on will. To explain the cyclothymic character of the behavior disturbances and their extension into manic states that are presented in Diathesis V, acupuncture points to the anatomy, the physiology and the pathology of the stomach meridian. Its secondary longitudinal channel, which ascends from the leg to the top of the skull and enters the brain, is particularly important. An excess of energy in this meridian corresponds to madness. The stomach fenglong point (luo point) indications are headache, dizziness, mental disorders and epilepsy. The patient is psychotic, sees ghosts, laughs and sings, gets undressed, runs around and wants to climb higher and higher.[90] This is typical of hypomania with its visual hallucinations.

The Syndromes

The syndromes presented by patients of this diathesis are digestive disorders, diabetic and prediabetic syndromes, sexual and adrenal malfunctioning, genital disorders, hypogonadism and obesity.

Digestive Disorders

Gastric and colic distension are part of the misadaptation diathesis and are prodromal symptoms of stomach ulcers and other non-organic and typically right-sided colitis.[91] These symptoms coincide perfectly with acupuncture theory, as we have shown in the case of ulcers[92] and functional colonopathies.[93] The excess or deficiency of energy in the spleen are two of the five main etiologies of these affections.

Diabetic and Orediabetic Syndromes

The pancreas is at the origin of diabetic syndromes in diathetic medicine as well as in acupuncture. Treatment entails needling the points of the spleen meridian, specifically the sanyinjiao point (SP-6). The hypoglycemic action of this point was demonstrated for the first time by Ionescu-Tirgoviste and his collaborators[94] and confirmed in part by our own hospital experience.[95]

Sexual and Adrenal Malfunction of Pituitary Origin in Children

Growth retardation, cryptorchidism and primitive enuresis[96] implicate the spleen, as it is the center of cortico-hypothalamo-pituitary disturbances. The sexual, endocrine and urinary impact of these mechanisms has already been explained. As far as enuresis is concerned, we have found only one publication, the modern Shanghai treatise of acupuncture,[97] that relates enuresis to a spleen malfunction and advises the needling of spleen points. It is also possible to relate prostatic malfunctions to the spleen; however, it is not the object of this work to expand on this field.

Genital Disorders

Genital disorders of genito-pituitary origin naturally belong to this diathesis. Among the disorders mentioned we find spanomenorrhea, frigidity, indifference and sexual impotence. The explanation of all these symptoms according to Chinese physiopathology centers around the spleen. These mechanisms, in particular the confirmation of a spleen etiology for impotence when associated with diabetes, will be explained in detail in the appropriate section of this book.

Hypogonadism with Obesity of Pituitary Origin

Another striking correspondence between diathetic medicine and acupuncture presented by this syndrome is the thickening of the connective tissue and the "endocrine obesity" during childhood which may persist into adulthood. This is related to the spleen, which is implicated in connective and adipose tissue, and the pancreas, whose role in obesity is more and more categorically confirmed in modern works and traced in glucose tolerance tests. In the *Su Wen* it is written that "sweets in excess damage the flesh."[98] In cases of true obesity, the physical and psychological profiles of the most recent psychological studies done by endocrinologists, with absence of aggressivity and lack of motivation, agree with the typical Earth profile described in the *Ling Shu:*

> Earth types have a yellow complexion, a big head, a round face, heavy shoulders and back, fat thighs and belly. Their hands and feet are small, they are calm and generous, although not very ambitious, and they do not aspire to high honors.[99]

As already noted, the spleen is also at the origin of the constitution of cellulitis.[100] It controls the flow of fluids. When the energy of the spleen is insufficient we find edema of the lower limbs. There is also a relation to the liver when there is poor circulation in the lower extremities as well as "water retention" or cellulitis.

Conclusions

Diathesis V relates precisely to the element Earth in all of its manifestations. The spleen, pancreas and stomach are the somatic poles. We can appreciate the value of acupuncture in this diathesis where the trace elements, with their limitations and contraindications, have so little to offer.

Conformation Conclusions

The correlation between the five diatheses as described by Menetrier and the school of diathetic medicine and the five phases of Chinese acupuncture seems to be apparent. It is easy to grasp their interrelationship. On the theoretical level, acupuncture brings to and perhaps beyond diathetic medicine and biology, the specific and still mysterious meridian pathways, whose real nature needs to be elucidated. This ''anatomical'' network describes specific identities of paired functions that are recognized as belonging to one or another of the five elements as well as to the corresponding diathesis. These identities represent two viscera conceived in a syncretic sense, that only the Chinese civilization with its particular binary and relativistic mode of thought could have developed.

All the correspondences defined within a phase are classified according to a Yin—Yang dialectic, ''which we only have to bring into play,'' in Granet's words, ''in order to understand or to take action.'' This, too, must also be operational. This is essentially the case in the laws of chronobiology determined by the positions and revolutions of the stars and calculated by the renowned Chinese astronomers.[101] From this chronobiology arise certain experimental or practical assumptions. One of the most logical of these assumptions is to calculate the best time of day to administer a trace element or any other pharmaceutical product.[102]

	Correlations between the Five Elements and the Five Diatheses			
	Diathesis	Phases	Trace Elements	Chinese Functions
I	Allergic Arthritic	Wood	Manganese	Liver-Gallbladder
II	Hyposthenic	Metal	Manganese-Copper	Lung-Large Intestine
III	Dystonic	Fire	Manganese-Cobalt	Heart-Small Intestine Pericardium-Triple Burner
IV	Anergic	Water	Copper-Gold-Silver	Kidney-Bladder
V	Misadaptation	Earth	Zinc-Copper Zinc-Nickel-Cobalt	Spleen-Stomach

Figure 7

Regarding therapy, we might suppose that acupuncture facilitates and complements the action of the trace elements. In practice, I personally find this to be the case. Diathetic medicine brings to the study of acupuncture a considerable body of research, carried out all over the world and concentrating on the enzymatic properties of the various catalysts. The conclusions of this research should be compared with the punctual action of meridian stimulation. We could, for example, measure the same biological parameters that are altered by manganese or sulfur when certain liver and gallbladder points are stimulated.

Diathetic medicine, because of its modern, scientific and rigorous observation of the facts and its non-clinical observations, has gained an official position. It brings to clinical medicine its own specific diagnostic method, confrontation between symptoms, morbidity and past family history. This original method helps the acupuncturist to easily and quickly gather and relate these symptoms to one another.[103] Thus, a precise knowledge of diathetic medicine helps the acupuncturist practice his art.

On the therapeutic level, the trace elements complement the effect of acupuncture treatment. In particular they enhance its efficacy by correcting deep diathetic malfunctions. Each treatment has its own properties and mechanisms of action: latency, speed, duration and depth. This is not the place for a comparison of the relative merits of the two systems except those directly concerned with our study of the treatment by acupuncture and trace elements for specific afflictions. In any case, this strategy is up to all of us and varies according to our own specializations. Based on my experience, I can state confidently that acupuncture and trace elements complement each other in a powerful way. This may be seen in the treatment of acute neurological and rheumatological pathology where both the efficacy of trace element therapy and the fast action of acupuncture are well known. This may also be the case in certain, more severe, even organic afflictions, against which, according to Menetrier, the trace elements alone are ineffective. Acupuncture is often effective in these cases and may bring results when classical medicine offers only symptomatic treatment. I believe this to be the case for treatment of cerebrovascular accidents.

Beyond the self-imposed restrictions on diathetic practitioners, what should stop us from fighting organic disease when attempting the combination of acupuncture and trace element therapy in association with traditional allopathic treatment? This association is all the more desirable since catalytic trace elements and acupuncture seem, more often than not, to potentiate each other. Before expanding the relationship of acupuncture, the trace elements, experimental medicine and the basic sciences, among which molecular biology and nuclear physics have their places, I must expand on the clinical comparison of the two medical systems so far introduced, concentrating on the classification by fives: the five elements, as traditionally represented in the *Ling Shu,* and the five diatheses. To go further in terms of comparison we must examine the concept of *temperament.* This we will do in the context of the six energies classification also described in the *Ling Shu.* By grouping the five elements (or diatheses) into pairs, we may attempt a comparison between the two classifications, the first by fives, the second by sixes. This will enable us to understand the diagnosis of two diatheses for a single problem or given behavior. These are common cases. This classification will lead to an original outlook that I feel is of some help in Chinese diagnosis, but which in no way alters the main principles inherent to diathetic medicine in clinical investigation.

Notes

[1] Let us recall that an internal branch of the liver meridian ascends to the brain (hay fever) and descends to the nose and the eye (conjunctivitis and rhinitis).

[2] Later we shall see the role the kidney plays in the etiology of depressions in Chinese medicine.

[3] See Table I, Part I.

[4] Sal (102), p. 39.

[5] Menetrier (46), p. 45.

[6] *Nei Jing Su Wen* (8), Chapter 5, p. 33.

[7] *Ling Shu* (8), Chapter 64, p. 511.

[8] Nguyen Viet Hong (68).

[9] Needham (54).

[10] *Ibid.* "Muscles, nerves and tendons belong to the liver" (*Nei Jing*).

[11] Nguyen van Nghi (67), p. 676.

[12] *Su Wen* (8), Chapter 8, p. 46.

[13] Nguyen Van Nghi (70), p. 676.

[14] Requena (86), pp. 97-109.

[15] Menetrier (46), p. 46.

[16] Taichong (LV-3) is indicated in the *Da Cheng* (8), p. 797, as treating all the nasal disorders. Nguyen Van Nghi and his followers use it for the treatment of seasonal rhinitis. We can similarly talk of the treatment of certain forms of eczema.

[17] *Ling Shu* (8), Chapter 10, p. 369.

[18] Nguyen Van Nghi (67), p. 123.

[19] They can be considered to be a liver meridian energy disorder of psychic origin, which Nguyen Van Nghi calls liver wind (gan feng) (67), p. 681.

[20] Shanghai (105).

[21] *Nei Jing* (67).

[22] Shanghai (105), p. 157. They remark, concerning hyperthyroidism, "Because of melancholy sentiments, the energies of the liver and the spleen cease to flow."

[23] *Su Wen* (8), Chapter 10, p. 150.

[24] Menetrier (46), p. 47. Thus asthma, eczema and rhinitis are seen in a patient, in his ancestors and in his children.

[25] *Ibid.*

[26] Sal (102), p. 39.

[27] Nguyen Van Nghi (67), p. 274.

[28] Menetrier (46), p. 48.

[29] *Ibid.*, p. 47.

[30] *Su Wen* (8), Chapter 7, p. 47.

[31] Nguyen Viet Hong (68), p. 217.

[32] Needham (54).

[33] Ectomorph schizoid type.

[34] *Ling Shu* (8), Chapter 64, p. 512.

[35] Menetrier (46), p. 48.

[36] *Ibid.*

[37] Nguyen Van Nghi (67), p. 201.

[38] Picard (75), p. 59.

[39] Menetrier (46), p. 52.

[40] Nguyen Van Nghi (67), p. 119.

[41] We shall understand its reasons during our detailed study of the temperaments.

[42] *Ibid.*

[43] Requena (83). Later, in Pathology of the Temperaments, we shall see what part the liver plays in this function.

[44] *Nei Jing* (8), Chapter 64, p. 511.

[45] Sal (102), p. 43.

[46] *Su Wen* (8), Chapter 62, p. 221.

[47] Nguyen Viet Hong (68), p. 216.

[48] Needham (54).

[49] This effectively depicts the cheerful, easy going attitude but not the passionate attitude that is so attached to its successive wishes and to their realization.

[50] *Nei Jing Su Wen* (59), p. 29-31.

[51] *Ibid.*

[52] This would be the tendinomuscular meridian if it is related to a cervical pain origin or the primary channel if related to the vascular and vasomotor disturbances observed in such cases as menopause.

[53] Menetrier (46), p. 52.

[54] *Nei Jing* (8), Chapter 10, p. 360.

[55] Nguyen Van Nghi (67), p. 119.

[56] Menetrier (46), p. 52.

[57] Fire melts Metal (large intestine).

[58] Sal (102), p. 45.

[59] A modern physiologic experiment proved that repetitive stress applied to rats led to the atrophy of the adrenal gland and kidneys. This is anatomically proven.

[60] *Ling Shu* (8), Chapter 64, p. 512.

[61] Nguyen Van Nghi (58), p. 16.

[62] "The kidney governs the will" *Su Wen* (8), Chapter 42, p. 221.

[63] This has already been discussed in the general introduction to acupuncture.

[64] *Nei Jing Su Wen* (59), pp. 34-35.

[65] Could we relate this remark and Menetrier's discussion of the sudden anergic stage that occurs in the middle age of the allergic (liver) who, from a lifelong euphoria switches to a depression? Menetrier (46), p. 55.

[66] The "celestial gui" or creative power.

[67] Compare with the renal biological disturbances met in this diathesis.

[68] *Nei Jing Su Wen* (59).

[69] Menetrier (46), p. 54.

[70] Requena (80).

[71] Nguyen Van Nghi and E. Picou (67).

[72] It is more specifically the kidney territory. The main meridian travels along the anterior vertebral bodies. The "heat" perverse energy may cause these infections, in particular osteomyelitis and meningitis.

[73] See the section, Introduction to Acupuncture. Wei qi relates to the lower burning space (liver and kidney).

[74] Chamfrault and Nguyen Van Nghi (10), p. 219.

[75] See Shao Yin.

[76] In acupuncture the marrow is the bone and the medullar marrows.

[77] Menetrier (46), p. 54.

[78] *Ibid.*, p. 57.

[79] Sal (102), pp. 45-46.

[80] *Su Wen* (8), Chapter 5, p. 34.

[81] *Ibid.*

[82] Menetrier (46), pp. 58-59.

[83] Sal (102), p. 46.

[84] It is the so-called English "spleen" (spleen is the word for the splenic organ too).

[85] Menetrier (46), pp. 58-59.

[86] This reminds the acupuncturist of the reticulo-endothelial splenic dependency.

[87] Nguyen Van Nghi (67), p. 109.

[88] *Ibid.*, p. 12.

[89] Menetrier (46), p. 57.

[90] *Da Cheng* (7), p. 357. See also, Nguyen Van Nghi (67), p 464.

[91] Menetrier (46), pp. 59 and 78.

[92] Requena (90), pp. 389-396.

[93] Requena (86).

[94] Hypoglycemic mechanism of point SP-6. *American Journal of Acupuncture,* Vol. 3, No. 1, March, 1975 (32), pp. 18-34.

[95] Requena (79).

[96] Menetrier (46), p. 58.

[97] Shanghai (105), pp. 223-226.

[98] *Su Wen* (7), Chapter 5, p. 34.

[99] *Ling Shu* (7), Chapter 64, p. 512.

[100] Requena (92) p. 192.

[101] Needham (54).

[102] This is in the light of the newly discovered Western chronobiology, a tendency that is currently expanding.

[103] This is because in ancient and modern treatises the pathology and the clinic are related according to a different logic, which values the specific form of energetic imbalance more than their grouping organ by organ (see the sections, Introduction to Acupuncture, Examination of the Patient).

The Psychology
of the
Six Temperaments

The Yin and Yang energies are variable, one may be more powerful than the other. We must subdivide them into three Yin energies and three Yang energies.

— *Guai Yu Zhu, Ling Shu, Chapter 66, "Study of the Cosmos."*

Generalizations

Five Constitutions and Six Temperaments

The five phase classification in acupuncture coincides with the five diatheses classification in Menetrier's catalytic medicine. This comparison reinforces the concept of typology found in the *Ling Shu* while it contributes to the definition of a precise psycho-physiological[1] constitution for each of the five categories. However, the ancient Chinese had another way of classifying natural and human phenomena. This classification was by six. As seen in the short quotation from the *Ling Shu* at the head of this chapter, the three Yin and the three Yang correspond in man to the six meridians: Tai Yin, Shao Yin, Jue Yin, Tai Yang, Shao Yang and Yang Ming. Each is divided into a pair of meridians, one in the upper part of the body, for example, shou tai yin, the lung, and the other in the lower part of the body, zu tai yin, the spleen. These six pairs are the twelve primary channels that participate in another paired relationship known as biao-li. This too is coherent with the five phases, as is explained in the *Su Wen:*

> There is an inner-outer lining relationship, a deep-superficial relationship between specific channels:
>
> In the leg: Tai Yang {bladder} and Shao Yin {kidney}, Shao Yang {gallbladder} and Jue Yin {liver}, Yang Ming {stomach} and Tai Yin {spleen}.
>
> In the arm: Tai Yang {small intestine} and Shao Yin {heart}, Shao Yang {triple burner} and Jue Yin {pericardium}, Yang Ming {large intestine} and Tai Yin {lung}.[2]

In the *Ling Shu* we are told that the heavenly cycle is characterized by the number six where the earthly cycle is characterized by the number five.[3] This distinction is intimately related to the human typology described in the *Ling Shu* that is based on these phases and energies. A whole chapter of this book is devoted to this explanation. In other words, the five phases and the six energies are inseparable and their physiology is closely related. By extrapolation, we could say that the symbol Earth, which is the fixed reference according to which we determine the five phases,[4] corresponds to the classification of five elementary physical types that are by nature stable. These are the five constitutions. The symbol Heaven, the reference for movement (the mobile, the energy, the immaterial), corresponds to the six energetic types that are by nature variable. These are the six temperaments.

Based on the correlations found between the five diatheses and the five phases we may associate pairs of diatheses, just as we associate pairs of phases within the six energies to describe six original temperaments. These temperaments correspond to the six energies and their specific psychologies and morbidities. In this way, we will be able to explain the frequent association, very common in practice, of prescribing two trace elements for a single patient or a single affliction.

Thus, we may distinguish between two sets of symptoms and two pathologies within a given diathesis, between those that evolve according to a Yin mode and correspond to a Yin temperament, and those that evolve according to a Yang mode and correspond to a Yang temperament. We have seen this already in the example of an arthritic (Diathesis I) patient who seemed to correspond to the pathology of the gallbladder, and thus to be related to the energy Shao Yang, whereas the condition of an allergic patient (also Diathesis I) corresponded to the pathology of the liver and to the energy Jue Yin. Such a distinction, however relative, is of considerable importance to acupuncture. If the therapeutic conclusion depends on this Yin—Yang distinction it will lead us to needle the points of one meridian rather than another. It has only a highly speculative importance in diathetic medicine, as the ion to be prescribed remains the same whatever the circumstances, provided the diathesis is the same. For example, manganese would be prescribed for both arthritic and allergic patients.

Psychology and Temperaments

Since the description in the texts is far from complete, it is necessary to compare what psychological factors we do know with a modern classification of biotypology or of psychology to arrive at a workable definition of the six temperaments in Chinese medicine. A review of the different biotypology studies shows numerous and varied theories. It is difficult, therefore, to define a subject morphologically or to relate behavior to a morbid state. The efforts of Pierre Janet, Sigaud, Pavlov, Bechteref and Ivanov-Smolenski, Corman, Sheldon, Pende and Vague, as well as the Middle Age alchemists and astrologists, are notable in this regard. However, the five constitutions obtained through the conformation of the five phases and the five diatheses are psycho-physiological. For reasons of descriptive continuity in our search for a model description of the six temperaments, these classifications are attractive.

Physio-psychological and psychological classifications are also numerous, including the schools of Kretschmer, Klages, Jung, Berger and others. I have chosen the school of the Dutch psychologists Heymans and Wiersma and the developments of their French disciples, Le Senne and particularly Gaston Berger.[5]

The Gaston Berger Test

The Gaston Berger Test is well known. Not long ago, it was systematically taught in the philosophy classes of French secondary schools. It makes questioning the patient easy and establishes his character type. There is no need for a specific apparatus or a psychologist. It is also easy to ask the patient to fill out the questionnaire at home if we want to have textual proof of his character type. Gaston Berger retained three fundamental factors in establishing this: activity, emotivity and resonance. These factors are well suited for the exploration of three different and complementary aspects of Chinese psychopathology.

96

Analysis of the Three Factors of the Berger Test

- **Activity**

The first of the three factors, activity corresponds to the global Yin or Yang aspect of the subject's behavior.[6] We are not interested in the quantity of the activity displayed by a subject, but in the facility with which he acts. Yang corresponds to movement, Yin to rest, to immobility. A Yang subject is apt to easily and willingly mobilize his energy, whereas a Yin subject will tend to have difficulty initiating movement and will be sparing of his activity. He needs to be motivated. A Yang person, by comparison, is frequently on the move for no reason at all. In Chapter 30 of the *Su Wen,* the words of Qi Bo confirm this description of Yin and Yang behavior:

> The limbs branch off from the Yang. When Yang is in abundance,
> the limbs are strong and able to climb up.[7]

With a little experience, it is not difficult to tell Yin subjects from those who are Yang. Those whose energy type is composed of two Yang bowel meridians are Yang and those whose energy type is composed of two Yin meridians are Yin. Tai Yang, Shao Yang and Yang Ming are Yang, whereas Tai Yin, Shao Yin and Jue Yin are Yin.

- **Emotivity**

This is the second factor according to which Gaston Berger classified his subjects:

> To be subject to an emotion is to be upset. Everybody is subject to
> emotions under certain specific circumstances. Circumstances of
> emotional intensity and arousal vary with the individual. We call an
> individual who gets upset when most people do not, and whose level
> of emotional arousal is above average, emotive. The emotive indivi-
> dual will be shaken over almost nothing and disturbed for a reason
> that he will be the first to agree is not worth the upset, but which is so
> real to him that he really feels his emotion and often suffers because
> of it.[8]

In Chinese medicine, the heart is the dwelling place of the five shen, the five vegetative souls: hun, po, zhi, yi and shen. The shen of the heart is the shen qi of the emotions. Subjects whose temperaments correspond to a Fire meridian may be considered emotive. As the French philosopher Pascal so simply said, ''The heart has its reasons that reason ignores.''

> {Non-emotive subjects are} ruled by reason, cold, discriminative and
> look with surprise on those who are swayed by their emotions, those
> who are shaken with passion. At best these subjects consider the
> emotive people as sick people who need help, or as drunks. To quote
> Voltaire, ''Enthusiasm is like wine.'' Vauven argues, ''Reason
> ignores the heart's interests.''[9]

97

In Chinese medicine, the vegetative soul, which corresponds to reasoning, to reflection, is the yi, the qi of the spleen and of Earth. Any individual whose meridian (temperament) belongs to the Earth will tend to be non-emotive.

In summary, the emotive subjects are Shao Yang (triple burner), Jue Yin (pericardium), Tai Yang (small intestine) and Shao Yin (heart). (See the Fire organs and bowels listed in Table I.) Tai Yin and Yang Ming are non-emotive.

• Resonance

The third factor of Berger's test, resonance is surely the most subtle and thus the most difficult to state precisely. The German psychologist Gross was the first to differentiate between primary and secondary intentions and their influences. Berger describes this factor as follows:

> All our impressions, or rather all our perceptions, have an immediate effect on us. This immediate effect is their primary function.
>
> The primary individual's life is directly dependent on the present events. The immediate excitation calls on his memory, and solicits the information best suited to appropriate action.
>
> For the secondary individual, the past does not serve only to support the present. It predetermines and orients and structures the present. He ignores certain aspects of the present, and extends the present into the future.

According to Berger, the primary individual focuses on what is happening; the secondary on what has happened and what will happen.

This parallels the distinction between introversion and extroversion or the relationship between the present moment and the world around us. "To pay attention to the immediate environment," writes Berger, "is to open outward, whereas the past is within."[10] These complex nuances make it more difficult to tell whether a person is "primary" or "secondary."[11] In Chinese medicine, the multiplicity of the vegetative souls recognizes this complexity and helps us to understand the difference between primary and secondary temperaments.

Ban Gu says that the hun is the Wood energy that pushes man outwards. It is the primary movement of the spring that wants to grow, to act here and now upon the future. Wood individuals are primary: Shao Yang, Jue Yin. The element Water corresponds to the trigram of immobility, to rest, to the time that prepares generation and renewal. It corresponds to a time of maturation preceding expression. Water individuals are secondary: Tai Yang, Shao Yin. The yi, reflective activity, and the po, ruling all that is perceived from the outside inwards (according to Ban Gu), can provoke either immediate or delayed responses, according to the circumstance. Thus, Tai Yin and Yang Ming individuals may be either primary or secondary. It may be said that in these temperaments it is Metal, the season of rest, of taking stock, of control of ideas, that will determine a subject's resonance.

Correlations

In summary, the eight temperaments described by Gaston Berger correspond to the eight temperaments of acupuncture as shown by Figure Eight. At first sight we notice the multiple correlations that exist between this classification and the aspects of each temperament, and the relation to the emotional qualities attached to the various viscera in Chinese medicine. We can easily imagine a correlation with Menetrier's psycho-physiological observations. For example, to the Wood constitution (Diathesis I) correspond Shao Yang and Jue Yin. Exuberant, irascible, furiously angry, Shao Yang is rightly called coleric or exuberant, and is completely different from Jue Yin who is timid, shy, fearful and who goes by the name of nervous. The name sentimental suits Shao Yin well. Energetically, it is the most Yin and contains the heart itself. Amorphous suits Tai Yin subjects, whose constitution is Earth, with its inertia and its lack of ambition. Apathetic fits Tai Yin subjects whose constitution is Metal. The closer we study the ancient Chinese texts and the more we learn about the psychological, morbid and physical characteristics of the temperaments, the more striking is their resemblance to Menetrier's experimental findings and to Berger's psychological profiles.

Correspondences — Phases and Diatheses			
Diathesis	**Phase**	**Trace Element**	**Chinese Function**
Allergic Arthritic	Wood	Manganese	Liver Gall Bladder
Hyposthenic	Metal	Manganese-Copper	Lung Large Intestine
Dystonic	Fire	Manganese-Cobalt	Heart Small Intestine Master of the Heart Triple Burner
Anergic	Water	Copper-Gold-Silver	Kidney Bladder
Maladaptive	Earth	Zinc-Copper Zinc-Nickel-Cobalt	Spleen Stomach

Figure 8: *Correspondences between the Gaston Berger temperaments and the six meridians*

Relativity of the Psychological Test

According to Gaston Berger himself, his test may give questionable results in about 25% of all cases. That is to say that one subject out of four will not agree with his personality description. This, I think, is owing to the lack of precision of a good many of the test questions.[12] This is why the test is out of fashion and is no longer taught in universities or used in practical psychology. Even though it has its limitations, I personally feel that it is a useful diagnostic tool for the assessment of a subject's emotivity, activity and resonance, and thus of his personality. Berger wrote:

> Le Senne's work has confirmed the findings of Heymans and
> Wiersma. Our own assessment of a good many cases leads to the

99

same conclusions: the emotivity, activity and resonance are the three basic factors of personality structure. They are like the body's skeleton. Muscles may add to the body structure, but they depend on the skeleton.[13]

These factors, with their combinations and interactions, enable us to determine eight character types. Though somewhat succinct, these represent eight specific psychological profiles among which we will have no trouble classifying a given subject.[14] Often there is no need to have a subject fill out the Berger test. If our examination of physical and intellectual behavior is as thorough as it should be and is complemented by an interrogation concerning general, physical and functional elements, as well as family antecedents, we may come to a precise idea of the patient's character type without the Berger test. The whole diagnostic investigation method developed by Menetrier comes into play, though an acupuncturist will add the nuances of the Chinese semiology and the examination will take on another dimension owing to the Oriental concept of energetic imbalances among the meridians. Our experience is that this technique facilitates Chinese diagnosis; that it adds to the traditional Oriental investigation, and enables us to cross-check the results of subjective factors such as the interpretation of the pulses.

Another comment concerning the diatheses and the Chinese temperaments is in order. Because of their intimate relationship, it is easy to comment on this diagnostic technique, as we did with catalytic medicine. For example, we often find patients whose personality is related to two or more character types, just as some belong to two or more diatheses with two or more associated or combined vulnerabilities. For example, an ulcerative colitis is often associated with Yang Ming (large intestine Yin-Metal: hyposthenia) and with Shao Yin (kidney Yang-Water: anergia). Such a patient displays an apathetic character, or is a mixture of phlegmatic and sentimental traits. This double aspect informs the acupuncturist that he must balance the large intestine meridian (zu yang ming) and the kidney meridian (zu shao yin). According to diathetic medicine, we must prescribe manganese-copper (hyposthenia) and copper-gold-silver (anergia).

These ambiguities may also be related either to some personal affective incidents, or to the phases of life: youth, maturity, menopause and old age.[15] Menetrier, who was probably most aware of such a difference, spoke of psychobiological personalities[16] and of simple, changeable and basic diatheses. In the same way, we differentiate between the concepts of constitution and temperament — the former permanent, the latter more mobile. We might speak of basic temperament, which includes the phase corresponding to the constitution, and transient temperament. It is important to note that following the discussion of behavioral traits dealing with energy types, the *Ling Shu* makes reference to a tendency toward energy imbalance that is specific to each type. We may, for example, notice that a Yang meridian has a natural tendency towards a pathology related to an excess of energy. Yin meridians have a tendency toward pathologies involving deficiency.[17] On Tai Yang it is written:

> When the Tai Yang subject is ill, one must not disperse his Yin, but rather his Yang, for if his Yin is dispersed, he will present signs of madness similar to those brought about by the excess of Yang.[18]

100

With this example, we see how this technique complies with the link between psychological behavior and an energy that the ancient Chinese describe between two meridians and their corresponding physiological vulnerabilities. We may also add to this link the whole set of semiological signs, illnesses and characteristics corresponding to the morbidity of these same meridians and organs. This is true if the energy imbalance is of emotional or somatic origin, whether it came about because of internal or external aggression, or whether it is influenced by climatic, geographical or seasonal factors, or by a change in living conditions, overwork, emotional shock, depression, illness, external trauma or surgery.

Now it is time to describe the psychology, physiology and pathology of the eight Chinese temperaments, which in my view represent the eight terrains of acupuncture. This description is based on the comparison of the traditional Chinese texts with the findings of diathetic medicine and with the character types defined by Gaston Berger.[19] As emphasized in the introduction, we must remain true to traditional Chinese semantics that best describe and name the movements of energy.

Behavior of the Shao Yang

Personality and Behavior

The Shao Yang is composed of the gallbladder meridian (zu shao yang), representing the element Wood, and the triple burner meridian (shou shao yang), representing the element Fire.

To define the temperament of Shao Yang subjects, who are of mixed Wood and Fire constitution, we must examine the characteristic traits of these two constitutions and confront them with the description of the Shao Yang temperament found in the *Ling Shu*. We must also compare this information with Menetrier's meticulous observations of Diathesis I (arthritic) and Diathesis III (dystonic) patients and also with the corresponding temperament defined by Gaston Berger. Shao Yang subjects are Yang. A good description of Wood subjects is found in the *Ling Shu*.[20] They are broad-shouldered hard workers. They are also agile, active and full of energy, which are also Fire traits. Of mixed constitution, the Shao Yang is described as a ''type'' by the physician Shao Shi:

> The Shao Yang subject is pretentious. This is typically a civil servant who behaves like a great minister. He likes to move around, and when he walks he swings his arms around. He has more Yang than Yin. His blood vessels are highly developed, he is all capillary. His energy, therefore, is consequently superficial.[21]

This is a good description of Yang subjects and fits in with certain common aspects of Shao Yang behavior. The Shao Yang are emotive people, owing to the Fire factor of their triple burner constitution. They are active, we might even say hyperactive, because of the Yang aspect of the two bowels that enter into their composition, one of which is the gallbladder, governing the muscles (Wood).[22] They are primary, since no inhibitory element (neither Water nor Metal) acts to restrict the hun, which, according to Needham, corresponds to the qi of neuromuscular activity.

Emotive, active, primary, the Shao Yang correspond to the temperament termed coleric by Gaston Berger, a temperament that bears its name well, for:

> Anger is the foremost symptom of energy imbalances involving the gallbladder.[23]

Anger, as we know, corresponds to the element Wood. Gaston Berger's description of the coleric temperament coincides with the one found in the *Ling Shu*, as it does with the psychological traits of the arthritic diathesis described by Menetrier. As Gaston Berger describes them:

> Generous, full of vitality, exuberant, optimistic, usually cheerful, they often lack taste and measure. Their activity is intense, febrile

and multiform. They are keen on politics, like people, believe in progress, they may be revolutionaries, are good speakers, are impetuous. They are leaders. Their dominating value is action![24]

The outstanding characteristic of Shao Yang subjects is indeed their action. We might add that they are incapable of resting immobile for a single minute.

Their pretentiousness, their grandiose airs, correspond to the impetuosity that makes them show off. As we often say, they roll their muscles. They are exuberant because their activity and emotivity are excessive and no secondarity works to balance them. Thus, they lack a sense of measure and sometimes they lack taste. They can't stop talking, giving orders, or offering advice. Soulie de Morant points out that in China, people who are audacious are commonly called "big gallbladders."[25] Shao Yang subjects tend to undertake many activities all at once. Victor Hugo is a good example. He was socially active, a politician and a writer; he had a wife, a big family and numerous extramarital affairs. "Fights are always good," Victor Hugo used to say. In love, the coleric subjects are not forgetful, but are "additive." They remain faithful and multiply faithfully. It might be said of the Shao Yang that they are possessed of a solid libido.

Conflicts do not disturb the Shao Yang. Gaston Berger says of the coleric subjects that these conflicts are "an opportunity for them to feel their force, and to manifest their power."[26] When they are interested in sports, the Shao Yang don't limit themselves to a single sport, but tend to practice two or three sports and sometimes more than that. Optimism is another trait that Menetrier attributes to the patients in Diathesis I. They are optimistically active, "even agitated, irritable and often emotive. . . On the borderline of the pathological," he writes, "they can show real aggressivity which may alternate with depressive moments."[27]

In Chinese medicine, when the energy in the gallbladder or triple burner meridians is in a state of imbalance, the patient may get overanxious. This is a typical feature of the diathesis (Fire), with its functional cardiovascular pathology.

Psychologically, what characterizes the Shao Yang is their outbursts of anger. Their hot tempers carry them away; they scream, shout, complain, are physically violent and may even assault people and break things. These moments of violence don't generally last long, but are frequently repeated. They are sorry afterwards and find excuse in claiming that it was only a moment of truth, during which they said everything they had on their chests. This is often true and is pathognomonic. The Shao Yang are frank; they hate lies and rarely hold a grudge.

Physically, the observations made by Menetrier hold true for the Shao Yang: they are tired in the morning, need activity, wake up with it and are euphoric in the evening.[28] The Shao Yang are not at all early birds. They tend to go to bed late and get up late in the morning. Staying up late is no problem compared to getting up early. This is explained in Chinese medicine by the trouble initiating movement caused by the stagnation of the Yang.

103

Morphological Features

Three facial features described in the *Ling Shu* can give us some idea of the morphology of the Shao Yang:

> If the subject has sideburns and an abundant beard, this means that the Shao Yang meridian is full of blood.[29]

We notice that the orbital cavities of the Shao Yang (pathway of the gallbladder meridian) are large and in an excess of energy in this meridian even the eyes tend to bulge and be mobile; in a deficiency of energy, they are small and deeply lodged. The *Ling Shu* relates that a high median nasal line indicates a healthy triple burner activity. The complexion of the Shao Yang is either green, as is classic for the wood constitution, or markedly red, as for the Fire constitution, particularly when the subject is angry. In Chapter 10, the *Ling Shu* is more specific:

> If there is grave trouble with the gallbladder, the face is wan, pallid, the body is dry.[30]

These disorders are most probably related to an excess of energy in the bowel, as this clinical situation is indicated in the *Da Cheng* for yangfu (GB-38), the dispersion point of the meridian.[31] The complexion of the Shao Yang is either congestive, especially from a certain advanced age onwards,[32] or more frequently greenish, matte, pale or pallid. This is the complexion of the Mediterranean peoples, particularly the Spanish, whose racial constitution seems to fit well in Shao Yang. Spanish folk dances, especially the flamenco, correspond to the Chinese description of this temperament (ample gesticulations with the arms). Among the Asian countries, the Japanese could be Shao Yang.

Physiologically, the *Ling Shu* points out that the Shao Yang is more Yang than Yin.

> When he is ill one must tonify his Yin and disperse his Yang, but only by bleeding his capillaries. Tonifying his Yin is absolutely indispensable, otherwise the treatment would be useless.[33]

These indications not only enable us to confirm the concept of temperament, in the physiological sense of the term, in the energetic sense, we might say, but bring us information on just how to treat this group of patients. Tonifying the Yin means tonifying the liver and the pericardium, which represent the Yin aspect of Shao Yang. We shall retain the following points that should be tonified: taichong (LV-3), ququan (LV-8), zhongchong (PC-9) and sanyinjiao (SP-6). We shall also bear in mind the physician Bo Gao's advice:

> If the subject is of the Wood type, we must balance the blood and the energy in the zu shao yang (gallbladder) meridian.

Behavior of the Jue Yin

Personality and Behavior

The Jue Yin is composed of the liver meridian (zu jue yin, Wood) and of the pericardium meridian (shou jue yin, Fire).

The Jue Yin temperament is not described in the *Ling Shu*. We therefore must seek out the characteristic liver and Wood constitutional factors, as well as the psychological factors and disorders, relative to these constitutions, which may be found in the ancient Chinese medical texts. Menetrier's observations of certain emotional symptoms connected with Diatheses I and III add to the Chinese material and we gradually form a profile that in many ways resembles the nervous temperament described by Berger.

The Jue Yin are Yin. Even though the Wood constitution might lead us to believe that they are hard workers, their activity is at least partly inhibited by the pericardium Fire that stirs up their emotions. If they are motivated, however, they can accomplish a great deal of work. As Berger wrote about the nervous subjects:

> Their work ability is irregular; they do only as they please.[34]

However, one trait that best characterizes the behavior of the nervous subject is what we commonly call nervousness. The nervous predisposition may express itself in an uncontrolled agitation and in violent or aggressive emotions that the individual can hardly hold back. Wood relates to anger, but too frequently the nature of the liver has been reduced to the phrase, "anger wounds the liver." This relationship between the liver and anger may in truth be found in the organ pulse theory. "If the liver pulse is frequent and tense, the patient is angry and swears easily... tense and frequent pulse is indicative of Yin (cold)."[35] This semiology corresponds to the excess of the liver energy (here, of external origin). We can also see the anger in its verbal manifestation: the patient swears.

Nonetheless, the Jue Yin subject's nervousness is more complicated than it might at first appear, if we limit our observation to the formula liver=anger. If we take the time and the care to read the texts more thoroughly, we find numerous reasons to modify our initial impression. This is the case, for example, in the text on the internal balance of blood and energy in which the Jue Yin and the liver, in particular, have an important role to play.

> When there is an excess of blood, the patient is angry. When the blood is deficient, he is anxious and fearful. If the blood ascends to the upper part of the body, and if the energy descends to the lower part of the body, the patient will have heart problems; he gets carried away and is easily angry.[36]

> On the other hand, if the blood descends to the lower part of the body,[37] and if the energy ascends to the upper part of the body, the patient will be delirious and will suffer from memory loss.[38]

105

Psychosomatic phenomena are not as simple as they might appear in aphorisms. The liver is responsible for a global movement of blood in balance with the energy in a vertical axis. This axis is the Jue Yin. According to the relative equilibrium of blood and energy which is closely related to the physiological state of the Jue Yin function, the subject will be somewhat coleric, or anxious and confused, and lacking in memory.

This last statement, and those previously made concerning the instability of the activity that varies according to the degree of motivation, may be related to Menetrier's observations concerning the behavior of Diathesis I subjects:

> Intellectually, the subject is neither stable nor constant; his memory is not sufficient. His efforts are discontinuous and his results look brighter than they are, as they lack consistency.[39]

Berger explains this attitude in the following way:

> The more the emotivity increases, the more vividly the conflict is felt. Those on whom it has the greatest effect are most probably the nervous subjects, whose emotivity is not controlled by secondary intention, and whose inactivity prevents the realization of their wishes.

He goes on to say that the reaction of the nervous subject who has a good imagination is to try to resolve his conflicts through symbolic escape, ranging from creative imagination to a pathological compensation such as mythomania or compulsive lying. We shall personally add that this escape may be somatized in a dystonic state or converted into hysteria.

The memory disturbances spoken of above are associated in another passage from the *Su Wen* with a host of other symptoms, which happen to be dystonic in nature:

> The Yellow Emperor asked, "What symptoms are displayed when the pulse of spring is in excess?"
>
> "When the pulse of spring is in excess," replied Qi Bo, "the patient is forgetful, angry, disordered in his head; he is uncomfortable and dizzy.[40]
>
> "Forgetfulness is caused by an imbalance in the liver. This energy in excess backwashes upwards."

This means an excess of energy upwards, of blood downwards. The etiology is thus the same as for anxiety and memory loss.[41]

Menetrier writes about the dystonic patient (Fire): "Intellectually, memory is impaired with temporary or permanent memory loss, which may even be total. One step further, and the patient is deluded."[42] The *Su Wen* adds that if the liver is deficient,

> The sight is disturbed, hearing disrupted and the patient has a feeling of great fear, as if someone were grabbing at him.[43]

Although not exclusively, anxiety is a symptom of a liver imbalance, with conflictive fear, fear of violence and memory loss. To sum up this two-sided emotional aspect of excess and deficiency, we may call to mind the phrase from the *Su Wen:*

> The liver is the dwelling of the hun {spiritual shen, advisor of the shen}.[44]

The shen, as we remember, is the qi of the heart. French popular expressions reflect this duality. It is said of those who are audacious and enterprising that they have "the heart in the belly." To be afraid, in French slang, is "to have the livers." This is also why, in the first chapters of the *Su Wen* that treat the relationships between the five elements, it is written that when the liver is ill, we become afraid and anxious,[45] and not angry, which obliges us to revise the notion of anger being the sole emotional manifestation of the liver.

Menetrier's Diathesis I symptoms include timidity, anxiety and panic, and fit logically beside the Diathesis III behavior in the Jue Yin profile, which include hyperemotivity, hypersensitivity to conflict and so on.[46] These symptoms, which may be grouped and associated with the "vagosympathetic dystonia"[47] pathology, fit in perfectly with the Chinese semiology. We have personally noticed that nervous or Jue Yin patients frequently suffer from one or more particular symptoms of the dystonia series, which show quantitatively the intensity of the functional or energetic disturbance of the liver or of the pericardium. These patients tend to have dizzy spells, tolerate the wind badly, are afraid of heights, get motion sickness,[48] are afraid of needles (intramuscular or intravenous injections, acupuncture needles), tend to have fainting spells, are claustrophobic, agoraphobic (afraid of crowds), perspire from the hands and feet, blush easily and have low tolerance to alcohol, which even in minute quantities may give them headaches, etc. Nonetheless, we must say one thing here that is true for all the temperaments: a Jue Yin subject in good health may present none of these symptoms at all!

On the Jue Yin mood changes, let us say that it also influences their affectivity. "Nervous subjects," writes Berger, "are emotionally unstable, easily seduced and easily consoled."[49] At the same time, they can be easily entertained. They need to enjoy life, to forget their problems and to have fun. They enjoy games and social entertainment.

One last psychological trait deserves to be mentioned. "Nervous subjects need something to excite them, to enable them to tear themselves away from inactivity, from boredom."[50] Little matter that this something be intellectual, affective or chemical, such as tobacco or alcohol. The important thing is that it puts them in shape, or lets them escape into "artificial paradise."

Morphological Features

Physically, the Jue Yin complexion is sometimes pale, sometimes pink, as if the subject were blushing all the time. His cheeks are flushed. The pale complexion is indicative of the Wood (liver) constitution of Jue Yin. The subject's skin is lusterless and sometimes covered with beads of sweat. He may look as if he were about to faint, even if this never actually happens. This is the complexion of the nervous subject who is anxious, who contains his anger and who may be spasmo-philic. The flushed complexion shows the domination of the Fire constitution (pericardium) and indicates a great lack of tonicity. The subject jumps at the slightest noise, laughs, then cries and is more than rarely hysterical.

The *Ling Shu* has two more criteria to add to the description of the Jue Yin morphology:

> According to the size of the eyes, we may measure the strength of the liver.[51]

As the Jue Yin meridian contains more blood than energy, we may say, as con-cerns male patients, "if there is more blood than energy, they will have very little beard."[52]

As far as national characteristics go, the Jue Yin temperament seems to best describe the French, as much in their abuse of stimulants as in their cultural sensi-tivity, love of the arts, their taste for lovely phrases, women, poetry, gallantry;[53] they are quickly seduced and even more quickly consoled and inconsistent in love. This is their reputation and their pride. In terms of pathology, Western semiolo-gists have taken it upon themselves to describe the typically French "minor hepatic insufficiency," that serves as a catch-all diagnosis. As soon as the French feel less than up to par, they accuse their livers. English hepatologists make great fun of this French "liver" mythology, but then, the English are Yang Ming, which might explain why they, on the other hand, accuse their stomachs for all their problems.

In conclusion, the Jue Yin temperament corresponds to subjects of the ner-vous temperament; the energy of the liver and that of the pericardium are respon-sible for this nervousness, the irritability, the anxiety, the memory problems, the imaginary escape, the dystonia and the hysterical behavior that we find in this tem-perament.

Behavior of the Yang Ming

Personality and Behavior

The Yang Ming is composed of the large intestine meridian (shou yang ming: Metal) and of the stomach meridian (zu yang ming: Earth). A description of the Yang Ming temperament, as was the case with Jue Yin, is not to be found in the *Ling Shu*. It is thus up to us to reconstitute this temperament, by noting the characteristic traits of the two constitutions, Metal and Earth, and by going through the Chinese texts to pick out all the psychological and psychosomatic factors that are associated with the organs, bowels and meridians of these two phases.

The Yang Ming are Yang and are therefore active. They are non-emotive, owing to the yi (reflection) aspect of Earth. They can be either primary or secondary, as we have seen in the introduction to this third part of our discussion, which leads us to distinguish between two different characters, the sanguine and the phlegmatic. The sanguine subjects are those Yang Ming whose constitution is related to Earth; the phlegmatic subjects are those whose constitution is related to Metal. This distinction is only important in determining the morbidity of these subjects, who have, in general, common vulnerabilities. The exceptions to this rule will be noted as we go along. A Yang Ming subject of constitution Earth can, for example, suffer from sinusitis (Metal pathology), in which case we will often find in his childhood a respiratory sensitivity associated with the hyposthenic (Metal) type.

The reverse may just as well be true, as a Yang Ming subject with a phlegmatic character (Metal) is every bit as vulnerable (or almost) to cardiovascular accidents as the sanguine. This distinction between behavior and character type will serve to distinguish the Yang Ming from the other temperaments, rather than to differentiate between the two types. This will also be the case with the Tai Yin.

To describe the Yang Ming, we may group together the *Ling Shu* descriptions of Earth subjects: calm, generous, not very ambitious, not out after honors;[54] and Metal subjects: humble, meticulous, clairvoyant, they make good judges. We may add to this a description of subjects who present a Yin—Yang balance:

> The patient whose Yin and Yang are in harmony is balanced in his constitution and in his mentality. He is normal; he is polite, humble, gay, with soft eyes. If he presents signs of excess, we must disperse. If he presents signs of deficiency, we must tonify. We must needle his jing points.[55]

We notice certain similarities in these three descriptions. We may already say that the Yang Ming are likely to be calm, polite, generous, humble and capable of ponderous thought. The common denominator is Earth, the element of the center, of equilibrium and which confers on the Yang Ming (as it does on the Tai Yin, as we shall shortly see) their qualities of harmonious balance. We might conclude that the underlying Yang activity, moderated by the preponderance of the yi, will be

109

characterized by harmony, tact and ponderous thought, giving the Yang Ming subject his well-balanced outlook and good mental health.

Berger's descriptions of the sanguine and phlegmatic character types confirm our impressions and add precision to the Chinese descriptions:

> Sanguine subjects are extroverts. They know how to make exact observations, and are remarkably practical. They enjoy company, are witty, polite, ironical and skeptical. They know how to manipulate others, and make good diplomats.
>
> Phlegmatic subjects enjoy their routine; they act according to the law; they are always on time, objective, trustworthy and well-balanced. Their mood is even lymphatic. They are patient and determined, although without pretense.[56]

We may notice even more similarities between sanguine subjects and phlegmatic subjects than between coleric and nervous subjects (Shao Yang and Jue Yin), although the only difference is one of primary or secondary intention. We shall also notice that the constitutional features are intermingled. The sanguine (Earth) Yang Ming shares some of the Metal features: the ability to judge, to make exact observations and be skeptical. The phlegmatic (Metal) Yang Ming shares some of the Earth characteristics: stable moods, impassivity, patience and a lack of pretense. Nonetheless, these two personalities are different from each other.

Earth Yang Ming

Particularly influenced by the Earth, the sanguine subjects, due to the absence of po, the qi of neurosensorial activity, tend to be extroverted, and are more practical than interested in theoretical speculation. According to Berger:

> {The sanguine is} liberal and politically open. They have little respect for institutions, but put great value on practical experience. They show initiative and flexibility, and are opportunistic. . .
>
> The sanguine, because they are primary, have something of the amorphous subject's lack of concern.[57] He is not easily upset and is not "burdened with conflicts," but actively dominates situations. He enjoys his company, sports and love life free of tragic passion. The law, the rules of the game, don't bother the sanguine, who considers that they are there to be learned, in order to exploit them and to get around them. He likes catchy phrases, puns and jokes and is "always on the lookout for better ones, for recipes and ways of playing cards better, hunting better or maneuvering politically to his better advantage."[58] The highest value for the sanguine subject is social success.[59]

In the context of Chinese energy theory, we may say that this behavior corresponds to the natural and relative excess of energy in the stomach and in its meridian. The sanguine is generally considered to be easy going and jovial. This natural good humor is characteristic of the element Fire and of the heart. The excess of stomach energy, which finds expression in the sanguine subject's good mood, is also visible in his complexion, and corresponds to the pulse:

110

A hard and stretched-out stomach pulse goes with a ruddy complexion.[60]

The complexion is the second correspondence with Fire. The name sanguine, attributed to Yang Ming, partly corresponds to Fire subjects.

The risk of cardiovascular accidents, to which the sanguine subjects are so particularly exposed, can be explained by the correspondence of the element Fire to the heart and the blood vessels. Cardiovascular symptoms are precisely a signal that the heart itself is ill; the heart whose qi is in relation with the blood vessels and whose visceral qi is the shen. The relationship between Yang Ming and the blood vessels is so close that we must not neglect the role played by the two meridians that compose the Yang Ming in this sort of affection. There is an anatomo-physiological unit that is common to the heart and to Yang Ming. This is the xu li, the great luo channel of the stomach, the link that enables us to explain the cardiovascular pathology commonly found among sanguine subjects. When the excess of the stomach goes beyond a certain point, cardiovascular problems begin.[61]

Metal Yang Ming

Phlegmatic subjects (Metal) are more secondary than primary and more rigid in their attitude and principles. Berger completes the description of the phlegmatic in the following way:

> They have a deep sense of civic duty; their religion is essentially moralistic. They have a lively sense of humor and are attracted to abstract systems. Their highest value is the law.[62]

This reminds us of the *Ling Shu* comment on Metal subjects, "They make good judges." According to the studies of the Dutch psychologist Heymans, the phlegmatic is the most objective of all character types.

The phlegmatic Yang Ming are usually cool, impassive, patient, determined and handle their problems calmly. "Thus," writes Berger, "they are almost never upset, except when circumstances are exceptional and in particular when the basic principles on which their lives are based are challenged."[63] This sometimes gives the phlegmatic a rigorous, strict outlook, whose sole argument is, "the law is the law." His meticulous, obsessional disposition, added to his moral rigidity, may lead him towards a more than implacable justice and may express itself psychologically through sadism and perversion.

Morphological Features

As far as the physical constitution related to the stomach goes, Qi Bo declares:

> A strong neck and a broad chest indicate a solid stomach.[64]

In daily clinical practice this observation is indeed found to be true of Yang Ming-Earth subjects. A long nose, according to Qi Bo, indicates a strong large intestine.[65] We find this also to be true among Yang Ming-Metal subjects who sometimes look somewhat like herons.

If we come back to complexion, the red cheeks of the sanguine subject are a distinction of the Yang Ming-Earth traits. Qi Bo says:

> When the face is hot, this is a sign that the zu yang ming meridian is affected.[66]

Another, more subtle trait is typical of the sanguine Yang Ming-Earth subject:

> If the capillaries of the neck of the foot are tense because of congestion in the region where we take the pulse of the stomach meridian {chongyang, ST-42}, this means that the stomach is affected.[67]

For the phlegmatic Yang Ming-Metal subjects, the examination of the forearms, along the pathway of the shou yang ming channel is of interest:

> If there is an accumulation of blood in the capillaries situated on the outside of the forearm {the "belly of the fish"}, this means that the shou yang ming is affected.[68]

We may remember that Yang Ming has plenty of energy and plenty of blood. Bo Gao indicates in the *Ling Shu* that a man who has a heavy beard and a fleshy face has strong blood and energy.[69] This information proves invaluable, since the Yang Ming tend naturally towards excess. Bo Gao is precise in his observation:

> If the blood and the energy of zu yang ming (stomach) are strong, the beard is abundant and silky.[70]

On the other hand, if a constitutional anomaly, owing to an innate deficiency or to exhaustion, causes the subject to be lacking in blood and energy, the subject's face will be lean and gaunt.[71] These observations bring us a wealth of information, about both diagnosis and treatment of our patients.[72] The English are the people who correspond most to the Yang Ming, especially the phlegmatic subjects. They have the reputation of respecting principles and of having a strong sense of civic duty. Although we might not immediately recognize the sanguine among the English, he is there in the person of Mr. Pickwick, and we only have to spend time in the English pubs to run into this jovial sanguine whose tongue has been loosened by beer, and whose language is not far from pagan. The sanguine type is the survivor of the original English temperament that has been inhibited by centuries of puritan conditioning, as we see in Shakespeare's Falstaff.

This correspondence is not void of interest in pathology. If hepatic insufficiency is French, the English often suffer from "indigestion and constipation." What the English call indigestion (stomachaches and dyspepsia) drives them to consume incredible amounts of eupeptic medicine.[73] Constipation is such a preoccupation that for the past forty years they have regularly consumed laxatives or bran.[74]

112

Behavior of the Tai Yin

Personality and Behavior

The Tai Yin meridian is composed of the lung meridian (shou tai yin) and the spleen meridian (zu tai yin).

The Tai Yin temperament is described in the *Nei Jing Ling Shu,* but this description does not cover all the specific psychological aspects of this temperament. Tai Yin subjects are Yin, therefore, they are non-active. They are non-emotive, too, because neither of their two meridians belong to the element Fire. If they are non-emotive, non-active and primary, they belong to the amorphous temperament and correspond to the Tai Yin-Earth temperament (or Tai Yin-spleen) and are the Yin equivalent of the sanguine type described in the preceding chapter. The *Ling Shu* description of the Earth constitution particularly applies to these subjects.

If they are secondary, they are the apathetic type and correspond to the Tai Yin-Metal temperament, the Yin equivalent of the Yang Ming phlegmatic subjects. The description of the Tai Yin found in the *Ling Shu* seems to fit these subjects, as do the remarks about the Metal constitution. We can describe not only two, but three different aspects of this temperament, although, as was the case for the Yang Ming, this serves more to distinguish them from the other temperaments than to establish distinctions among them. For lack of a better term, the third type will be called the mixed type.

We must also stress that the distinction between the three psychological Tai Yin types does not exclude the intermingling of their mental characteristics, as for the Yang Ming, just as in pathology, it is almost impossible to dissociate one meridian disorder from another. In terms of behavior, it is difficult to define someone as being only Metal or only Earth without introducing some of the other characteristics into his personality.

Tai Yin-Metal

The Tai Yin-Metal type corresponds to the Metal type, as described in Part II, and to the Diathesis II type (hyposthenic). The Tai Yin description given by Bo Gao in the *Ling Shu* suits him well:

> The Tai Yin is crafty and perfidious. His complexion is always dark. He is extremely polite, bowing down before everybody else. He is tall and slim, with long legs. He is more Yin than Yang, as his Yang hardly exists at all. His blood, the most Yin of energies, is impure. His defensive energy functions badly, his skin is thick, his muscles slack. When he is ill, it is important to disperse his energy rapidly.[75]

At first glance we notice that the Yin dominates these subjects who belong to the highest Yin. In other words, they are the most passive and nonactive of all. The name apathetic suits them well. Berger defines them as follows:

113

> The apathetic react with inertia; their independence is defined by the resistance of their habits to change. Their way of adapting to change is to ignore it, to leave it alone, to play dead.[76]

Their force is thus the force of inertia.

Psychologically and physically the Tai Yin-Metal fit the Metal descriptions found in the *Ling Shu:*

> Metal types have a white complexion, a small head, narrow shoulders, tiny hands and feet. They are plain, meticulous and wise, and make good judges.[77]

Somber, taciturn, crafty, perfidious, but also plain, meticulous, perspicacious: this is a general description of the Tai Yin and, more specifically, the Tai Yin-Metal. Some of these personality traits pertain to the mixed Tai Yin, who will have to be considered separately. Among these traits, the ones we've found best describing the Tai Yin-Metal include taciturn, perspicacious and meticulous. Berger's observations concerning the apathetic subjects echo the Chinese: "Closed in about themselves, secretive, introverted, but without an exciting inner life, somber," and we find the same terms, "taciturn, they hardly ever laugh." He adds, "Slaves of their habits, they are conservative. Tenacious in their emnity, they are difficult to reconcile. The least talkative of all, they like to be alone."[78]

The simplicity and precision of Metal and the calm nature of Earth can also be found in Berger's definition of the apathetic:

> Even though social life does not interest them, the apathetic subjects are usually honest, trustworthy, reliable, and their main value is their tranquillity.[79]

We have personally noticed that the purest Tai Yin-Metal agree with this description, but that they are not, as the *Ling Shu* would have us believe, crafty or pernicious. This trait belongs to the mixed type.

The somber, taciturn and often begrudging side of the Tai Yin-Metal personality remains an element of importance. It may be caused by an excess of sadness, the Metal emotion, which gives the subject reason to talk little and laugh even less. Or it may be caused by an excess of introversion (secondary intention) which brings on obsessional behavior. Precision in this case becomes meticulousness and exaggerated scruples. Excessive sadness, the lung mood, corresponds to the element Metal and to the fall. This frame of mind, specific to the Tai Yin-Metal, has been beautifully worded in verse:

> *Les sanglots longs des violons de l'automne, bercent mon coeur d'une langueur monotone.*

This translates, as does most poetry, with difficulty:

> The long sobbing of the violins of autumn, rock my heart with a monotonous languor.

The genius of this poetry is contained not only in the words, but in the sounds and rhythms, suggesting the slow pace of life in such an atmosphere. Intellectually and physically, the apathetic is slow and tends to live in slow motion as if time were suspended.

Menetrier says of his hyposthenic subjects that they are "hindered in their youth by difficulties in concentrating, in fixing their attention."[80] He says that because he is distracted, the hyposthenic child stands a good chance of becoming dyslexic, since according to certain Western specialists dyslexia is as much a hearing or listening problem as it is one of expression.[81] Menetrier continues his description of the hyposthenic's intellectual behavior by saying:

> He can find his own intellectual capacities limited by a chronic tendency to be distracted, and has trouble expressing himself. Later in life, he will seem to be deeply knowledgeable, rather than brilliantly intelligent.[82]

I believe this difficulty in concentrating, in listening and in speaking, as well as this lack of intelligence, suggests a disorder of the po, the vegetative qi of the lung, the qi of neurosensorial activity. It is perhaps because the afferent sensory messages are perceived too intensely. If a stimulus is too strong, it may bewilder an individual who is predisposed to inaction. His imagination constructs a world of images or ideas around the delayed sensorial message thus removing the individual from the real world, because he is too sensitive. He becomes physically slow, as we are told of the Tai Yin-Metal subjects. Although they are usually punctual, often rigidly so, their movements are slow, their speech is delayed and sometimes their voices are hardly audible. They chew their food so slowly that they upset their neighbors, who have finished their dessert, while they are only starting the main course. This physical condition has a physiological basis.

We remember that Menetrier described the hyposthenic subjects as being easily fatigued by even the slightest effort. Their slowness is their insurance against fatigue and represents a saving of useless action in order to economize on their energy capital. Menetrier noticed that the hyposthenic needed much rest, sleep and holiday. "The older he becomes, the more his sparing of activity becomes a part of him, and in maturity he becomes a wise man who knows the difference between activity and agitation."[83] This is a perfect definition of the Tai Yin-Metal subject. In Chinese medicine, the lung (metal) rules over the energy. A specific lung weakness leads naturally to chronic asthenia. This is what is written between the lines in their energetic description: "They are more Yin; their Yang hardly exists."

Tai Yin-Earth

Although this type essentially corresponds to the Earth type (and to the comportment of Diathesis V, maladaptation) that has already been studied, it is wise to reiterate:

> The earth types have a yellow complexion, a big head, round face, fleshy back and shoulders; the thighs and the belly are large, the hands and the feet small. They are calm, generous, not terribly ambitious and do not look for glory.

115

The psychological aspects of this description correspond to the amorphous description given by the psychiatrist Berger:

> Disengaged, conciliating, tolerant through indifference, they are the perfect example of passive and tenacious obstinacy. Dominating value: pleasure.[84]

Berger adds to this a certain number of other traits to complete this portrait, which well establishes for all practical purposes the Tai Yin-Earth corresponding to the amorphous type:

> On the whole, it is said of this type that they have a good temper. Careless, prone to indolence, they completely lack punctuality. They are indifferent to the past, as much as to what portends, and often show an aptitude for music and drama.[85]

Such is the psychological presentation of the Tai Yin-Earth type, when in equilibrium. "Complaisance" might well be the term that comes to mind to describe these insouciant, jovial subjects. A popular French expression goes that laughter splits ones sides, or, literally, dilates one's spleen. Among the verbal manifestations given for organ affections in the *Su Wen* are "shouting for the liver, sobbing for the lung. . . singing for the spleen[86] Happy-go-lucky, cheerful, the amorphous often sing. As composers, they understand how to create a music of exquisite gentleness and sweetness, of which perhaps the most genial example might be the music of the amorphous Mozart.

Their non-emotive and non-active quality is what permits the amorphous Tai Yin-Earth types their lightness of character, their ability to remain unburdened by the weight of any conflict, which is often inversely proportional to their weight and the volume of their physique. On the other hand, one might say that it is to remain insensitive to this burden of conflict that the amorphous are driven to eat, and the distinction between obesity due to constitution and reactionary obesity is difficult to discern. On the mental level, their indulgence, according to Berger, renders the amorphous unstable, apt to yield to every impulse.

Because of these character traits, the amorphous seems inclined to numerous weaknesses. Yet these weaknesses may, to the contrary, constitute his strength. Faced with a conflict, the amorphous reacts, according to Berger, in the manner of the reed in the fable. He seems to yield in the face of the storm, yet is afterward found in his place. He bends, but does not break.

The character of Tai Yin-Earth is quite credibly compared with the trigram ☷ that represents Earth. The three traits of the three levels are broken, representing Yin, the greatest Yin. In the symbolism of the *Yi King (I Ching)* the trigram Earth represents the female, the mother. On a practical level, women are particularly exposed to the pituitary-pancreatic or pituitary-genital misadaptation.

Intellectually, according to Menetrier, the episodes of misadaptability that are part of Diathesis V may be expressed as a temporary intellectual vacancy, frequently manifest as "light headed" feelings due to hypoglycemia, driving the Tai Yin-Earth subjects to eat between meals, which fits the 11 a.m. and 5 p.m. craving for food that Menetrier describes, and which is also described in the *Su Wen*.

116

On the physical side, the asthenia is typical. It is a cyclical fatigue when the problem is merely functional, but if the disorder becomes organic, the fatigue may turn to prostration. This may be explained by the physiological properties of the extraction, transformation and distribution of the energy coming from the nutrients, which is the role ascribed to the spleen-pancreas in Chinese medicine.

We must note that Tai Yin-Earth men are sometimes effeminate, and sometimes lean towards homosexuality. In any case, whatever the secondary temperament may be, Tai Yin-Earth will ever be present. Certainly, their gonado-pituitary misadaptation is at a maximum, and in a way causes the sexual inversion. In Berger's test, a high Venus score suggests this misadaptation in the Tai Yin-Earth male.

Tai Yin-Mixed

Generally, the two types we have described above are easy to recognize. The Tai Yin-Metal is slow; the Tai Yin-Earth is soft. Both belong to what was formerly called the lymphatic type. However, there is another way of identifying the Tai Yin. When we examine patients to determine their dominating temperament, we are sometimes surprised by an intangible aspect of their personality that is hard to define and that disorients us. Experience shows that this curious feeling leads more often than not to a Tai Yin diagnostic. In the logic of Chinese theory, this is explained by the fact that the Earth corresponds to the center, to that which is neutral, to nothing specific or characteristic. Similarly, the mild flavor that corresponds to Earth may be sweet, but it may also be insipid or almost tasteless.

To this feeling of neutrality, of the indefinable, we add the results of our investigation of the antecedents of morbidity, and the study of our patient's behavior, to arrive at a conclusion of Tai Yin-Earth or Tai Yin-Metal. Occasionally, the results remain ambivalent, the feeling remains ambiguous. Thus we arrive at a categorization of these remaining subjects as Tai Yin-mixed. These subjects have a look in their eyes that seems indifferent, disabused, absent, or else inquisitive and thoughtful, giving the person who regards them the impression of being a mouse before a cat. It may be for this reason that the *Ling Shu* calls them crafty and perfidious. In fact, sometimes appearances accord with reality, and we can say of these people that they are "too polite to be honest."

Sometimes the Tai Yin have another look in their eyes that is not at all perfidious, but rather hard and metallic. We can say of these subjects that they "have an iron hand in a velvet glove." They remain cool and reserved in all circumstance, they are non-emotive and insensitive (the opposite of the pure Tai Yin-Metal), they are implacable judges, who enjoy carrying out the law and are at times on the fringe of perversity which constitutes, as an undertone, their psychiatric decompression.

Morphological Features

The physical aspects of Tai Yin-Metal and Tai Yin-Earth are clearly distinguishable. The *Ling Shu* is explicit: for Metal, the complexion is pale, the head small, the shoulders narrow, the hands and feet slender; for the Tai Yin, a tall frame with long legs. This description fits well with the schizoid ectomorph type.

The Tai Yin-Metal are usually tall and slim, or even skinny; their eyes are frequently blue. In Europe, this type might be of northern or Anglo-Saxon origin.

On an energetic level, a remark is in order regarding the narrow shoulders. If we compare this constitutional factor with the comments on the morphology associated with the lung in the *Ling Shu* chapter, "Teachings of the Ancient Masters," where Qi Bo affirms that broad shoulders indicate strong lungs,[87] we may conclude that the Tai Yin-Metal have weak lungs. But weak means vulnerable, not energetically deficient. Sadness is a sign of excess of energy in the lungs. We must not confuse the concepts of weakness, vulnerability and deficiency.

In regard to Tai Yin the *Ling Shu* specifies characteristics that correspond well to Metal: the defense energy is weak, the skin thick, the muscles loose. We find in practice that the Tai Yin skin is either white and thin, or dark and hard as leather, as if it were stretched over the bones.

In sharp contrast, the Tai Yin-Earth are frequently short and tend to obesity. They have thick skin and flesh, with full cheeks. Women of Tai Yin-Earth constitution are often portly, with almost global cellulitis. Diagnosing the Tai Yin and differentiating between them in a physical aspect is simple if we are dealing with a Don Qixote or a Sancho Panza type. But in reality, the Tai Yin is not always obvious; the indefinable aspect of the Tai Yin-mixed might hide Earth or Metal, and might present psychological characteristics of the amorphous, the apathetic, or even both. It is not rare to encounter subjects of slim and tall stature, apathetic throughout their lives, who suddenly begin to put on weight at middle age, or even at the time of puberty, and who genuinely become the corpulent amorphous type. One can also see thin subjects who equally exhibit this typical amorphous comportment.

As far as the secondary Tai Yin features are concerned, the soft characteristics of the hair are determined since the Tai Yin meridian contains more energy than blood. "If there is more energy than blood, the beard is shorter and less abundant."[88] As the Tai Yin has more Yin than Yang, and as the blood is impure, it is said, "If blood and energy are lacking, there is little or no facial hair, and there are many wrinkles."[89] Often, Tai Yin men, and Earth type more than Metal type, have little facial or body hair.

Though some of the peoples of central Europe are Tai Yin-Metal, the Tai Yin in general, and more specifically the Tai Yin-Earth, are best exemplified by the Chinese. The Chinese themselves called their land the "middle country," and Earth is the middle. A morphologic characteristic of the Earth type is a round face; the color of Earth is yellow. The word "Chinese" in the French language is frequently related to the rationalist side of that populace, in relation to the yi, the Earth qi, the vegetative soul of the spleen. The verb "chinoiser" in French means to split hairs, in a sense, and the adjective "chinois" relates to those who are excessively subtle. Poussah, the mythical personage in the folk tradition of China who since ancient times has embodied happiness, is the characteristic representation of the amorphous character and philosophy. The Chinese people instinctively chose the Buddha, a sage who embraced the middle road, in the amorphic image of Poussah.

118

Behavior of the Tai Yang

Personality and Behavior

The Tai Yang meridian is composed of the small intestine meridian (shou tai yang) and the bladder meridian (zu tai yang). The description of this temperament is given by the *Ling Shu*.

The Tai Yang are Yang and are therefore active. They are emotive because of the element Fire in the shou tai yang meridian and they are secondary because of the Water in the zu tai yang. Emotive, active and secondary, they are the passionate type described by Gaston Berger. Here is Bo Gao's description:

> The Tai Yang type is presumptuous and arrogant, his back and his head are straight almost to the point of being thrown backwards. He is more Yang than Yin. When he is ill, one must not disperse his Yin, but rather his Yang, for if we disperse the Yin of a patient whose Yin is deficient, he will show signs of madness similar to those created by an excess of Yang.[90]

This description, as sober as it may seem, resembles the paranoid personality.

At the other end of the spectrum, Berger describes the Tai Yang subject as one who is "ambitious, who works, has a tense personality, and directs his activity towards a unique goal. Domineering, a natural leader, he knows how to dominate, and to use, his aggressiveness. . . He is good company, courteous, helpful, a good speaker. He considers country, religion and family to be serious matters. He has a deep sense of grandeur and knows how to reduce his organic needs to a minimum, even to the point of asceticism. His main value is accomplishment."[91] This attitude is not surprising, coming as it does from the greatest Yang, the Tai Yang. We may recognize in this portrait certain famous personalities who have been leaders of the arts, of schools, of nations and even of empires. Berger mentions Napoleon as an example of the passionate type, but we may also mention Julius Caesar and General de Gaulle, with his ideal of "national sovereignty."

Two specific personality traits, according to Berger, are typical of the passionate behavior and correspond to Tai Yang also. These are termed "integration" and "spirit of sacrifice." Integration refers to the supreme goal that the subject has fixed as his purpose in life. It is the quality that pushes him to subordinate to that goal all other tendencies that risk leading him astray. Driven towards the realization of his ambition, the Tai Yang forces himself to integrate all his efforts and to maintain a system of "hierarchical subordination," as Berger says, enabling him to integrate all other tendencies. Even though this might sometimes represent a real or apparent setback, it enables him to progress towards his goal.

119

Sacrifice, the second personality trait described by Berger, is best illustrated by the theater of Corneille. Again he refers to the supreme goal, the work to be done, the "cause":

> The deliberation is dramatic, because the subject is an emotive who suffers because of what he neglects, and pays with his own happiness the success of his undertakings.[92]

The Tai Yang who is torn between two alternatives must sacrifice one of them so that the other may prevail. He is not one to put off the choice until later, not one to make compromises.

Psychologically, this combination of personality traits (emotive, active, secondary) which makes the subject among the most efficient, destines him to the most moving of combats. In the symbolic Chinese frame of reference, the Tai Yang (the greatest Yang) is the temperament best suited for action and for creation, but at the same time is split between Fire in its most Yang and most passionate aspect, and Water in its most Yin and its most inhibitory aspect of sacrifice and sublimation.

Intellectually they are usually bright, but those who are fit to succeed and to create are also those most apt to be subject to the most tragic of sentiments. During their childhood, they were difficult, as they were restless and vulnerable. During their first years, they had to bear their nervous system's hyperexcitability, the despotism of their passions and the repression of those around them. Gradually they had to learn how to control and refrain, at high cost, their violent emotions which already brought many grievances and dramatic conflicts with their entourage. In later years, having outdone themselves in the task they have fixed as a goal, they take on the air of superiority of those who have managed to dominate themselves and are unpitying.

Nevertheless, behind this mask there lies a hypersensitive heart. Damaged in the past, because of the feelings of rejection that their superior attitude brought about, the Tai Yang come to see the whole world as hostile. Because of this misinterpretation owing to an excessively harsh judgement, they feel more or less persecuted and this moral pain that they feel forced to hide makes them become harder, more rigid, and drives them all the more to transcend.

Anatomically, the Tai Yang meridian is located in the most Yang part of the body which it outlines: the back and the head. It is closely tied to the spine and to the du mai and enters the brain at the point baihui (GV-20). The natural physiological tendency towards an excess of energy in that meridian explains the physical and psychological tension and rigidity. Their neurological hyperexcitability may lead to the best as well as to the worst, to intellectual and creative, even genial, tendencies and to sleeping difficulties, convulsions, epilepsy (Julius Caesar) and madness.

In psychiatry the Tai Yang decompensation leads to paranoia. This is precisely the pathology that Heymans, Wiersma, Le Senne and Gaston Berger link with the passionate temperament.[93] The symptoms of the anergic diathesis (Diathesis IV, copper, gold, silver), corresponding to the element Water, may be expressed as an episode of deep, dark depression. Menetrier showed the cyclical quality of this anergic asthenia and psycho-asthenia as paradoxical outbursts of aggressiveness and elation,[94] which may easily be understood within this context. The Tai Yang depression is usually well controlled, hidden and sober. He holds his head high but one may read his misery in his tragic look and fixed expression. This is the classic behavior of the exile that many great Tai Yang have exhibited during the course of history.

Morphological Features

In the context of the blood-energy duality that determines certain physical features, Tai Yang always contains more blood than energy.[95] We can read in the *Ling Shu,* in the chapter devoted to the condition of blood and energy according to certain physical features, that one feature helps in the diagnosis of an excess of blood in the Tai Yang: if the eyebrows are thick it is because the Tai Yang meridian has plenty of blood.[96] On the physiological level, the Tai Yang and specifically the shou tai yang (or small intestine meridian) play an important role in the regulation of the blood.

This same chapter contains another indication relative to this meridian. In our study of the Yang Ming we have mentioned that a man whose energy and blood are strong has a full face and a strong beard. If his face is gaunt, he doesn't have enough energy. The *Ling Shu* adds:

> In the same way, according to whether the palms of the hands are
> thick and full or slack and fleshless, we can tell if we must balance
> the energy in the shou tai yang {small intestine meridian}.

The chapter entitled "Teachings of the Ancient Masters" mentions two more features that are characteristic of the Tai Yang:

> Both lips are thick, and the upper lip is long, suggesting a strong
> small intestine. The orifice of the nostrils, if they are slack, suggests
> that the bladder functions poorly.[97]

These features will vary towards excess or towards deficiency according to the physiological tendency of these two viscera.

Among the famous literary examples of Tai Yang, theatrical characters aside, we may mention numerous characters out of the romantic Russian literature, such as those in the works of Dostoevsky. The Slavic temperament seems incarnate in the Tai Yang, with a sense of grandeur that we associate with the great leaders as well as to the land itself, its theater, arts and legendary heroes, whose passionate character is renowned for their conquering airs and who are transformed into sentimental beings by the music of the gypsy violins.

Behavior of the Shao Yin

Shao Yin is composed of the shou shao yin (heart meridian) and the zu shao yin (kidney meridian).

Personality and Behavior

The Shao Yin is Yin. Therefore these people will be inactive. The heart is the dwelling place of the shen, the qi of the emotions. Shao Yin people are extremely emotive. The kidney is related to Water, to the trigram of stillness — the Shao Yin personality is thus. Emotive, nonactive and secondary, these individuals exemplify the sentimental type described by Gaston Berger. The *Ling Shu* describes the Shao Yin as follows:

> The Shao Yin type is jealous and gloats over other people's problems. He always looks cold. He can never stay still. When he walks, he holds his head down. He has more Yin than Yang. His stomach is small and his intestines are overdeveloped. His six bowels are not in harmony. His stomach pulse is weak and small. His Tai Yang pulse is ample. When he is ill, one must not disperse his energy, but rather balance it, as both his blood and his energy are weak.[98]

These two physiological drawbacks intimate why their inactivity leads them to be introverted and withdrawn. As we have said in the Introduction, Yang temperaments tend towards a pathology of excess and Yin temperaments tend toward pathologies of deficiency. The *Ling Shu* description confirms this.

Insufficiency of the two viscera will lead to deficiency of the related visceral qi, the shen and the zhi. Deficiency of shen, the great fire that normally orders the confusion of the sentiments, will lead to an emotional explosion. The zhi, will power, the affirmative power of life, is excessive in the Tai Yang personality and makes natural leaders. Zhi is deficient in the Shao Yin individuals and leads to inhibition and an incapacity to realize ambitions. In Chinese physiology the Shao Yin represents the fundamental axis of man. I agree with Nguyen Viet Hong when he says, "For the Chinese, the psyche is spread all over the whole body by the two main organs, the heart and the kidneys." This helps explain an exact correspondence with Berger's sentimental type. As he says:

> The sentimental are ambitious, but don't go beyond the stage of aspiration. Thoughtful, introverted, schizothymics, they often are melancholic and unhappy with themselves. Shy, vulnerable, scrupulous, they feed their inner life with their rumination of the past. They have trouble relating to others and easily become misanthropic. Maladroit, they resign themselves to what could still be avoided. Individualistic, they have a great feeling for nature. Their dominating value is intimacy.[99]

When we compare the two descriptions we notice that these people are unhappy with themselves. They cannot take the action that would fulfill their motivations and fully justify the "cold outlook" and "envious personality" that the Chinese attribute to the Shao Yin, who are shy, vulnerable and walk with their heads down.

Those who enjoy others' misfortunes are those who cannot manage to attain their own happiness. While they cannot be blamed any more than the aggressive Shao Yang, the proud Tai Yang or the frivolous Earth-Tai Yin, the Shao Yin feel guilty. Contrary to the Tai Yin, when a Shao Yin temperament is perverse, there is no regret for others' misfortunes, but rather enjoyment of them! The strong feeling for nature, the need for intimacy and the shy and fearful attitude suggest characters such as Jean Jacques Rousseau, whose confessions bear witness to such an intimate nature. Rousseau was, by the way, an accomplished herbalist. Stendhal was also a sentimental writer. The shy, fearful attitude is typical of zhi deficiency and is related to fear, the psychic attitude of Water.

On the physiological level, this may be related to the kidney (adrenal gland). We could say that adrenalin is the Tai Yang fighting hormone and the Shao Yin hormone of escape. Fear inhibits and paralyzes the Shao Yin. The Shao Yin is not a coward, but when he fights it is rarely face to face. This does not suggest that his methods are questionable or dishonest. The sentimental Shao Yin is the type of person who keeps a diary. "The sentimental," writes Berger, "coils himself in his loneliness, which he cultivates, even though he finds it painful."[100] The Shao Yin cultivates reflective techniques and psychological analysis, the only means to escape loneliness. Of all the subjects we have described, this is the one who best knows his weaknesses and tries to change his personality. In Chinese philosophy, he is the one whose shen has the deepest communication with itself.

For Berger, the reflection gives the sentimental person the chance to compensate for failure by providing an ideal justification for lack of action. The pain suffered thus confers a real grandeur and lucidity is his claim to superiority over the active subjects, whom he sometimes envies all the same. Just as fear is the sentiment linked to the kidneys, joy is linked to the heart. Joy means the ability to be moved, the common human desire to feel emotions and satisfactions, a desire that Taoist wisdom invites us to dominate in order to keep the heart serene and empty — the opposite of those who fail to live long because "they think only of satisfying the heart." For the Taoist sages, any feeling that wounds the heart wounds also the shen, the qi of all our metabolisms.

The Shao Yin are vulnerable not only in their shen, but also in their zhi (vitality). According to the texts, "Sadness, anguish and fear can wound the heart and if joys and angers are not under our control, or if heat and cold are in excess, the zhi will be damaged." Trapped between hypersensitivity and hyperemotivity, the Shao Yin choose to withdraw, to hide, to avoid their intolerable vulnerability. Occasionally, a Shao Yin type may overcome vulnerability. As Berger said, "Sometimes the sentimental try to make themselves insensitive, and if they fail, at least they manage to look insensitive and to act like the phlegmatic people around them." Thus the Shao Yin psychological portrait is easy to recognize: sentimental, shy, vulnerable, upset over nothing, inhibited, cowardly, intimate, deep. While these meditative qualities afford the chance to overcome emotivity at least partly, "his cold bearing" is the sign of victory over himself. "It is often difficult," reminds Berger, "to tell which part of his victory is due to his courage and which part is due to his weakness."

We should not consider the Shao Yin to be useless and unable. They are able and superior, as compared to the showy, irregular Jue Yin. The Shao Yin tries to hide his emotions, to go beyond his limits and change. The flashy and emotive exhibitionist is the Jue Yin; more controlled, Shao Yin tries to hide his feelings and may be deeply moving if we manage to get inside his defenses. It is not rare to find Shao Yin persons who are self-effacing (one of their greatest qualities), efficient, tenacious, serious, moral, constant and, above all, modest.

As far as mood is concerned, Shao Yin's main risk is depression, the purest manifestation of zhi deficiency and the kidney meridian (zu shao yin). The close relationship between this Water shen and Menetrier's anergic diathesis recalls the emotional aspects Menetrier described as "loss of interest for life, wish to die or to commit suicide, feeling the absurdity of existence, the desire to give up, to rest." This reflects the deficiency of zhi, of the will to live and to procreate, of the individual's instinct of survival and of the species. "What's the use?" ask depressed and discouraged patients. This is an attitude we find common to Shao Yin, the anergic diathesis and Berger's melancholic type. The shen of the heart plays a role in this attitude; the symptom of energy imbalance of the heart is sighing.[101] The depressed Shao Yin frequently sigh, moan and complain. This behavior is of course common to any depressed person, but is greatly intensified in the Shao Yin, who cries easily.

In a state of normal health, the Shao Yin have a moist, moving and charming look. The most famous Shao Yin caricature is Charlie Chaplin. It is among the Shao Yin that we find the mourning neuroses, the neuroses of failure. These individuals are caught in a painful destiny and we may wonder if they don't cultivate misfortune. Like widows and orphans, they are inconsolable and endlessly victimized. Fate seems to be after them.

Morphological Features

On the physical level the anergic asthenia is global. This is explained by the insufficiency of the kidneys and the resulting deficiency of jing qi, the essential energy that the kidney distributes. The Shao Yin physiological sensitivity mentioned previously in the *Ling Shu* confirms this. Not only are the "six bowels" not harmonious, which brings about certain assimilation disorders in relation to these Yang viscera, but the pulse of the stomach is weak and small. In studying the Yang Ming physiology we see the extent to which the stomach pulse is proportional to the energy assimilated and to the deeper state of health. As the *Ling Shu* points out, for the Shao Yin, both blood and energy are weak. This constitutional, global deficiency, which is so specific to this temperament, explains why these people are very sensitive to the cold and may wear a sweater even when the weather is fine.

Frivolity, when it is severe, is a pathognomonic sign of Shao Yin or is at least due to a kidney disease. On the morphological level, the Shao Yin complexion is usually rather black, especially around the eyes. This reminds us of the Middle Eastern complexion and suggests renal insufficiency. The eyes, in addition to the wet look, may be red, as if tearful. In the chapter of the *Ling Shu* entitled "The Teachings of the Ancient Masters," we read: "The Shao Yin accordingly have small and narrow shoulders."

The condition of the ear informs us of the condition of the kidney.[102] In regard to racial characteristics, the Middle East temperaments seem to be most easily related to Shao Yin. There is an exacerbated sentimentalism in these cultures that is not always easy to understand. It expresses itself in the arts, in love and in the Islamic and Judaic religions. Israel includes in its culture the history of a persecuted people. In Jerusalem, the Wailing Wall is a characteristic tradition of the religion. The country's current behavior illustrates the tenacity and sustained activity that the Shao Yin may have when they realize their ideal. Finally, the Shao Yin temperament is the one that is associated most often with another temperament to form mixed temperaments, the most common of which is Jue Yin-Shao Yin.

Notes

[1] "Pyscho-physiological" is the word used by Menetrier himself for his diathesis. See Menetrier (45).

[2] *Su Wen* (28), Chapter 24, p. 147.

[3] *Ling Shu* (28), Chapter 66, p. 249.

[4] Earth is also linked to the concept of matter, stillness and permanence. We quote Granet, "To Heaven belongs the personality, to the Earth the individuality that depends on the infinite variety of the spaces" Granet (22), p. 331.

[5] Since my Doctorate in Medicine thesis I have been interested in the possible application of Gaston Berger's psychological profiles to acupuncture. (79), p. 54.

[6] See Chapter 3, part I.

[7] This answer is given to Huang Di's question on the unmeasured agitation and physical excess in hypomania, in the chapter concerning Yang Ming. *Su Wen* (28), Chapter 30, p. 163.

[8] Gaston Berger (2), pp. 42-43.

[9] *Ibid.*, p. 44.

[10] *Ibid.*, p. 48.

[11] That is why we have to apply tests in medicine to compare physiological and morbid equivalents with psychological outlook.

[12] We see this again when I introduce my own TC40 which explains Berger's temperaments in forty questions and gives decreasing scores for the eight characters for a given person.

[13] Berger (2), p. 72.

[14] We have to mention that Berger's test is usually completed with a questionnaire that determines the secondary factors such as insight, polarity, greed, sensorial interest and tenderness, that strongly tint the basic personality. In summary, these profiles are easy to manipulate in the context of a functional pathology and are less significant than the psychiatric ones. Our TC40 test acts in the same way. We have to think of the physician's reluctance to accept the psychiatric label of his patient's personality. Berger tests seem to apply to "normal" people. However, they represent some serious psychiatric pathology and functional morbid profiles. For example, the passionate individual, or Tai Yang, may turn to paranoia. The acupuncture relationship is total, as proved by the Tai Yang description in Chapter 72 of the *Ling Shu,* where the attitude resembles that of the paranoid personality.

[15] That may be related to the assumptions in *Su Wen,* Chapter 1, on the expansion and decay of the viscera every seven years in women and every eight years in men.

[16] Menetrier (45).

[17] Even though it is only a draft, it does help acupuncture prevention and in particular preventive attitudes, and confirms pulse diagnosis.

[18] *Ling Shu* (8), Chapter 72, p. 529.

[19] Like this writer, with some nuances, we could not resist relating constitution and national origins. As already suggested, there may be national morbid features.

[20] *Ling Shu* (8), Chapter 64, p. 511.

[21] *Ibid.* Chapter 72, pp. 529-530.

[22] The yanglingquan (GB-34) is the specific gallbladder point and the hui point of the muscles.

[23] *Su Wen* (8), Chapter 23, p. 102.

[24] Berger (2), p. 52.

[25] Soulie de Morant (107), p. 570.

[26] Berger (2), pp. 65-66.

[27] Menetrier (46), p. 45.

[28] See Wood constitution and Diathesis I.

[29] *Ling Shu* (8), Chapter 65, p. 515: "Shao Yang always contains more energy than blood."

[30] *Ling Shu* (8), p. 369.

[31] *Da Cheng* (7), p. 564.

[32] During old age Menetrier relates that to the transformation in the dystonic diathesis (Fire-manganese-cobalt)

[33] *Ling Shu* (8), Chapter 72, pp. 529-530.

[34] Berger (2), p. 53.

[35] *Ling Shu* (8), Chapter 4, pp. 325-327.

[36] *Su Wen* (8), Chapter 62, pp. 222-224. Husson precisely translates, "The heart creates and suffocates irritability."

[37] This fits with pelvic congestion or shan (san khi) of liver origin.

[38] *Ibid.*

[39] Menetrier (46), p. 45.

[40] *Su Wen* (66), Chapter 19, pp. 287-289.

[41] The therapeutic implications are essential as we see in Jue Yin pathology.

[42] Menetrier (2), p. 52.

[43] *Su Wen* (28), Chapter 22, p. 143.

[44] *Su Wen* (28), Chapter 23, p. 146.

[45] *Ibid.*

[46] Sal (102), p. 43.

[47] Menetrier (46), p. 52.

[48] Travel sickness is caused by a vestibulary hypersensitivity that brings about dizziness and may cause confusion. This may be caused by the wind.

[49] Berger (2), p. 53.

[50] *Ibid.*

[51] *Ling Shu* (8), Chapter 29, p. 436.

[52] *Ibid.*, Chapter 64, p. 512.

[53] Berger (2), p. 60-61, defines the nervous people according to their apparent dilettantism, refinement, estheticism, etc.

[54] *Ling Shu* (8), Chapter 64, p. 572.

[55] *Ibid.*, Chapter 72, p. 530.

[56] *Ibid.*

[57] *Ibid.*, pp. 57-59.

[58] *Ibid.*

[59] Compare to the amorphous Earth-Tai Yin, who prizes pleasure, and is devoid of ambition and desire for honors.

[60] *Su Wen* (28), Chapter 16, p 118.

[61] See *Ling Shu* (8), Chapter 10. According to Berger, the manic attack is a morbid psychiatric correspondence with the sanguine character type. (See Psychiatry of this temperament.)

[62] Berger (2), p. 58.

[63] *Ibid.*

[64] *Ling Shu* (8), Chapter 29, p. 437.

[65] *Ibid.*, Chapter 4, p. 330.

[66] *Ibid.*, Chapter 29, p. 437.

[67] *Ibid.*, Chapter 4, p. 330.

[68] *Ibid.*

[69] *Ibid.*, Chapter 65, p. 514.

[70] *Ibid.*, Chapter 64, p. 512.

[71] *Ibid.*

[72] The dark complexion is found in the pathology of Yang Ming.

[73] Rennies, Alka Seltzer, Bisodol, Bicarb of Soda, Milk of Magnesia.

[74] On the market since at least 1940, sold under the name of "All Bran" ("helps keep you regular"). Noticeable consumption of agar agar (Agarol) as well.

[75] *Ling Shu* (8), Chapter 72, pp. 529-530.

[76] Berger (2), p. 53.

[77] *Ling Shu* (8).

[78] Berger (2), p. 53.

[79] *Ibid.*

[80] Menetrier (46), p. 48.

[81] Tomatis (109).

[82] Menetrier (46), p. 48.

[83] *Ibid.*

[84] Berger (2), p. 53.

[85] *Ibid.*

[86] Nguyen Van Nghi (59), p. 216.

[87] *Ling Shu* (8), Chapter 29, p. 437.

[88] *Ling Shu* (8), Chapter 64, p. 512.

[89] *Ibid.*

[90] *Ling Shu* (8), Chapter 72, p. 529.

[91] Berger (2), p. 52.

[92] *Ibid.*

[93] *Encyclopedia Universalis* (113), p. 783.

[94] Menetrier (49), pp. 52-56.

[95] *Ling Shu* (8), Chapter 65, p. 515.

[96] *Ibid.* We may think of the eyebrows of someone like George Clemanceau or Charles de Gaulle.

[97] *Ling Shu* (8), Chapter 29, p. 437.

[98] *Ibid.*, Chapter 72, p. 529.

[99] Berger (2), p. 53.

[100] *Ibid.*, p. 62.

[101] *Su Wen* (8), Chapter 23, p. 102.

[102] *Ling Shu* (8), Chapter 29, p. 436.

Pathology
of the
Temperaments

Shao Yang

Physiology of Shao Yang

Several comments concerning the function of the gallbladder are in order before discussing the pathology of Shao Yang. The triple burner will be spoken of throughout the course of the chapter. The gallbladder, for several reasons, is one of the most important viscera in the Chinese medical paradigm. In the sixty year cycle, the gallbladder relates chronologically to the first celestial stem and to the first terrestrial branch, known as jia yi.[1] It is thus the first phase. Within the nyctohemeral period, the first phase corresponds to the passage from night to day. It is midnight, the zi hour, which lasts from 11 p.m. to 1 a.m. Yin is then at its apogee, which is the opposite of noon, when Yang is at its apogee (the hour of the heart). At midnight, Yang is at its low point, at its minimum of intensity, but at the same time, at its maximum concentration and ready to grow. In the cycle of energy circulation, Yang growth passes first through the liver, then to the lung.[2] In other words, the gallbladder is the first viscera. According to Zhang Zhi Cong:

> The gallbladder corresponds to jia-Wood, classed first among the five phases and the six energies. This is why, when the energy of the gallbladder increases, the other energies follow spontaneously.[3]

Shao Yang is known as "the first Yang." The gallbladder meridian connects with the liver meridian. In chronological order, the gallbladder meridian comes first, followed by the liver, then the lung meridian and so on. In Chapter 8 of the *Su Wen,* entitled "On the Secret Treatises Stored in the Emperor's Treasure House of Books," dealing with the physiological identity of the viscera, Qi Bo states:

> The liver is the general from whom strategies are derived. The gallbladder is the impartial justice from whom judgements are derived.[4]

Despite the considerable importance of the liver, it is the gallbladder that makes the decisions.

A comparative study of this aspect with our Western physiological knowledge of the gallbladder proves interesting. The gallbladder is on a shunt off the main pathway. It stores and concentrates the bile secreted and excreted by the liver. When food enters the duodenum, the gallbladder contracts and aids digestion by increasing the emulsifying power of the pancreatic fluid.

In Chinese medicine, the "spleen-pancreas" is the sea of the five organs. We can measure the importance of the absorption of energy by the liver, which is influenced by the action of bile, to the rest of the body. Bile is composed of bile A (sodium, chloride, potassium, glucose, cholesterol) and of bile B (biliary salts, bilirubin, and hormones and foreign compounds that are inactivated and excreted by the liver). The biliary salts themselves are by-products of cholesterol oxidation. Constantly synthesized by the liver cells and reabsorbed by the intestine, the

133

biliary salts thereby regulate their own production. Their job is to stabilize the bile and to maintain cholesterol in the state of micellae, to prevent gallstones and to digest the non-water soluble fats. These fats are cholesterol, fatty acids and so on. Bile thus aids in the absorption of cholesterol, fatty acids and also liposoluble vitamins (A, D, E, K). We shall see the role of vitamin A in our study of opthalmological pathology in relation to the treatment of the Shao Yang points. The liver meridian passes through the eye, the sensorial organ of the element Wood, and gives it energy. The gallbladder meridian originates in the eye socket.

Vitamin D promotes the absorption of calcium and phosphorus in the intestine, as it does their fixation in the bones. Its sterol nucleus relates it to cholesterol; its molecular structure to the corticoadrenal hormones. Vitamin D3, of animal origin, is the 7-dehydrocholesterol.

In Chapter 10 of the *Ling Shu* we read that the zu shao yang (the gallbladder meridian) imbalance is involved in "all bone disorders." Among the complications of hyperthyroidism, we find osteoporosis and note that hyperthyroidism is related to an imbalance of Shao Yang.

The vitamin E found in wheat germ as alpha and beta-tocopherols is considered to be a testicular and ovarian hormonal precursor that affects the libido. Vitamin E deficiency is responsible for female sterility and male azoospermia. Zu shao yang is linked with dai mai and with the uterus, and although their relationship does not automatically imply sterility, it is involved in many forms of dysmenorrhea. One complication of hyperthyroidism is impotence and frigidity. In such cases the Shao Yang libido is deficient. A vitamin E deprivation lasting more than a year may cause muscular degeneration and paralysis. In the *Su Wen* it is written that "The liver rules over the muscles and the fascia."[5]

Vitamin K (phytonadione, menaquinone and menadione) is important in the formation of prothrombin by the liver. In the *Su Wen* we read, "The liver produces the blood."[6]

The gallbladder — or at least the biliary function of the liver and the bile ducts that collect the bile — plays a considerable physiological role, by way of the bile salts, in the absorption of all these vitamins. It is considered to be one of the "curious" bowels, the "irregular" bowels, as Husson calls them, or "miscellaneous" bowels, as they are sometimes referred to in English. These bowels are energized by the jing qi that flows throughout the eight miscellaneous channels and is the purest of energies. In the eleventh chapter of the *Su Wen,* we read:

> Six organs are born of the terrestrial breath: the brain, the marrow,
> the bones, the blood vessels, the gallbladder and the matrix (uterus).
> Located in the region of Yin, they are in the image of the earth and
> do not excrete. We call them the irregular receptors (jiheng).[7]

The gallbladder, therefore, has a part to play in the formation of jing qi and in its distribution. From the gallbladder stems the miscellaneous meridian dai mai, the belt meridian encircling the six meridians Tai Yang, Shao Yang, Yang Ming, Tai Yin, Shao Yin and Jue Yin.

134

The dai mai key point is zulinqi (GB-41). This channel passes through ming-men (GV-4), which is the receptacle of yuan qi, the original energy, and between the two kidneys, which store jing qi. This may all be related to the strategic molecule in endocrinology whose basis is sterolic, namely, cholesterol. Bile contains cholesterol, which permits intestinal absorption of fatty acids. These, in turn, allow the production of certain elements of cholesterol by the liver. The phospholipids, which are essential brain stem[8] and myelin constituents, are mainly secreted by the liver. Cholesterol is also at the origin of the production of sexual and corticoadrenal steroid hormones.

This links the gallbladder with the adrenal gland. In Chinese medicine, the kidney is composed of the kidneys and the adrenal gland and stores jing. It circulates jing at the body's command. The intermediate compound between cholesterol and the sexual hormones is pregnenolone, which may turn into progesterone. Another possibility in the adrenal gland leads us to aldosterone and to cortisol, which regulates the production of glucose in the liver, increases neoglycogenesis and elicits muscular proteolysis. Cortisol acts on collagen and is a vector of the bones (a curious bowel). Aldosterone favors the reabsorption of sodium. The serum sodium level rises and the potassium serum level falls. In excess, aldosterone is responsible for water retention and hypertension. This represents a link between the blood vessels (a curious bowel), the adrenal gland (as the dwelling place of jing qi) and the gallbladder.

Progesterone gives way to D4 androstenedione, the precursor of the testosterone secreted by the testes or precursor of the estrone and the estradiol secreted by the ovaries. And the ovaries are, along with the uterus, the last of the curious bowels.

The alkaline phosphates (each of which may be isolated and distinguished)[9] are another bond between the six curious bowels. They are secreted not only by the microvilli of the bile ducts, but are present as well in the bones, the intestines, the kidneys and the placenta.[10]

An excess of cholesterol causes atherosclerosis. The enzymatic intravascular endothelial role that cholesterol plays demonstrates another relationship between the jing and the blood vessels.[11] Cholesterol is closely linked to the Chinese jing and is one of its Western physiological equivalents. It must be added that vitamin A participates in the biogenesis of the genital hormones, as Grangaud[12] has shown. The testis function is also thyroid-dependent. A severe hyperthyroidism may impair the pituitary gonadotrophic function. We shall discuss the relationships between the thyroid and the gallbladder further on, as we have already spoken about them in our discussion of the correlations between Diathesis I and the element Wood, concerning hyperthyroidism. Vitamin A or E deprivation may lead to the atrophy of the testes canaliculi and of the interstitial cells of the testicles. This reminds us of the testicle degeneration observed in rats who were totally deprived of manganese, which establishes a correlation between liposoluble vitamins A and E, the gallbladder, the thyroid, the testes and manganese. In summary, we may say that the role of the gallbladder function is critical. The liver function is also important, in that it is responsible for the secretion of bile and may be related to the endocrine, skeletal, neurological and vascular systems.

The spasm and shrinking of the gallbladder is not yet fully understood physiologically. We know that a pneumogastric nerve branch innervates the gallbladder. The contractility of the organ is the key factor to the bile excretion when food enters into the duodenum. This excretion is related to the Oddi sphincter, which is normally synergistic to the gallbladder. When fatty matter penetrates into the duodenum, this triggers the sphincter aperture and the contraction of the organ. These two factors are more or less independent. There is no apparent subordination of the sphincter relaxation to the gallbladder contraction.[13] Cholecystokinin (chole=bile; kystis=bladder; kinein=to move), a hormone that is secreted by the duodenum, plays an important role in the mechanics of the phenomenon. Apart from this mechanical role, the gallbladder acts chemically to concentrate the bile (there are five times as many pigments as in hepatic bile). The gallbladder reabsorbs the water and certain lipids with it, perhaps even the cholesterol. This activity is again hormonally dependent on cholecystokinin and may be compared to this statement in Chapter 12 of the *Ling Shu,* "Zu shao yang brings in clear water from outside, and transports it to the gallbladder in the form of bile."[14]

There are several reasons to think that the Chinese considered the gallbladder to be far from passive. First, we have the position given to the gallbladder in the celestial chronology. Second, the role of the "judge who decides" is conferred upon the gallbladder by antiquity, and above all, the title of nobility that is confirmed in the *Nan Jing:*

> It is an error to consider the bowels, even though they are Yang, as viscera that contain pure matter; indeed, the *Nei Jing* has pointed out that the gallbladder alone is a pure bowel.[15]

As Qi Bo said, it is the gallbladder that makes the decisions, and "the liver agrees with the gallbladder, because the latter is a bowel containing the vital essence of the middle of the body."[16] In the *Su Wen,* Qi Bo says:

> There is one more important point. This is the yanglingquan point (GB-34). It rules over the heat and the cold (the Yin and the Yang). All these energies are important, but it is the gallbladder that makes the final decision, as it is the ruler of all the energies that begin to take form.[17]

This text may relate to the gallbladder mu collecting point (GB-24), riyue, reminding us that its translation means "sun and moon." The cosmic symbols of Yang and Yin that signify this gallbladder point are like medals of honor that tell us of the importance of this viscera in Chinese energetic physiology.

Cardiovascular Pathology

Functional Cardiac Disorders

The Shao Yang temperament is dominated by Wood and Fire, though most often by Wood. Menetrier says, in speaking of the corresponding diathesis, "Diathesis I is the diathesis of the young, of individuals in good health." Optimistic and active, Shao Yang types suffer in general from benign functional disorders in the early part of their lives, which give rise to complications and more serious disorders only in their fifties. At this time they may be considered as Diathesis III patients, governed by Fire, and they will suffer from palpitations, heartburn and cardiac rhythm problems. In the functional stage, a Shao Yang imbalance produces heartburn and short-lived substernal pains.

In the *Su Wen* chapter on the symptomology of the six unit meridians according to the seasons, it is written:

> For the Shao Yang: pain in the heart and in the thorax. The Shao Yang is in overabundance that manifests in the heart (Shao Yang, fire minister; heart, imperial fire). By the ninth month, Yang is exhausted and Yin is in full blossom, whence come the pains in the heart and thorax.[18]

We understand, in reading this text, the relationship of the Shao Yang (lesser Yang), representing the Ministerial Fire, the thorax and the heart. Excess in this meridian can disturb the ministerial energy in the thorax, thus provoking precordialgia and the disturbance of cardiac rhythm problems.

The *Ling Shu,* in Chapter 10, confirms this semiology specifically for the gallbladder meridian: "The heart and the sides of the chest are painful."[19] Thus it is an excess of the gallbladder meridian that is responsible for the symptomology that we have described. Nguyen Van Nghi calls this a surging of the fire of Wood, or of the gallbladder, a phenomenon that may as easily occur in the liver. The interior pathway of the Shao Yang meridian explains the surge of energy. The shou shao yang, the triple burner meridian, runs from the collar bone (quepen, ST-12) into the thorax, passes through shanzhong (CV-17), shangwan (CV-13), zhongwan (CV-12), xiawan (CV-10), which are the sea of energy points, through the mu of the triple burner (sanjiao), and from there arrives at the gallbladder itself, to leave the interior of the body at riyue (GB-24), the point known as "sun and moon," the mu point of the gallbladder.[20]

In the case of excess, the energy moves upwards, against the normal flow, and disturbs the circulation of energy in the thorax.[21] In this way, Shao Yang can surge upwards and disturb the energy of the heart. The same mechanism, as we shall see further on, is likely to cause dyspnea and asthma. This physiopathology usually coincides with a full radial Shao Yang pulse. "When the Shao Yang pulse is visible, it is sometimes frequent, sometimes rare, sometimes long, sometimes short."[22] This is characteristic of cardiac rhythm problems, which may take on the form of tachycardia or tachyarhythmia. Qi Bo, in the chapter "Relationships between the Meridians and the Arteries," defines the Shao Yang pulse: "It is sliding, which is not to say full."[23] Although sliding, it is a moderate pulse that does not attain the extreme characteristics of Yang Ming, which is ample and superficial. In practice, we notice that this cardiac erethism can be tolerated for a long time without any ischemic accident and that angina pectoris, the real infarction, if it does occur, will do so only later in the patient's life. The Shao Yang, nonetheless, is an ideal terrain for cardiac rhythm disorders and non-necrotic conduction disorders.

Zu Lien, in *La nouvelle science de l'acupuncture et des moxas,* agrees with all the classical authors in pointing to fengchi (GB-20) as the best way to disperse the

137

meridian in cases of tachycardia or palpitations.[24] This point, which seems to have a sympatholytic action as much on the erection as on the dilation of the pupil and on nasal vasomotricity gives us some idea of the general deregulation caused by excess of the Shao Yang meridian. Along with fengchi, there are two other dispersal points: yangfu (GB-38) to disperse zu shao yang; and tianjing (TB-10) to disperse shou shao yang. The symptomology for these two points is found in the *Da Cheng*. For yangfu we read, "pain in the heart and in the sides"[25] and for tianjing, "pain in the heart and in the chest, swollen legs."[26] The *Ling Shu* points out, however, that we must not forget to tonify the Yin, or the treatment will be ineffective.

Shou shao yang is coupled with shou jue yin (pericardium) which acts on the vascular parasympathetic tonus. According to the *Su Wen,* the zu shao yang energy cleft points are tianchi (PC-1); the mu point of shou jue yin, riyue (GB-24), which is the mu point of zu shao yang; and zhangmen (LV-13), which is the triple burner cleft point.[27] These are the points to consider when we are called on to treat cardiac erethism and tachycardia in Shao Yang individuals.

The main points to be retained in the treatment of functional cardiac disorders in the Shao Yang type are as follows: GB-20, GB-24, GB-38; TB-10; PC-1; LV-13.

There is a direct correlation with the Diathesis I (Wood) described by Menetrier. He speaks of cardiac instability, "anginoid states" without electrical modification. "Allergic behavior is commonly observed along with functional cardiac disorders. Manganese, iodine and cobalt are usually effective and primary precordialgia is almost always improved through manganese-cobalt treatment."[28] It is nonetheless important with these patients to regularly keep an eye on their blood pressure and to have them undergo regular electrocardiograms, in order to catch any real coronary disease at the beginning.

High Blood Pressure

Variations in blood pressure are a complex acupunctural phenomenon and involve almost all the meridians. Once again, it is most important to understand the individual patient, his temperament and his case history, and to analyze with care the different factors that may play a part in causing high blood pressure. This is why our classification of the six temperaments is so important, as is also true in the case of dysmenorrhea or colonopathies.

Shao Yang patients frequently suffer from high blood pressure; their clinical profile reveals the disorder. Within a clinical profile of cardiac erethism, hyperthyroidism, hot flushes and of frequent outbursts of anger, the high blood pressure is usually of the Shao Yang type. Its development is similar to that of the cardiac disorders previously examined and the dynamics have been known to Chinese medicine for thousands of years. Without giving the phenomenon the modern name of high blood pressure, Qi Bo explained in the *Su Wen:*

> Violent anger wounds the Yin; too much joy wounds the Yang. If the breath is blocked,[29] it backs up and fills the vessels and separates mind from body.[30]

138

When Qi Bo speaks of vessels in this passage, he means meridians. However, within the meridians flow both blood and energy — the relationship between meridians and arteries is a close one in the framework of Chinese medicine, as we have already seen. This is why, in Chamfrault's translation of the same work, we may read, "These two energies in excess cause hypertension and damage the forms."[31] Nguyen Van Nghi (59), p. 96, translates: "The surge of energy causes the overflow of the vessels, which is harmful to the form." Anger and joy cause jue, or blockage, followed by a surge of energy with the risk of "separating body and mind" or of coma, owing to a cerebro-vascular accident (see Yang Ming). Anger primarily causes jue in Shao Yang, joy in Yang Ming.

Modern Shanghai physicians know of five etiologies for high blood pressure, two of which are related to Wood. The first of these two is "flourishing of fire of the liver and gallbladder," and the other is "the agitation of the wind of the liver."[32] These are not new concepts and, among others, Nguyen Van Nghi has spoken of the rising fire of the liver and the gallbladder in relation to high blood pressure.[33]

High blood pressure syndromes that are caused by Shao Yang imbalances will be severe and poorly tolerated by these types, as we will see further on in our study of cerebrovascular accidents (Yang Ming). Owing to the relationships between Shao Yang and the eyes and ears, the symptoms that accompany Shao Yang high blood pressure are: dizziness, tinnitus, hypoacusis, blurred vision and headaches. Here the upward surge of energy concerns the passage of energy from the thorax into the encephalon and indicates an imbalance in the "windows to the sky," which, like safety valves, blow under the energy pressure. The *Ling Shu* advises us to "needle the point tianyou {TB-16, Shao Yang window to the sky} in cases of sudden deafness or loss of visual acuity."[34] The context of this passage makes it obvious that this is advised for transient cardiovascular accidents (sudden hypoacusis, amaurosis).

According to modern Chinese physicians, the protocol for the treatment of high blood pressure caused by fire in the gallbladder and liver — considered to be typical of the Shao Yang temperament — calls for use of yanglingquan (GB-34), the he point with a specific action on the gallbladder, and taichong (LV-3) and xingjian (LV-2) to calm the fire in Wood, in the organ and in the bowel.[35] Fengchi (GB-20) is used consistently in such cases. Used in dispersion, it "hides the Yang of the gallbladder" and shunts the Yang into the miscellaneous channel yang wei mai that passes through this point. Yifeng (TB-17) is also referred to by these modern authors. Its name means "bothered by the wind,"[36] and the semiology of the point in the *Da Cheng* reads: "becomes suddenly mute, mouth and eyes are distorted."[37] This is typical of hemiplegia with facial paralysis. Concerning the point tianyou (TB-16), which means "heavenly window," we read "face swollen by the wind, becomes suddenly deaf, pain in the eyes, visual distortion."[38] Chamfrault, citing the advice of the ancient authors, claims that use of moxas on this point is likely to aggravate facial and palpable edema.[39] Elsewhere, Soulie de Morant, in his translation of more recent texts, indicates the use of the point tianjing (TB-10), dispersion point of the meridian shou shao yang, as well as daling (PC-7), dispersion point of the meridian shou jue yin, for treatment of high blood pressure.[40]

139

Acupuncture treatment of high blood pressure is usually effective and long lasting, especially when there is no complication of arteriosclerosis. It is important to know the temperament of the patient in order to determine the physiopathology involved. In treating Shao Yang patients for high blood pressure, the points to keep in mind are the following: GB-20, GB-34; LV-2, LV-3; TB-10, TB-16, TB-17; PC-7; and BL-45.

Menetrier, in his description of Diathesis I (Wood), writes, "Ill tolerated primary hypertension (with headache, blurred vision, dizziness, tachycardia and precordialgia)."[41] He adds that these symptoms are commonly found in the passage from Diathesis I, in young patients, to Diathesis III, during the passage to andropause or menopause. He writes that "the action of manganese and iodine is consistent with signs of blood pressure problems." He feels that it is more important to alleviate the suffering of patients with high blood pressure than to bring down the reading itself, if the patient can tolerate his condition. As acupuncture is effective in treating this problem, there is an obvious interest in associating the two treatments synergistically. One last remark is that manganese-cobalt is effective in cases of high blood pressure among the elderly.

Varicose Veins and Phlebitis

This pathology is described in the chapter on Jue Yin.

Chronic Obstructive Arteriopathies of the Lower Limbs

The symptomology of these disorders is particularly well explained in the chapters that deal with Yang Ming and Tai Yang. To summarize briefly here, we may say that circulatory obstruction in the lower limbs is related to an excess of Yang energy that, instead of flowing downwards (from head to toe), has a tendency to flow upwards, abandoning the lower territory. The primary channels are in excess, but so are the luo vessels. The small amount of Yang energy that does flow downwards in the primary channel tends to flow back upwards from the luo point and through the longitudinal luo, bypassing the transverse luo, which would ordinarily lead it to the coupled Yin meridian.

Meridians represent the dynamic vectors of the blood. In the *Ling Shu,* a paragraph in Chapter 60 alludes to the transverse luo channels and to their close relationships with the precapillary arteriovenous anastomoses:

> The main capillaries enable man's energy to pass by the shortest route
> from a Yang channel to a Yin channel, or the other way around, and
> to circulate energy all over the body, in the skin, in the muscles and
> so on. On the meridians there are main capillary points. These are
> the collateral meridian points {the luo channels}.[42]

Thus we have not only to regulate the energy in the Yang meridian, but also to open the revascularization pathways by needling the luo of the Yang meridian and the yuan point of the coupled Yin meridian.

Once again, the patient's temperament, his psychophysiological behavior, will enable us to establish more precisely if we are dealing with a Yang Ming, a Shao Yang or a Tai Yang excess. In our opinion, this is the order of frequency.

140

In the tenth chapter of the *Ling Shu,* concerning the semiology of the luo of zu shao yang (gallbladder), we find, "The legs are frozen."[43] We are thus called on to disperse guangming (GB-37) and to tonify taichong (LV-3). The *Da Cheng* confirms this semiology. For guangming we read, "Pain in the calves that prevents the patient from standing up for too long," and for taichong, "Numbness at the tips of the toes, pain in the calves and in the internal malleolus, frozen feet."[44]

Two other points will be retained in treating chronic obstructive arteriopathies of the lower limbs: zusanli (ST-36; see arteriopathy and preventive treatment of Yang Ming cerebrovascular accidents) and xuanzhong (GB-39). The correlation in diathetic medicine for these two points is represented by manganese-cobalt in these disorders. Menetrier also prescribes a combination of iodine and sulfur,[45] the catalysts of Diathesis I (Wood). Xuanzhong, furthermore, is related to the Wood element.

The main points to remember in treating Shao Yang patients for arteriopathies are the following: GB-37 and GB-39; LV-3; and ST-36.

Respiratory Pathology

Asthma

In acupuncture, there are two types of asthma: "excess asthma" and "deficiency asthma."[46] These two forms of asthma and the parallel drawn with "exogenous asthma" and "endogenous asthma," as described by the science of diathetic medicine, are explained in the chapter that deals with Tai Yin. In cases of excess asthma, we often discover an excess of Wood energy. There are also two types of Wood excesses. An excess of liver affects the more nervous Jue Yin subjects. Fortunately, it is less frequently that we find a gallbladder excess, which affects Shao Yang subjects.

In the *Ling Shu,* Qi Bo states, "Shao Yang is linked to the kidneys and the lungs, and depends on these two organs."[47] This establishes a physiological relationship between the kidney of the lower burner and Shao Yang, and between this meridian and the lung of the upper burner. We believe this relationship to be metabolic rather than circulatory and will expand on it elsewhere in this work. This view is supported by Huang Di, who declares, in the *Su Wen:*

> Shao Yang, which plays the role of mediator between Yang and Yin, going back and forth between one and the other, is not in accord with the lungs. When Shao Yang energy connects with the lungs, the ren ying and qi hao[48] pulses become like wire, contracted and floating, as if suspended. If the energy of Shao Yang cannot manage to dissociate itself from the Yin {the lungs}, it means death.[49]

There is thus a close physiological relationship between Shao Yang and the lungs, but certain rules of exclusion must be respected, or else the patient may become severely ill. We read, however, in the *Nan Jing,* concerning Difficulty Number 11:

> Breathing in acts on the energy of the lower burner, in the liver and
> the kidneys, and makes it flow deeply inwards. Breathing out acts on
> the energy of the upper burner, in the heart and lungs, and drives it
> outwards.[50]

We show elsewhere[51] that Shao Yang completely traverses the thorax and the lungs. The origin of the lung meridian is in the stomach and it passes through the three mu points (lower, middle and upper) of the triple burner, xiawan (CV-10), zhongwan (CV-12) and shangwan (CV-13). We may therefore understand why stagnation of energy in Shao Yang can bring on a pathology that is extremely difficult to control by usual therapeutic means. This may be the symptomology that Qi Bo is trying to describe in Chapter 7 of the *Su Wen:*

> Suffering in the lesser Yang (Shao Yang) makes one breathless, with
> a tendency to coughing and diarrhea, subsequently leading to a pul-
> ling pain in the heart and blockage of the diaphragm.[52]

Acupuncture is very effective in these cases. We must needle all the points through which the interiorized energy of Shao Yang passes: jianjing (GB-21), shanzhong (CV-17), shangwan (CV-13), zhongwan (CV-12), xiawan (CV-10), riyue (GB-24), in that order. These points may cause a temporary aggravation of the attacks and the patient should be informed of this. Certain other points on the Shao Yang meridian are indicated in the *Da Cheng,* with a specific pulmonary semiology. The *Da Cheng* indicates the master points of dai mai and of yang wei mai miscellaneous channels in rapport with Shao Yang, zulinqi (GB-41) and waiguan (TB-5). Needling these points proves to be a safer way of shunting the energy blocked in the thorax.

Zulinqi (GB-41) is effective in the case of labored breathing when walking, excess in the chest and pleurisy.[53] Soulie de Morant adds to this translation, "sluggishness, slowness, the functions are slow, cervical lymphadenitis, fear of cold, frequent dental caries."[54] This corresponds to the description of the Metal hyposthenic type (see Tai Yin and Yang Ming). In other words, zulinqi (GB-41) is a point that is effective for both excess and deficient asthma with intermingling of liver and lungs (Tai Yin), which corresponds to the mixed diathesis that Mene-trier termed "arthro-infectious" (see Jue Yin). This contributes to the suitability of zulinqi in the treatment of pleurisy, be it tubercular or secondary to a long term pulmonary disorder.

Waiguan (TB-5) is indicated by Soulie de Morant for asthma.[55] For "asthma attacks,"[56] he also suggests the gallbladder dispersal point, yangfu (GB-38). In cases of "coughing with the feeling of energy flowing towards the upper part of the body and purulent expectoration," the *Da Cheng* mentions the triple burner dispersal point, tianjing (TB-10).[57] These are two points that are indispensable for treating cases of excess asthma attacks among Shao Yang patients. We must also indicate giuxu (GB-40), xiaxi (GB-43) and zuqiaoyin (GB-44), points with similar pulmonary indications.

In summary, Shao Yang asthma does exist and is not rare, although it is much less frequent among Jue Yin or Tai Yin individuals. Shao Yang asthma patients are usually fiery people, whose anger and aggressiveness aggravate their condition, as does the wind. This explains the interest of the point zuqiaoyin (GB-44), a Metal point that helps Metal control the nefarious effects of wind, anger and the excess of Wood that turn against it.[58] There is not necessarily an aggravation of this condition in the springtime.

The main points to be retained in treating Shao Yang asthma are the following: GB-21, GB-24, GB-38, GB-40, GB-41, GB-44; CV-10, CV-12, CV-13, CV-17; TB-5 and TB-10.

As concerns treatment with trace elements, manganese must be prescribed with care when the asthma is exogenous. H. Picard has detailed the protocol for such treatment.[59] In cases of asthma among Shao Yang types, we are logically led to prescribe iodine and sulfur and manganese-cobalt for the elderly.

Digestive Pathology

The triple burner, or san jiao, consists of three levels. Anatomically, the upper level is represented by the lungs and the heart, the middle level is represented by the spleen and the stomach, the lower by the kidneys. Physiologically, the three levels are the upper, middle and lower parts of the stomach, represented by shangwan (CV-13), zhongwan (CV-12) and xiawan (CV-10). Here, Shao Yang is only concerned with the physiology of liver and the bile ducts, because the meridian, shou shao yang, is distinct from the Shao Yang organ, the triple burner, san jiao.

Dyskinesia and Cholelithiasis

The specific excess of energy in zu shao yang and in the bowel, the gallbladder, will frequently give rise to functional disorders, the first among which is biliary dyskinesia. The *Ling Shu* tells us that anger is harmful to the liver, also that it is a symptom of energy imbalance in the gallbladder. This shows the psychological and physiological interaction in the disturbance of this bowel, of which Shao Yang types are victims.[60] Chapter 10 of the *Ling Shu* describes the symptomology of zu shao yang:

> The mouth is bitter, the patient sighs often, his heart and the sides of
> his chest are painful, he cannot turn over.[61]

This depicts the physical discomfort felt by the patient whose gallbladder is disturbed and who suffers most from biliary colic.

In the *Ling Shu,* we also find a description of an attack of biliary dyskinesia on the behavior of the cholelithiasis victim:

> A patient who displays the symptoms of frequent vomiting, spitting
> up of bile, sighing, anguish (as if someone wanted to catch them and
> put them in prison), has a diseased gallbladder. The stomach is also
> affected.[62] It is as if there were a leak in the bile secretion; this is why
> the patient's mouth is always bitter. In this case we must needle the
> point zusanli {ST-36} as well as the points located beneath it.[63] If the
> energy of the stomach is disturbed, we must needle the points located

143

on the small capillaries of the gallbladder meridian to balance excess and deficiency and in this way the perverse energy will be expelled.[64]

We may note that even here, in an internal condition, perverse energy is to blame. It follows that the temperament is a predisposition to accommodate perverse energy — here wind and heat, or heat alone. We may also note the relationship established between the gallbladder and the stomach and that the ancient Chinese understood the gastric role of the gallbladder, which our semiologists finally discovered twenty odd centuries later. Qi Bo makes it clear:

> The symptoms of the diseases of the gallbladder are as follows: frequent belching, bitter taste in the mouth, vomiting of bitter water from the gallbladder; nervousness and fear as if being tracked down; obstructions to the throat that create a frequent desire to spit out. Such diseases should be treated by all the points of the lesser Yang meridian of the foot (the gallbladder meridian). And also moxibustion therapy should be applied to treat depressions in the same meridian. Yanglingquan (GB-34) should be used to treat cold and burning sensations.[65] It is also clear that the treatment must be adapted to the symptoms and to the intensity of the suffering.

Concerning the sighs spoken of in the *Ling Shu*, we have seen time and time again that Shao Yang patients sigh as if they were frustrated or bothered by something. They blow air out through tensed lips, making a sound that makes it seem as if they were chasing away an excess of wind. This is different from the sighing of the kidney or of the lungs in Shao Yin or Tai Yin subjects, in whom the vocal chords are used to make a sad sound.

At its worst, a gallbladder disorder can take the form of hepatic colic (pathetic) and the patient will find it impossible to move. There is a risk of angiocolitis and fistulization. This is the organic stage of the disorder and is, therefore, serious. It may be taken for jue (energy blockage), the most severe complication in energy imbalances and the main cause of casualties. The symptoms of energy blockage in the gallbladder meridian are described in the *Su Wen:*

> The symptoms of the upstream disease of the lesser Yang include: a malfunctioning of the machinery {the joints} which means that the loins are unable to move, the patient cannot turn his neck to look back; intestinal carbuncle, which should not be treated by this meridian {the gallbladder meridian} nor by acupuncture; and death of the patient if he is also in shock.[66]

Every medical doctor has learned the pathos of hepatic colic, for the pain is such that the patient is incapable of moving. This impossibility to move is given as one of the characteristic features of Shao Yang in the following chapter of the *Su Wen,* which gives the symptoms of the disease. Along with pain in the heart and thorax, as we said in dealing with cardiac pathology, we find, "Inability to turn over in bed; the Yin makes people reserved."[67]

These observations are firmly established as pertaining to the hepato-biliary attack in the chapter of the *Su Wen* that deals with coughing:

144

All the viscera, zang {solid} or fu {hollow}, may be said to cause
coughing, not only the lung. . . when the liver cough passes to the
gallbladder, the patient vomits bile. . . The liver cough hurts on both
sides beneath the ribs, and may hurt so much as to prevent the patient
from turning over."[68]

We are led to think that the above symptoms of energy blockage in the gallbladder
with intestinal abscess represent the angiocolitis and its fistulization.[69] Western
anatamo-physiological research has shown the existence of cough reflexes in the
liver.[70] We will also note that the strapping shoulder pain is related to the right
gallbladder meridian pathway that runs through this region and is homolateral to
the viscera. When this symptom occurs, we must treat the liver and gallbladder
divergent channels, especially the jing-well points (GB-44 and LV-1) on the left or
opposite side.

Cholelithiasis is related to a Shao Yang temperament, a perverse energy (heat)
and an elimination disorder that is located in the triple burner and on which we
will expound when dealing with urinary lithiasis. This elimination disorder is
often aggravated because of the errors of nutrition of Shao Yang subjects who are
given to eating much meat and drinking wine.

In our discussion of the treatment of dyskinesia and cholelithiasis, we may
once again quote from the *Su Wen:*

The Yellow Emperor asked, "Some people suffer from bitter taste in
the mouth which is treated by the yanglingquan point {GB-34}.
What is the name of the disease that causes bitter taste in the mouth?
What causes the disease?"

Qi Bo replied, "The name of the disease is hot gallbladder.[71] The
liver is the general and receives judgements from the gallbladder.
The throat is the servant of the liver and the gallbladder {because
both the liver and the gallbladder meridians reach the throat}; and if a
person is frequently indecisive, his gallbladder will be in deficiency,
with bile overflowing upstream causing the bitter taste in the mouth.
It should be treated by the gallbladder gathering and transport points,
namely the riyue {GB-24} and the danshu {BL-19}."[72]

To summarize, we must needle yanglingquan (GB-34) and apply moxas to
danshu (BL-19) and riyue (GB-24). For the treatment of gallstones, Zu Lien, in
La nouvelle science de l'acupuncture et des moxas, adds the shu points of the principal burner, sanjiaoshu (BL-22), shenshu (BL-23) and also qihaishu (BL-24), as
well as the point zhangmen (LV-13), the point at which the internal gallbladder
meridian emerges.[73]

The main points used in the treatment of biliary dyskinesia and cholelithiasis
are: GB-24, GB-34, GB-44; BL-19, BL-22, BL-23, BL-24; LV-1, LV-13; and
ST-36 or CP-152.[74]

We again find a direct correlation with the theory of diathetic medicine, in
that Menetrier lists lithiasis and specifically cholelithiasis among the symptoms of
Diathesis I.[75] Picard writes that the association of manganese and sulfur, with or

without manganese-cobalt (according to the specific case), may help the patient to suffer less from gallstones and to avoid painful attacks. This treatment is particularly effective in treating primary biliary dyskinesia.

When surgery must be delayed or avoided, the synergism of acupuncture, trace element therapy and phytotherapy is highly effective. When the gallstones are of small or medium size, consistent results are obtained with this therapy, as we have witnessed personally in clinics in Shanghai, where the expulsion of gallstones is common practice.

Gastralgia and Stomach Ulcers

Excess or heat in the gallbladder is apt to bring on gastric symptoms. This happens due to the phenomenon of control of the stomach by the gallbladder (the controlling cycle): Wood triumphs over Earth. We may also come up against atypical gastralgia, as well as very real ulcers caused by an excess of gallbladder energy. This etiology is spoken of by all the classical authors, ancient as well as modern.

In practice we sometimes, but not always, find such gastralgia associated with biliary dyskinesia. Occasionally, the psychological profile alone allows us to make a correct diagnosis. The *Trung Y Hoc* of Hanoi, which we have frequently quoted,[76] attributes ulcers to the element Wood in three out of six etiologies. These are clarified in the chapter on Jue Yin. However, the fifth etiology of ulcers — stagnation of blood with excess heat — implicates gallbladder involvement. This is an emergency case, in which the perforation is the first sign of the ulcer. In this case we may speak of energy blockage in the stomach bowel (either gallbladder energy or stomach energy, but most often both) with accumulation and compression of this energy, which is transformed into heat and causes the "stagnation of the blood," an ancient term that designates ischemia.

The *Trung Y Hoc* describes it as:

> Acute, stabbing abdominal pain, hematemesis or melena, polypnea,
> perspiration, facial congestion, the tongue is red or has red edges and
> a yellow coating, the pulse is tight and rapid.[77]

The text advises us to "cool the blood" and to strengthen it, to stop the hemorrhage. In China, treatment of perforated ulcers has been effective for the last twenty years and surgery has been avoided 218 times in a series of 316 cases (69).[78] The points to be treated are: zusanli (ST-36), neiguan (PC-6), tianshu (ST-25) and zhongwan (CV-12).[79] Shao Yang types are the most susceptible to this progression of ulcer pathology.

Functional Colonopathies

To our knowledge, no classical text, be it ancient or modern, describes the physiopathology of functional colonopathies. We have taken it on ourselves to describe this pathology elsewhere and have come up with five profiles of morbidity that relate to this disorder.[80] The fifth of these profiles corresponds to "excess of gallbladder."

146

Just as Wood can impinge upon Earth, Wood may also turn against Metal and thus attack the colon. A diagnosis of colonopathy due to an excess of gallbladder may be made in the presence of the following symptoms: severe abdominal pains located in the left and especially in the right colic angles (pains that come and go, leaving the patient free of pain between attacks), constipation (sometimes alternating with diarrhea), epigastralgia, bilious vomiting, frontal and retro-orbital headaches, opthalmic migraines, hemorrhoids, insomnia or, in short, one or more Shao Yang symptoms.

X-rays show the gallbladder to be dilated and slow to evacuate. The treatment is the same as in the case of biliary dyskinesia, with the addition of the point dadun (LV-1), especially if the patient suffers from hemorrhoids. We may also needle "zusanli {ST-36} and the points that are beneath it," as we saw above, in cases of dyskinesia, that is to say shangjuxu (ST-37), xiajuxu (ST-39), etc.

Once again, we find a direct correlation between acupuncture and trace element therapy. Among the symptoms described by Menetrier, concerning Diathesis I (Wood), we find, "intestinal disorders, of the right colitic type."[81] In Diathesis III (Fire), we also find, "gastralgia, abdominal swelling, right-sided colitis. . . "[82]

The treatment of predominantly right-sided colonopathies among Shao Yang patients involves the following points: GB-24, GB-34; ST-36, ST-37, ST-39; LV-1; and BL-19.

Constipation and Hemorrhoids

Constipation may be isolated or associated with a colonopathy. Typical constipation in Shao Yang subjects involves both the gallbladder and the triple burner, the latter in its body fluid function (with the spleen and the kidneys, it involves the middle and lower burners).

The success in the treatment of hemorrhoids and constipation depends on the diagnosis of the affected meridian and on the chosen points. When the Shao Yang type has these problems, the context is one of elimination problems with oliguria. This is why zhaohai (KI-6) and zhigou (TB-6), the latter being the concentration point of shou shao yang, are chosen. As for constipation, this is more often than not related to a colonopathy that must be diagnosed and treated. The gallbladder meridian pathway, with the passage through the baliao[83] and changqiang (GV-1), the perianal and master point for hemorrhoids, explains the influence of the gallbladder in cases of thrombosis.[84] The correlation with manganese-cobalt (Fire), which is indicated in certain cases of constipation and hemorrhoids, should be clear.

Bone, Joint and Ligament Pathology

Body Fluid Physiology

In the tenth chapter of the *Ling Shu*, concerning the semiology of the gallbladder meridian zu shao yang, we read, "In cases of bone disease, we must needle the points of this meridian."[85] Elsewhere, Qi Bo says of the triple burner

147

(san jiao), "The triple burners serve to irrigate the organism, and are the sources of all the 'sea routes' of the organism."[86] The famous Chinese physician Zhang Zhi Cong made the following commentary on this text:

> Within the human body, the outside is Yang, the inside Yin. The stomach is Yang (middle burner), the kidneys are Yin. The kidneys are the gateway to the stomach. They communicate through the intermediary of the lower burner. The lower burner brings the nutritive fluids to the intestines, from there to the kidneys by way of its internal channel.[87]

The san jiao (triple burner), represented by the meridian shou shao yang, plays an important part in the regulation of body fluids. This is confirmed by Zhang Jing Yao:

> Energy is the mother of water. If we understand the reasons for which energy is transformed, we understand already the better part of how the general movement of water in the body is regulated.[88]

The viscera in control of the transformation of energy is the san jiao, or more exactly the organs that it represents, as "the triple burner is an immaterial bowel and is coupled with no organs."[89] These organs are the heart and the lungs, for the upper burner, the spleen, stomach and liver for the middle burner and the kidney for the lower burner. The transformation of body fluids here, as well as their metabolism, is especially related to the kidneys and the liver. However, the stomach, the spleen and the lungs also play a considerable part. In other words, one of the multiple physiological concepts that is included in the term san jiao, or triple burner, is the principle of transformation. This may be understood as anabolism (specifically spleen and stomach) but also as catabolism.

A constitutional disturbance of this function due to excess (or heat) means evaporation of the fluids and in the vocabulary of physiology we might express this as increased concentrations of urinary and blood catabolites. Oliguria, a symptom of heat, goes right along with insufficient detoxification.

The osteo-articular pathology of Shao Yang subjects is explained by their defective metabolism of body fluids in general and more specifically of those that affect the bones. "The synovial fluid is of ying {or rong} origin, when it is secreted in the articulations beneath the skin, it is called za."[90]

Arthralgia, Polyarthralgia and Gout

We shall leave aside the endocrine role of the gallbladder, which will be dealt with further on. Within the osteoarticular pathology of the Shao Yang meridian, we shall thus expect to find disorders related to metabolic misfunction and deficient elimination. We expect to find mobile and erratic arthralgia, gout, polyarthralgia and osteochondritis.

Indeed, in "Difficulty Number 38," the *Nan Jing* sheds light on the metabolic functions of the triple burner and on its circulatory physiology:

> The triple burner possesses all the qualities necessary to control the functions of transformation of the energy of the organs and the bowels. Its meridian spreads its energy throughout the body.[91]

This subtlety of energy circulation is inherent in the anatomical character of Shao Yang:

> The first Yang {Shao Yang} wanders throughout all the parts of the body. The first Yang {gallbladder} forms six lateral and intermediary lines that distribute the qi throughout the body.[92]

And as far as the distinction of bone disease goes, the *Su Wen* is even clearer, as we will see in the chapter on Shao Yin. For the moment we shall concentrate on the paragraph that concerns Shao Yang: "If the pain is not localized in a precise spot, it is preferable to needle the yangjiao {GB-35} points."[93] We see that Qi Bo suggests treating a point on zu shao yang, which is related to yang wei mai, for inflammatory arthritic pain among Shao Yang subjects (Diathesis I, the arthritic diathesis defined by Menetrier, corresponding to the element Wood in Chinese energy theory). The lesions associated with this sort of rheumatism or those of synovial origin, compared to arthritic pain, are mainly located in the cartilage.

Shao Yang subjects are sensitive to heat, but are also sensitive to the wind, which is in relation to the Wood constitution. Qi Bo states, in the chapter that deals with bi,[94] "if wind dominates, the pain will be erratic."[95] He goes on to say, "if the wind dominates, we have a better chance of curing the patient."[96]

There is reason to believe that yin qiao mai and yang qiao mai are involved in disorders affecting body fluids. Their relationships with the urinary tract are well codified:

> The yin qiao mai is an annex of the kidney primary channel. It corresponds to the energy of the Earth. Consequently, it flows upwards and brings energy to the eyes. Yang qiao mai is an annex of the bladder primary channel. It receives the energy from yin qiao mai at the point jingming and from there descends towards the lower extremities. These two meridians, yin and yang qiao mai, are very important. Yin qiao mai is especially important for women, as it brings the energy from the kidneys to the upper part of the body. Yang qiao mai is important for men, as they receive their energy from the kidneys.[97]

It is precisely their relationship with body fluids that confers on these two channels their central role in this pathology. Huang Di explains:

> When a patient feels pain that he cannot localize, we must needle the points of yang or yin qiao mai located over the malleolus. We will needle the yang qiao mai when the patient is a man, and the yin qiao mai when the patient is a woman; but never the contrary.[98]

The rest of the clinical profile associated with the semiology of zu shao yang is found in Chapter 10 of the *Ling Shu:*

> Wherever the meridian passes, there is pain, especially at the articula-
> tions. . . if the problem is serious, the upper part of the foot is very
> warm.[99]

To summarize this pathology, in cases of excess heat in Shao Yang, whether among patients of the Shao Yang temperament or not, we find "evaporation of body fluids," especially in the synovia. These subjects are more sensitive to the penetration of the wind that blows through Shao Yang throughout the body, caus- ing pain, especially in the meridian zu shao yang (gallbladder). The feeling of heat in the feet, even in the big toe (liver meridian), comes from Shao Yang.

Western pathology has described pharyngitis and phlebitis to be of gouty ori- gin. These are obviously disorders related to Shao Yang. Gouty iritis and con- junctivitis are also frequent. In these cases, the eye, the sensory organ of the ele- ment Wood, is the first to be stricken by perverse wind and heat, and displays the imbalance in body fluids.

> It is in the eyes that the ancestral meridians yin qiao mai and yang
> qiao mai meet. This is the path for the elevation of the fluids.[100]

To treat, or avoid, this complication we must needle zhaohai (KI-6) or shenmai (BL-62) according to the sex of the patients, and jingming (BL-1) when there are visible symptoms. The treatment for gout and erratic arthralgia is complemented by needling yangjiao (GB-35) and dadun (LV-1), as well as the points located along the Shao Yang pathway.

We may also needle the ting-Metal point to disperse both heat and wind. Zuqiaoyin (GB-44), the ting point of zu shao yang, is indicated in the *Da Cheng* when a patient finds it impossible to lift his arm, when his elbow is in spasm and especially when his hands and feet are quite warm but do not perspire.[101] Guan- chong (TB-1) is indicated for severe pain in the arm and elbow.[102] This acupunc- ture treatment is perfectly capable of reducing and eliminating pain associated with this pathology.

Chinese medicine makes a definite distinction between this superficial pathol- ogy and the altogether different pathology of bone degeneration. Theoretically, superficial pain is Yang, whereas deeper pain is Yin.

The main points to remember in treating arthralgia, polyarthralgia and gout among Shao Yang patients are the following: GB-35, GB-44; BL-1, BL-62 (with male patients); LV-1; TB-1; KI-6 (with female patients); and the ahshi points.[103]

The correlation between Shao Yang and Diathesis I is once again perfect, as much so for erratic arthritis that is painful, dry, non-deforming, non-stiffening and chronic as for cases of gout.[104] Menetrier prescribes manganese and sulfur in all these disorders. The gallbladder is so strongly linked to the arthritic phenomena that we are tempted to split Diathesis I into distinct parts: arthritic when associated with the Shao Yang temperament and allergic when associated with Jue Yin. In any case, we may clearly establish the link between arthritis and the gallbladder, a link that has never before been made in Western physiology.

Lumbago

Shao Yang lumbagos, when they occur, are severe, sudden and typical. In Chapter 41 of the *Su Wen,* which is devoted to lumbago, a paragraph is reserved for Shao Yang lumbagos:

> When the meridian of the zu shao yang (gallbladder) is attacked, it can also provoke pain in the renal area, giving the sensation as if one has been pierced by needles. One can neither bend forward nor backward, nor turn his head from side to side. This is because the gallbladder meridian traverses the neck, the shoulders and the sides of the body. In this case, it is necessary to puncture and bleed the point that is found just below the tip of the bony prominence {the region of the yanglingquan point, GB-34}, except in summer {because the lesser Yang is in harmony with the liver that reigns in spring and begins to decline in summer}.[105]

Further on in the same chapter, the yang wei meridian, which was also involved in erratic arthralgia, is linked to lumbago.

> When the miscellaneous channel yang wei mai[106] is diseased, the kidney region is suddenly swollen; we must then needle the point jinmen {BL-63}, the point of origin of the meridian yang wei mai, and the point yangjiao {GB-35}.[107]

This treatment has shown excellent results in practice and often one or two sessions are sufficient. The main points here are: GB-34 and GB-35; BL-63; and the ahshi points.

According to Menetrier:

> Arthralgia with periodic evolution, which is influenced by the climate and the geography, and which is accompanied by various pains in the joints, in the back, though having a normal x-ray, is typical of the allergic behavior. This is accompanied by asthenia, morning stiffness and various equivalents (migraines, eczema, asthma, etc.).[108]

Manganese and sulfur are, of course, to be prescribed.

Gonalgia

A semiological description of gonalgia is given by Qi Bo in Chapter 60 of the *Su Wen:*

> If the knee may not be straightened yet may be bent, we must needle the points below the knee: in this case it is a muscular disorder.[109]

> If the knee is stiff when extended, we needle the "pushbolt." If the knee is painful when sitting down we needle the "mechanism." If the patient feels as if the bones were about to dissolve and has hot sensations when standing up, we must treat the "skeletal barrier." If the pain in the knee gains the big toe, we needle the popliteal fossa, weizhong {BL-40}. If on sitting down the patient feels pain, as if

something were hidden inside, we needle the "gate." If the pain in the knee causes inability to bend and to extend, we needle the point in the back of the neck, dazhu {BL-11}. If the leg feels as if it were about to break up, we needle the point in the bone hollow in the middle of Yang Ming {sanli of the stomach}, and the rong points of Tai Yang, tonggu {BL-66} and of Shao Yin, rangu {KI-2}. If sore pain with weakness involving the tibia occurs, along with the inability to stand up for very long, the "link" of Shao Yang, guangming {GB-37} should be treated. It is located five osteo units above the lateral ankle.[110]

The joint cavities are subsequently localized. "The pushbolt, jian, is located beneath the condyles and above the pubis: biguan {ST-31}."[111] This point is located between the muscles *vastus internus* and *vastus externus* at the apex of the scarpa triangle and means "the gate of the hip." The symptomology described in the *Da Cheng* is, "Muscular stiffness of the lower limb that cannot bend; spasms of the thigh that prevent flexion; cold and insensitive knee; sensation of paralysis of the legs; insensitivity of the foot; inability to stand up."[112] This is the semiology of knee disorders treated by needling the "pushbolt," biguan. This first of nine etiologies broadly covers all coxalgia.

The "mechanism," ji, encircles the coxal bones — huantiao (GB-30). This is the point to needle in the second etiology, pain in the knee sitting down. This is not a muscular disorder, but a deep lesion, which is Yin by nature and causes the patient to suffer, even while at rest. The *Da Cheng* gives this description:

> Rheumatism in the knee that is immobilized: the patient can move neither leg nor foot. Edema of the lower limb from humidity.[113]

This etiology covers the painful knee found in coxitis; it is only logical to needle the point on the hip.

The "skeletal barrier," haiguan, is the point yanglingquan (GB-34).[114] This point is needled when the bone feels as if it were about to melt when the patient is standing up. This third etiology corresponds to the acute gonalgia that tends to strike Shao Yang types and describes very well an acute and primary arthropathy. It may correspond also to a metabolic disorder such as gout or osteochondritis. It fits logically into the Wood constitution. For the point yanglingquan, the *Da Cheng* iterates: "Pain in the knee that may not be bent, knee of the heron {rheumatism in the knee}.[115]

The fourth etiology corresponds to sciatic pain, "Pain in the knee that gains the big toe." Weizhong (BL-59) is needled.

The fifth etiology is related to gonarthrosis. "If sitting down causes the patient to feel as if something were hidden inside. . . " we needle the gate. This is the "mobile part over the popliteal crease."[116] This point seems to correspond to fuxi (BL-52), which means just that: floating point. Its semiology includes muscular spasms in the calf, blockage of the hip joint and immobility.[117]

The sixth etiology, the "inability to bend and to extend," is a good description of arthrosis. It signals a bone disorder. It is only logical that the treatment calls for needling dazhu (BL-11), a point with special action on the bones.

The seventh and eighth etiologies correspond to muscular pain in the leg consecutive to an arterial deficit of the lower extremities (arteriopathy). "If the leg feels as if it were about to break," it is the equivalent of our Western description of stabbing pain. Zusanli (ST-36) is the point to needle (see Yang Ming). Another way to conduct the energy is to needle the cold point of zu tai yang, tonggu (BL-66), as the meridian is in excess, and also the heat point rangu (KI-2), as zu shao yin is deficient. We have already talked about guangming (GB-37), the luo point of zu shao yang, in relation to the excess of the luo, whose symptomology is explicit in the *Ling Shu:* "Lower extremity and foot are frozen."[118]

This discussion shows once again how important it is to study the Chinese texts in detail and how precise were the observations of the ancient Chinese in their effort to understand the mechanisms at work within the human body.

In cases of acute pain in the knee, we will retain the point GB-34.

Coxalgia and Coxitis

Shao Yang passes through the hip, huantiao (GB-30) and at the knee, yanglingquan (GB-34). In general, coxitis occurs late in the second half of a patient's life, when the shen, the qi of Fire of the metabolism, begins to diminish (see Tai Yang and Shao Yin). This is the Diathesis I-Diathesis III transformation spoken of by Menetrier, that calls for treatment with manganese-cobalt.

Shao Yang weakens first in the triple burner (shou shao yang), corresponding to the viscera that have metabolic activity. This explains the presence of degenerative rheumatisms at this stage. The hip seems to be the first target for Shao Yang subjects, as well as for those subjects whose anatomical constitution or external traumas have contributed to the weakening of this joint.

In any case, zu shao yang is affected. Its passage through the knee enables us to explain the gonalgia of coxitis without having to look for other causes. The treatment is simple and effective, easing the pain often totally and, if not permanently, at least for a long time, particularly when the problem is taken care of in the early stages.[119] We may follow the technique given in the *Su Wen:*

> If the perverse energy {humidity or cold} is lodged in the collateral channel of the zu shao yang {gallbladder meridian}, there may be pain in the articulation of the hip; we must then needle right in the middle of the articulation, the point huantiao {GB-30} with a long no. 7 needle, and leave it in place for a long time, according to the moon.[120]

We may add to this treatment yanglingquan (GB-34) whose semiology is "bi of the Yin in the hip and the knee."[121] This treatment may be augmented with moxibustion and trace elements, which prolong the results.

Often we may want to needle xiaxi (GB-43), the tonification point, and the point zulinqi (GB-41), the master point of dai mai which is also the shu point that combats humidity (Wood triumphs over Earth).

The main points indicated for coxarthritis are: zulinqi (GB-41), huantiao (GB-30), yanglingquan (GB-34), and xiaxi (GB-43).[122] Along with the basic

153

treatment, we should associate manganese-cobalt, fluoride, potassium, phosphorus, magnesium, etc.[123] The two forms of treatment in combination are most effective, even in advanced cases.

Osteoporosis and Bone Pain

Although we are not yet in a position to establish a precise correlation between Western physiology of the bile (vitamin D, liposoluble) and the semiology of the *Ling Shu,* which states that the gallbladder is involved in all problems relating to the bones, we must nonetheless admit that elderly Shao Yang types do suffer from bone mineralization problems, with the associated pain commonly known as rheumatism. This is especially the case when the gallbladder itself is diseased. We notice that young women who undergo cholecystectomy seem to display bone degeneration earlier than normal; degeneration that is remarkable in its intensity as well as in its precocity. They show also spinal column disorders, especially cervical (fengchi, GB-20) and lumbar (dai mai), and the pain and discomfort are as considerable as the disorder is difficult to treat (see Shao Yin for treatment). The same may be said for women who undergo hysterectomies (see Jue Yin).

Urinary Pathology

Kidney Stones

Renal lithiasis is a problem in from 10 to 30 percent of all cases of gout. When we are confronted with a patient who has gout, we must always look for kidney stones and vice versa.

Shao Yang subjects have a constitutionally weak triple burner function (see Gout, above). Remember Qi Bo, who said, "The triple burner serves to irrigate. . ."[124] This passage is translated by Chamfrault in the following way: "The triple burner is like a dam gate that is used to maintain the level."[125] In Chapter 2 of the *Ling Shu* we may read:

> Shao Yang is in relation to the kidneys and the lungs. It depends on both organs. The triple burner is related to the bladder, it is a solitary bowel.[126]

Solitary means that it is not coupled with another organ according to the biao-li relationship, as are all the other bowels. We may conclude that the triple burner-bladder relationship is one that is almost as privileged as the other biao-li relationships. Qi Bo calls Shao Yang the "axis" that controls the flow.[127]

All these links between the triple burner and the urinary tract predispose the Shao Yang individual in such a way that he is vulnerable to oliguria, to cystitis, to renal lithiasis and especially to urolithiasis.[128] With age, these disorders tend to get worse.

In the chapter of the *Ling Shu* that deals with exudates and edemas, Qi Bo describes the deficiency of the triple burner by saying that the skin is slack and swollen.[129] This is often the case among patients over fifty who have serious circulatory problems in the legs, problems that concern the veins more than the arteries, sometimes with monstrous malleolar edemas.

The deficiency of Tai Yang complicates the problem even more; not only zu tai yang, which represents the bladder and is coupled directly with the triple burner in urinary elimination, but also shou tai yang, the small intestine meridian, which is also concerned with regulating the body fluids (see Tai Yang). Let us quote once again Zhang Zhi Cong:

> The kidneys are the gateways to the stomach. Indeed, the stomach communicates with the kidneys through the intermediary of the triple burner, which brings the nutritive fluid to the intestines, and then from the intestines to the kidney through its internal canal.[130]

This explains, on the one hand, the symptomology given by Qi Bo for disturbance of body fluids caused by the small intestine, ". . . swelling in the loins that extends to the region of the kidneys."[131] This symptomology reminds us of a renal colic. On the other hand, we may understand the crucial role played by the small intestine, by its energy and by the points of its meridian in a renal colic attack and in its treatment.

What Western medicine calls reflex paralytic ileus may be translated into Chinese as the origin of the imbalance that causes oliguria and the acute attack of renal colic.[132] In more severe cases, there is anuria. This is explained by Qi Bo in the chapter entitled, "Meridian Imbalance Due to Perverse Energy":

> When the triple burner is affected, the belly is swollen, but the groin is swollen even more: anuria. If the water overflows, edemas form, and we will see the symptoms in the skin over the collateral channels of Tai Yang and Shao Yang. In this case we must needle weiyang (BL-53).[133]

This point, weiyang, is the special action he point of the triple burner. Anatomically it is located on the bladder meridian, close to the special action he point of the bladder, weizhong (BL-54), which shows, once again, the close ties between these two viscera.

In the special chapter, "Exudates and Edemas," all fluid overflow problems are treated by needling zusanli (ST-36) — the stomach being the organ that synthesizes fluids and passes them to the inferior burner — as well as the three mu points of the triple burner and the mu point of the small intestine:

> In cases of swelling we need only needle zusanli (ST-36), and, in recent cases, a single session is sufficient. In chronic cases, we need only three sessions if we manage to touch the energy. If we get no results, which is rare, we must needle the energy points, that is, those located over and under the navel: shangwan {CV-13}, zhongwan {CV-12}, xiawan {CV-10}, guanyuan {CV-4}. If we manage to draw the energy, the patient will surely be cured.[134]

To sum up this discussion, minor fluid disorders that affect Shao Yang types can lead, sooner or later, to gout or urolithiasis. With age, the triple burner function tends to become even more deficient, especially if the patient has a tendency to overeat.

The accompanying circulation difficulties, principally affecting the veins rather than the arteries and generally affecting the legs, aggravate the renal edema of these lithiasis patients. In Chapter 23 of the *Su Wen,* devoted to the symptoms displayed by patients with diseased viscera, we read, "The sign of imbalance in the inferior burner is edema."[135] We may add the comment by Ma Shi, quoted by Nguyen Van Nghi, "If the energy of the lower burner loses its function, the water will overflow and will cause edema."[136] To treat this condition, we will needle BL-39, ST-36, CV-13, CV-12, CV-10 and CV-4, as well as the symptomatic points, in case of attack, and the etiological points (see Lithiasis, Shao Yin chapter, and Urinary Infections, Jue Yin chapter). This discussion of physiology will help us to understand the correlations between Diatheses I and III described by Menetrier. Among the symptoms associated with Diathesis I are "Lithiasis, especially biliary lithiasis, and primary urinary disorders linked to acidity."[137] Part of the pathology associated with Diathesis I is biliary and renal lithiasis. Relative oliguria figures among the symptoms of Diathesis III.[138] This supports our statement that urinary lithiasis generally appears later in life and is associated with a metabolic disturbance.

Without going into enzymology, manganese acts upon insufficient elimination (manganese-cobalt).

The physiological logic specific to acupuncture enables us to split Diathesis I into two different groups: the arthritic subjects in one group and the allergic subjects in the other. The coleric arthritic subjects are Shao Yang, whereas the nervous allergic subjects are Jue Yin and are altogether different.

Picard describes his urolithiasis patients as being "optimistic, aggressive, oriented towards leadership."[139] Serane and Pean describe them as "enterprising, sociable, taking pleasure in getting together with friends for dinner. The lithiasis of these patients seems determined by their worries, especially economic worries."[140] For Picard, this is the moment of passage between Diatheses I and III. From our point of view, this is the moment of the failure of the triple burner excretory bowel, already constitutionally weak among Shao Yang subjects, even if young and still Wood.[141] Worries are harmful to the heart and to its "qi of all the metabolisms," the shen, thus causing the failure of the Ministerial Fire, the triple burner.[142]

We are grateful to Menetrier for defining the parameters of increases in urea and urate levels according to blood-urea clearance texts, which vary proportionally with Ambard's formula. Such urinary syndromes presented by elderly patients, along with oliguria, electrolytic imbalances and even variations in the phospho-calcium equilibrium, are a part of the aging commonly experienced by these patients as they pass from Diathesis I to Diathesis III.

These syndromes are forestalled, diminished and stabilized with a prescription of manganese-cobalt if treatment is early, or with an alternation of manganese and manganese-cobalt when there are signs of vesical calculus.

This treatment can be associated with acupuncture and we will choose to needle the beishu and mu points of Shao Yang and Tai Yang. Another option is to needle the following Shao Yang and Shao Yin points: sanshu (BL-19) and riyue (GB-24), sanjiaoshu (BL-22) and shangwan (CV-13), zhongwan (CV-12), xiawan

(CV-10) or shenshu (BL-23) and jingmen (GB-25), yinjiao (CV-7), xiaochangshu (BL-27), xinshu (BL-15) and guanyuan (CV-4). It is also possible to alternate the use of these points with moxibustion on the following points: BL-19 and GB-24, BL-22 and CV-13, CV-12, CV-10, CV-5, CV-7, BL-23 and GB-25, BL-27 and CV-4, BL-15.

Genital Pathology

Dysmenorrhea, fibroma and Shao Yang link the dai mai, the gallbladder and the uterus. This pathology is developed in Jue Yin.

Endocrine Pathology

The endocrine pathology of Shao Yang focuses on three targets: the thyroid, the parathyroid and the ovary. We will study the first of these three; the other two are to be found in the Jue Yin chapter.

Hyperthyroidism

Graves's disease, or exophthalmic goiter, is contracted particularly by women, subsequent to emotional shock. It is often linked to genital episodes (puberty, pregnancy, menopause). The emotional factor in these episodes affects the liver and the gallbladder (see Jue Yin).

None of the Western texts have described the Chinese physiopathology of hyperthyroidism, but the modern Shanghai authors have interpreted this disease as being "due to melancholy[143] of the sentiments, because of which the energy of the liver and the spleen lose their circulation."[144]

In fact, the element Wood as a whole is involved in this illness, and it is perhaps in this sense that we may understand what the *Su Wen* has to say: "Coagulation in Jue Yin and Shao Yang will cause soreness in the larynx."[145] In any case, we find that Shao Yang and Jue Yin patients are those who suffer most often from hyperthyroidism, a condition clearly betrayed by its symptoms. The swelling of the eyeball, exophthalmia, shows the excess of Yang in the eye, which is the sensory organ of the element Wood.

Loss of weight, although the patient maintains a good appetite,[146] calls to mind the gallbladder semiology referred to in the tenth chapter of the *Ling Shu:* "When the disorder is serious, the body is dry."[147]

We find rapid tachycardia in these cases, from 110-120 beats per minute to even higher rates in emotional situations. The patient feels palpitations and we witness the whole range of cardiac erethism — which we discuss in the sections concerning cardiovascular pathology among Shao Yang and Jue Yin (pericardium) patients.[148]

157

The myasthenia that is responsible for the patient's fatigue is attested to by the "symptom of the stool" — a difficulty in rising from a low stool. They cannot get up if we make them squat. This is a Shao Yang trait. The *Da Cheng,* published centuries before Froment, described the symptom of the stool, and has this to say of the semiology of xuanzhong (GB-39): "The patient is unable to rise from a sitting position."[149] This myasthenia is in contrast with the muscular excitability, the spasms and the contractions from which the patient suffers and which are visible in the shortening of the Achilles tendon reflex. This may even lead to amyotrophia (see Shao Yang neurology).

Motorial diarrhea is evidence of the fact that the gallbladder "insults" the large intestine and controls the spleen. This reminds us of the etiology of right-sided colonopathy (see Digestive Pathology). This affliction of the spleen results in a high rate of glycemia and causes a secondary excess of zu yang ming (stomach meridian), aggravating the vascular erethism of the goiter blowing through renying (ST-9),[150] and which is observed as a thrill.

The emotional symptoms witnessed among these hyperthyroid patients, irritability, aggressiveness, agitation, anxiety and excitation, give them an identifiable "personality" that is a mixture of Shao Yang and Jue Yin traits. We may present two caricatures of female patients who dominate this pathology. The first is somewhat like a drill sergeant, authoritarian, with a low voice. She is Shao Yang. The second is more like a mouse: timid, trembling, easily frightened, not at all outgoing; she is the model of the hyperthyroid Jue Yin patient. Among biological disorders, apart from all physiological consideration, we find hypocholesterolemia.

Several protocols of treatment are suggested. The modern Shanghai authors balance Jue Yin and the spleen (Tai Yin) by needling jianchi (PC-5), sanyinjiao (SP-6), as well as neiguan (PC-6) "for tachycardia," and taichong (LV-3) "when the patient is impatient and the face red with fire."[151] It is also suggested to needle renying (ST-9), the carotid point, and jiaosun (TB-20), for exophthalmia.[152] Soulie de Morant points out that Abrams determined a direct relationship between the thyroid and the sixth and seventh cervical vertebrae.

Zu Lien, in *La nouvelle science de l'acupuncture et des moxas,* indicates the regional points: tianzhu (BL-10), fengchi (GB-20),[153] dazhu (BL-11),[154] dazhui (GV-14), shenzhu (GV-12). For goiter, he indicates the local points: renying (ST-9), as well as tiantu (CV-22), lianquan (CV-23), shuitu (ST-10). For exophthalmia, the points tongziliao (GB-1) and sibai (ST-2). As general points, he suggests daimai (GB-26), zhongzhu (KI-15) and wailing (ST-26).[155]

These last two points are located on the same horizontal line as yinjiao (CV-7) and all four are indicated for gynecological disorders. Yinjiao (CV-7), a mu point of the triple burner, may be translated as "the crossing of the Yin," and the associated semiology is:

> Irregular menstrual periods, or of abnormally long duration, hemorrhage, leukorrhea during the period, fainting after giving birth, unceasing flow of black blood after giving birth, sterility, metritis, pruritis vulvae.[156]

158

The same goes for daimai (GB-26), whose name means "belt meridian" and which links zu shao yang to the miscellaneous channel dai mai. This point is "specific for gynecologic affections."[157] This all bears witness to the fact that Shao Yang, the gallbladder, dai mai, gynecology, cholesterol (and hormonal steroids)[158] and hyperthyroidism are all closely related. It is not surprising to discover that hyperthyroidism affects women more than men and specifically at crucial moments in their genital lives.

We will note in passing that Zu Lien chose to needle dazhu (BL-11), the he point of the bones, against the risk of bone complications such as osteoporosis that we sometimes find associated with hyperthyroidism.

The number of points mentioned for cases of hyperthyroidism is impressive: PC-5 and PC-6; GB-1, GB-20, GB-26 and GB-39; BL-10, GB-11; TB-20; SP-6; LV-3; ST-2, ST-9, ST-10 and ST-26; KI-15; GV-12 and GV-14; and CV-22.

Menetrier declares that the action of manganese, in cases of hyperthyroidism, is often "clear and long lasting. Iodine (as a trace element) is a good substitute for opotherapy in most cases."[159] This shows the preponderance of Diathesis I (Wood) in this pathology. He adds that copper seems to be an excellent regulator of dysthyroidism. Since he relates copper to the spleen (see Tai Yin), our quote from the modern Shanghai authors at the beginning of this discussion takes on importance. It is no doubt the diencephalohypophyseal regulatory aspect of this organ that brings Menetrier and the Shanghai authors together.

Except for thyroid adenoma, of course, trace element therapy is most effective against this disorder. Associated with acupuncture, this treatment is worth all the tranquilizers and betablockers put together.

Neurological Pathology

Tics, Muscular Spasms and Contractions, Blepharospasms, Facial Hemispasms

We read in the first chapters of the *Su Wen* that the liver, the organ linked to the element Wood, corresponds to the muscles and the nerves. This correspondence may be explained by the liver's role in glycogenesis and in the synthesis of phospholipids.

"How can the five viscera cause atrophic paralysis?" asks Huang Di of Qi Bo in the chapter devoted to paralysis. The wise doctor answers, concerning the liver:

> The liver governs the muscles and the fasciae. When the liver is hot,
> a trickle of bile makes the mouth bitter, the muscles and the fasciae
> are dry, and in the tight muscles an atrophied jin wei develops.[160]

This symptomology corresponds to jin wei amyotrophy of Wood origin. It is specifically the case with conditions such as hyperthyroid amyotrophies.

159

In Chapter 49 of the *Su Wen,* which is devoted to explanations of the channels, we find that along with pains in the heart and thorax and with difficulty turning over, which we have already seen related to Shao Yang, we also find:

> In more severe cases, spasms in the ninth month, the subjects are weakened, the incubative period is over, the qi leaves the Yang for the Yin; if there is an abundance of Yang in the lower part of the body, there are spasms in the legs.[161]

This remark, with the comment on the jin wei, allows us to say that the excess of Shao Yang leads to a neuromuscular hyperexcitability, likely to cause cramps and contractures in the lower limbs, as well as all along the pathway of the meridian.[162] This is also the case of facial tics or of trismus, which may cause various forms of facial neuralgia (see Pathology in Stomatology).

Among points indicated for the treatment of facial tics, which Zu Lien compares to chorea and to abnormal movements,[163] we find fengchi (GB-20) and wangu (GB-12). Facial hemispasm is one of the more dramatic abnormal facial movements. It can begin progressively, first a tic and then a spasm of the orbicular region, and gain one whole side of the face in a spasmodic contracture that is painful. This pathology is practically specific to Shao Yang patients.

Treatment calls necessarily for needling yangfu (GB-38) and tianjing (TB-10) to disperse Shao Yang, as well as fengchi (GB-20), jiaosun (TB-20) and other local points, after needling the key points zulinqi (GB-41) and waiguan (TB-5) on the opposite side. Craniopuncture is of considerable value in these cases.

Myoclonia

The main symptom is epilepsy, which is possible among Shao Yang subjects. The points to be considered are GB-40, GB-20, GB-12, GB-38, TB-10, GB-20 (again), GB-41, and TB-5.

Epilepsy

The muscular contractures may be of central nervous system origin and generalized, corresponding to the clinical picture of epilepsy. In this case, the excess of Shao Yang penetrates into the brain by way of the complex and highly developed meridian network in both cerebral hemispheres.

The physiopathology of epilepsy is multiple in Chinese theory (see Tai Yang). We may say here that the two master points involved in epilepsy are found on Shao Yang and specifically on shou shao yang (triple burner meridian), in relation with the temporal lobe. These are huizong (TB-7) "meeting of ancestors"[164] and tianjing (TB-10) "celestial well," which are linked with "five sorts of epilepsy."[165] There are no others.

Among the local points on the skull and neck, six points of zu shao yang (gallbladder) are indicated for epilepsy. These include: shangguan (GB-3), hanyan (GB-4), benshen (GB-13), linqi (GB-15), fengchi (GB-20) and jianjing (GB-21). Also useful are three distal points on the lower segment of the meridian: huantiao (GB-30), guangming (GB-37), and xuanzhong (GB-39).

160

Qi Bo gives the following therapeutic advice:

> In cases of epilepsy, we must disperse the lung meridian five times, the bladder meridian five times, the heart meridian once and three times the point guangming (GB-37), situated five osteo units over the malleolus.[166]

The main points to be retained in treating Shao Yang epilepsies are: TB-7 and TB-10, GB-3, GB-4, GB-13, GB-15, GB-20, GB-21, GB-30, GB-37 and GB-39.

As for trace element therapy, Menetrier states that cramps and spasms call for "testing uresis, cholesterol and all the other tests of excretory disorders." This shows his preoccupation with the passage from Diathesis I to Diathesis III (Fire). Manganese-cobalt (Fire-triple burner) and sulfur (Wood) alleviate these symptoms.

As far as epilepsy is concerned, manganese-cobalt and cobalt have a positive action. Manganese-cobalt here is synonymous for us with Shao Yang (triple burner), Tai Yang (small intestine) and with Shao Yin (heart), etc. Copper-gold-silver is often useful as well. Menetrier believes it is important to look for a manganese-copper diathesis (Metal), which is often subjacent and which implies the lungs and corresponds to what Qi Bo had to say. The Chinese etiological diagnosis is complex and shows once again the importance of determining the temperament of a patient before choosing the points to treat.

Sciatic Nerve

In the general semiology of the gallbladder meridian, it is written, "Pain all along the pathway of the meridian; the fourth and fifth toes are paralyzed."[167] It is important to remember that sciaticas often result from an imbalance in the energy of this meridian. In these cases, the patient is disturbed by the wind. Menetrier advises the prescription of manganese to treat this syndrome. (See Treatment of Sciatica, Tai Yang.)

Migraines and Headaches

The etiologies in acupuncture are multiple and are summarized in the Tai Yang chapter. It is important to note that the real migraines, opthalmic migraines and fronto-orbital headaches that involve the temporal region, indicate an imbalance of the element Wood and of the Shao Yang meridians (gallbladder as well as triple burner) and Jue Yin (liver). This is clearly set forth in the *Ling Shu:*

> In cases of migraines with pain in the temporal arteries, with crying and moaning, we needle and bleed the artery in excess, then we balance the energy in zu jue yin (liver).

> In migraines with atrocious pain, the arteries in front of and behind the ears[168] are very tight. We must disperse and bleed them, then we needle the points of zu shao yang (gallbladder).[169]

Thus Shao Yang and Jue Yin are involved, most often together, and both liver and gallbladder are imbalanced.

161

The problem is more complicated than it may appear, and involves the liver-gallbladder alternative, as well as their relative excess or deficiency compared to the blood[170] in their respective meridians.

> When Shao Yang is in excess, this indicates excess of energy and lack of blood. This will cause troubles in the muscles[171] and swelling in the sides.[172] If Shao Yang is deficient, there will be trouble in the liver.[173] If there is excess of energy with heat, there will be congestion of blood and symptoms of wind.[174] If there is excess of blood and lack of energy, the patient will have pain in the eyes and contractures.[175]

In the corresponding Jue Yin pathology, we find, "If there is a lack of energy and excess of blood, there will follow pains in the groin from accumulation of qi {shan qi}."

Husson's translation of this passage is more subtle: "If the meridian Jue Yin is too fluid: wind of Shan of the fox." This corresponds to pollakiuria (see corresponding discussion in the chapter on Jue Yin). Husson continues, "If there is a lack of fluidity: accumulation of qi in the groin." In other words, the liver and the gallbladder are related through Jue Yin and Shao Yang, with a coagulation of blood, or in other terms, a deregulation of the factors of coagulation related to genital activity and the hormonal steroids.

The pathology of shan qi corresponds to all the causes of pelvic congestion (see Jue Yin) and among women with dysmenorrheas whose etiology is "dark liver," with clotted blood during menstruation.[176]

This "lack of fluidity of Jue Yin and Shao Yang" causes pelvic congestion in Jue Yin and muscular twinges and episodic ocular pain in Shao Yang. This is why we consider opthalmic migraines and Arnold's occipital neuralgia, with or without dysmenorrhea, as being specifically Shao Yang disorders. These migraines are Yang, which means they are brutal and throbbing, coming on suddenly with photophobia and often on the same side. Patients suffering from this sort of migraine are generally Shao Yang (coleric).

Jue Yin migraines are less specific; they go from side to side, or are bilateral fronto-orbital headaches, attacking the forehead and likely to radiate to the occiput. They are deeper, less brutal and come on more progressively. The crying and moaning described in the *Ling Shu* are signs of a nervous and dystonic temperament and these patients may go so far as to be hysterical. We often find accompanying pelvic congestion, dysmenorrhea (with or without nausea) and bilious vomiting.

These headaches follow many women's periods, coming on in the second half around the moment of ovulation and in the days that precede menstruation. They are part of the so-called allergic symptoms of dysmenorrhea, sometimes associated with cutaneous eruptions of Quincke's edema, with nausea and with vomiting (see Jue Yin). In other patients, the rhythm is associated with other factors that bring on the migraines (a car trip, emotional upsets, etc.). One factor, found in Shao Yang patients more than Jue Yin patients, is the wind, which brings on or aggravates the pain:

If the patient fears the wind, we must needle the points located around the eyebrows.[177]

These points are sizhukong (TB-23), tongziliao (GB-1) and taiyang (M-HN-9).

In treating migraines, as well as fronto-orbital headaches, we will needle the points of Shao Yang and Jue Yin indiscriminately, as the two meridians are involved. Other than the local points we have just indicated, we will needle fengchi (GB-20), yanglingquan (GB-34), zuqiaoyin (GB-44), dadun (LV-1), taichong (LV-3) and ququan (LV-8).

Beyond the points listed above, we will needle the ting points, dadun and zuqiaoyin, on the opposite side if the migraine is unilateral; fengchi (GB-20), as it hides the Yang (see high blood pressure); yanglingquan (GB-34), as it is the special action he point on the gallbladder; taichong (LV-3) as a point that disperses the liver, and that is related to its cephalic development;[178] and ququan (LV-8), the he point corresponding to the element Water-cold. Needling this last point is like adding water to the blood, increasing its fluidity. This is indispensable.[179]

In cases of pelvic congestion, we are to needle several more specific points: daimai (GB-26), wushu (GB-27), weidao (GB-28) (see Jue Yin).[180]

We should no longer allow so many women to suffer, contenting ourselves with the diagnostic of dysmenorrhea or migraine of psychosomatic origin, since the results of acupuncture treatment in these cases are consistent, excellent, definitive and long lasting.

To recapitulate the points: GB-1, GB-14, GB-20, GB-26, GB-27, GB-28, GB-34 and GB-44; TB-23, taiyang (M-HN-9), LV-1, LV-3 and LV-8.

Menetrier classifies these "traditionally hepatic" migraines among the symptoms of Diathesis I. The prescription of manganese and manganese-sulfur is automatic.

Cerebrovascular Accidents

Related to a jue, in Shao Yang, cerebrovascular accidents are discussed in detail in the chapter on Yang Ming.

Neuromuscular Deficits

We must remember that Wood corresponds to the muscles. On the zu shao yang meridian, yanglingquan (GB-34), the special action he point of the gallbladder, is at once the special he point of the muscles. This is why we read, in Soulie de Morant's treatise, among the indications for this point:

> Weakness of the muscles, the patient cannot rise from a sitting position,[181] muscular pains, cramps, contractures, chorea.[182]

Aside from these indications, in neuromuscular pathology we may read, "Slack muscles, flaccid hemiplegia," corresponding to the vascular etiology of muscular deficit.[183]

For yanglingquan, Soulie de Morant indicates "atrophy, myelitis, poliomyelitis (makes muscles grow)," which corresponds this time to the neurological etiology of muscular deficit. This last indication is related to multiple sclerosis, whose physiopathology is studied in Jue Yin.

Psychiatric Pathology

Reactional Neurosis and Nervous Anxiety

The psychiatric pathology of Shao Yang can be divided into two different syndromes, one being due to excess of Shao Yang, the other to deficiency of the meridian.

An excess of Shao Yang, particularly of zu shao yang, the gallbladder meridian, accompanied by an excess of hun,[184] intensifies the feverish behavior of these coleric subjects as well as their overexcitation. They just can't stay still for a minute, as if they had springs under their feet. Their overactivity is accompanied by an intense and multiple psychological preoccupation. They have so much to do that there is not enough time. This is accentuated by thoracic oppression and functional cardiac symptoms and causes anxiety.

Shao Yang types, who are enterprising, feverish ("great gallbladder," as the Chinese say of those who are audacious),[185] are prime victims of reactional anxiety, which may take on the proportions of truly neurotic behavior. The excess is at its height when their complexion turns "ash white, the eyes are circled with black, they have a bitter taste in the mouth in the morning, their mouths are dry."[186] There are fits of anger that are often brutal and violent.

Concerning the "role of the mind," Qi Bo says, in Chapter 8 of the *Ling Shu,* "Anger may cause death."[187] The psychiatric symptomology of guangming (GB-37) is, "Becomes suddenly crazy."[188] This brutal explosion of anger, according to the Chinese translations of Soulie de Morant, may possibly cause a fatal cerebral accident. "Indignation, rage, likely to cause apoplexy," is the semiology of xuanzhong (GB-39), which is a point to be needled in priority, along with zusanli (ST-36), among patients stricken with arteriopathy of the lower limbs and who are thus in danger of a stroke (see Yang Ming). A transitory deficiency of energy inevitably follows these excess anger attacks,[189] and Shao Yang is deficient. However, the trouble is far from over. This inhibition of activity (hun) is often accompanied by an intolerable intensification of anxiety; the patient is paralyzed, incapable of doing anything.

It is worth noting the direct link made by the Chinese between the physiological role of the gallbladder and its psychological manifestations. Physiologically, the gallbladder acts as a judge and "makes the decisions."[190] Qi Bo states that "The eleven warehouses make the decisions of the gallbladder."[191] In Chapter 47, he goes on to describe the physiological properties of this bowel:

> The liver is the general who commands the interior. The decisions are made by the gallbladder and promulgated by the throat.[192] If a subject meditates for a long time without making a decision, the

gallbladder is deficient, the qi overflows and the mouth is bitter. This may be treated by needling the mu {collector} points and the shu points of the gallbladder.[193]

In other words, an excess of gallbladder means an excess of decision, and a deficiency of gallbladder means a deficiency of decision with inhibition. This inhibition is accompanied by a characteristic anxiety that is obsessional and conflictive:

A patient who acts as though someone were out after him, to try to catch him and put him in prison, is diseased in his gallbladder.[194]

Dreams, which have been studied by Chinese medicine since the most ancient times, are revealing. A whole chapter of the *Ling Shu* is devoted to dreams. "When the gallbladder is deficient, we dream of fighting, of lawsuits, of suicide."[195]

Gaston Berger and the Dutch school of psychology felt that the coleric and nervous temperament corresponded to hysteria and to what was called then by Dupre, "emotive psychoneurosis."[196] This is, more or less, the modern reactional neurosis, and coincides perfectly with Shao Yang.[197]

When these personality disorders are not too deep-rooted, acupuncture treatment is effective, especially against anxiety and reactional neurosis. The points to treat are: GB-20, GB-34, GB-37, GB-38, GB-39, LV-2, LV-3, LV-8, PC-6, CV-17 and GV-20.

Menetrier described Diathesis I allergic subjects as being nervous, irritable and likely to alternate periodically between aggressivity and depression.[198] This description matches Shao Yang subjects perfectly.

Primary anxiety may be treated with manganese. The evolution towards the dystonic diathesis (*i.e.*, the progression of menopause, andropause), necessitates a prescription of manganese-cobalt.[199] It is often useful to associate sulfur and iodine, as well as lithium, with this treatment.

Insomnia

Insomnia often accompanies the preceding behavior, but may also be an isolated problem.

The excess of fire of the liver and of the gallbladder that surges to the head is well known and has already been discussed.[200] However, there is also insomnia caused by deficiency of Shao Yang, with worry and apprehension. This is the semiology of xiaxi (GB-43) tonification point, indicated along with an "incapacity to make decisions" that signals the inhibition characteristic of deficiency of zu shao yang.

Treatment of the Wood insomnia, caused by excess or deficiency, follows the same course as that of anxiety; the two points that are crucial are fengchi (GB-20) and yintang (M-HN-3).

165

Menetrier includes the difficulty in getting to sleep among the allergic and dystonic diatheses.[201] It is characteristic of the Wood behavior as we defined it in the beginning of the chapter. Manganese, manganese-cobalt, sulfur, iodine and even aluminum, are the trace elements indicated as effective by Menetrier.

Dermatological Pathology

Sweating and pruritis dominate the dermatological pathology among Shao Yang subjects.

Sweating

In general, it is true that Shao Yang patients perspire profusely. Some, on the other hand, do not perspire at all. These imbalances are related to the physiology of the triple burner, which, as we have seen, depends on two organs: the kidneys in the lower burner and the lungs in the upper burner.[202] If the renal emunctory functions poorly, it can affect the lungs. Perspiration is an effort to compensate for this situation and we must remember that the skin is linked with the lungs.

In the discussion of the symptomology of the primary channels in the *Ling Shu,* we find, for shou shao yang and for zu shao yang, there is "abundant perspiration."[203] Thus not only the triple burner, but also the gallbladder is involved in the elimination of the three "burners" (san jiao). The whole of Shao Yang is related to this function.[204] Let us not forget that "the meridian zu shao yang brings in new water from the outside, and brings it to the gallbladder in the form of bile."[205] If we follow the Chinese reasoning, excess of Shao Yang is the equivalent of an excess of Fire (fire of wood, fire of the triple burner) that evaporates the body fluids.

The renal and biliary emunctory functions are then disturbed, and this is seen as oliguria and a risk of biliary and renal lithiasis (see Lithiasis). The organism, in an effort to defend itself, tries to eliminate through perspiration. It's as if the upper burner were coming to the rescue of the lower burner.

The miscellaneous channel, dai mai, which shunts into Shao Yang, links the kidneys and the gallbladder. Treatment consists of opening dai mai by needling zulinqi (GB-41). The symptomology of this point is found in the *Da Cheng:* "Abundant perspiration."[206]

We must next treat the general imbalance and disperse Shao Yang by needling the dispersal points tianjing (TB-10) and yangfu (GB-38). The *Da Cheng* says of tianjing, "Abundant perspiration," and of yangfu, "Abundant perspiration that flows from the kidneys as if one were sitting in water."[207] This treatment aims not only to dry up the hypersudation, but above all, to correct the emunctory function of Shao Yang to avoid the precipitation of gallstones and bladder stones.

We sometimes, but rarely, find the opposite: absence of perspiration. The upper burner fails to perform correctly and fails to inhibit growth or formation of stones. A single point is indicated here, qiaoyin (GB-11) "cavity of yin". This is an important point, according to Chamfrault, as it is the point of the "essence of the energy of the gallbladder meridian." It is also considered to be the intersection of the bladder and triple burner meridians.[208] This explains the name "cavity of yin." As we have indicated in the beginning of the chapter, the gallbladder is an irregular bowel, stemming from the Earth. The nature of its essence, bile, is thus Yin.

It is probable that the Chinese attribute to the bile and to the gallbladder a major role in the interior equilibrium of body fluids, coupled with the triple burner.

Pruritis

Pruritis is common in cases of jaundice caused by extrahepatic retention. It is caused by the increase in conjugate bilirubin and in bile salts in the blood. The jaundice in these conditions is green, the color of Wood (liver and gallbladder),[209] or dark. Among the etiologies that will interest us[210] are choledocholithiasis,[211] and, of course, the "non-surgical" jaundices resulting from hepatic excretory disorders including hepatitis, cholestasis due to medicines such as chlorpromazine, methyltestosterone, etc., benign and chronic intrahepatic cholostasis (rare). For the most part, these etiologies respond well to acupuncture treatment.[212]

Three specific etiologies attract our attention. The first is cholostasis from overmedication, an overprescription of methyltestosterone. An excess of this sexual hormone has a noxious effect on the catabolic function of the hepatocyte. The second etiology is cholostatic jaundice observed in contraceptive treatment with synthetic estroprogestational hormones, which attracts our attention to the repercussions on the biliary function of "the pill." The third is the cholestatic jaundice observed among pregnant women during the third month which is benign and moderate.

These three etiologies illustrate once again the link between the gonads, the pelvis, the adrenal gland and the gallbladder, by way of the belt meridian, dai mai. Here the jing function of the gallbladder, a "curious" bowel, is of great importance.

In Western medicine, there is no specific treatment for pruritis, outside of cholestyramine, which must be administered with care. In acupuncture, the treatment of pruritis must be etiological to be effective. However, we may always needle zulinqi (GB-41), the dai mai master point, as well as fengshi (GB-31), which is the specific point for pruritis and whose semiology is "itching all over the body."[213] This point is indicated in all three etiologies presented here and also in pruritis and urticaria of external origin, *i.e.*, allergies. Fengshi means "city of wind" and is related to the perverse wind that is likely to bring on all the allergic manifestations that are signs of spring. It is indicated in the *Da Cheng* for "attack of feng."[214] It may be associated with etiological treatments whenever there is pruritis.

In Chapter 9 of the *Ling Shu,* we read, "In case of itching, we needle superficially, as itching is Yang by nature."[215]

Menetrier states that allergic patients are most apt to have urticaria. He also says that manganese and sulfur are effective against this affection, as they are fast-acting and long lasting. This shows us once again that there is a definite correlation between Diathesis I and the element Wood.

167

Onychopathy

Here, let us quote Qi Bo in the chapter of the *Ling Shu* devoted to "the organs":

> The liver, which is linked to the gallbladder, is represented on the outside by the muscles. But the liver is represented on the outside also by the fingernails. If they are greenish, this indicates that the liver is affected. If they are black and lined, this means that the gallbladder is blocked.[216]

Eye, Ear, Nose and Throat Pathology and Stomatology

Presbycusis and Deafness

According to the *Su Wen,* the ear is the essential organ belonging to the kidney. We are tempted to jump to the conclusion that hearing problems involve the kidney and, therefore, Shao Yin types. Although this is true to a certain extent, it is not always the case.

The ear receives much of its energy from Shao Yang, equally from shou shao yang and from zu shao yang. One pathway flows through the ear. It starts at fengchi (GB-20), passes through yifeng (TB-17), pierces the ear and ends in ting-gong (SI-19). This last point is essential in treating the ears, because of its link with Shao Yang. Energy imbalance in Shao Yang is thus likely to affect acoustic acuity.

We find reference to this in the *Yi Xue Ru Men,* where we also find an indication concerning laterality:

> A patient is deaf in the left ear when anger and unhappiness have troubled the fire of the gallbladder. He is deaf in the right ear when the fire of his desires and his license have troubled the fire of his conscience.[217]

Among the etiologies of Shao Yang deafness we may include that which is caused by cochleovestibular arteriosclerosis and is accompanied by dizziness and tinnitus, evolving quite rapidly.[218]

Shao Yang deafness is referred to in the most ancient of texts, the *Ling Shu,* in a discussion of the symptomology of the primary channel of shou shao yang:

> The disorders of shou shao yang, the triple burner, are deafness and a sore throat; in these troubles caused by energy imbalance, we must needle the points of this meridian.[219]

Another paragraph in the same work, in a chapter devoted to "various illnesses," makes the picture even clearer:

> In deafness without pain, we needle zu shao yang. If there is pain, we needle shou shao yang.[220]

In other words, deafness without pain corresponds to the internal etiology, cochleovestibular arteriosclerosis, and thus to the fire of anger and of the gallbladder. This is the risk run by coleric patients, who, in old age, often suffer from this type of presbycusis, with a series of tinnitus that bothers them a great deal.

Deafness with pain corresponds to the external etiology, whose origin is infectious: shingles, mumps,[221] and other viruses, as well as acute or chronic labyrinthitis and bacterial otitis complications.[222] We can also include here post-operatory labyrinthitis, a complication of otospongiosis surgery.

These acute Shao Yang disorders that cause deafness are also dealt with in the *Su Wen*. Qi Bo describes them along with other symptoms in "Energy Blockage Disorders," or jue:

> When Shao Yang is affected, auditive acuity is disturbed, the cheeks
> are swollen, there is fever with pain at the sides of the body.[223]

We believe that this semiology may refer both to mumps and to the various localizations of shingles: geniculate, intercostal, sciatic. It is not clear whether the text intends to describe the different symptoms of a single disease, or all the possibilities resulting from a single energy imbalance, "troubles of Shao Yang."

The contexts of the other references to the jue of Yang Ming, Jue Yin and Tai Yin tend to support both interpretations, making it difficult to establish direct correspondences between the symptoms presented in the text and the illnesses discussed.

In the chapter of the *Ling Shu* on "Energy Circulation Disturbances," we find:

> In the disturbance of energy, if the patient becomes deaf, we must
> needle the points located around the ear. If he complains of ringing
> in the ears, we needle over the artery, in front of the ear.[224] If there is
> pain in the ears, because of suppuration, we must not needle.[225] If
> there is only energy imbalance, we needle guanchong {TB-1}; then
> we needle the meridian zu shao yang in the foot.[226]

This text makes no reference to the distinction of deafness with or without pain, concerning zu shao yang or shou shao yang. We are led to believe that we must only know in which meridian the major imbalance occurs, to needle it first. The whole of Shao Yang is to be treated in cases of acute deafness. This enables us to understand the choice of points recommended by Zu Lien in his *General Treatise on Acupuncture,* including "poor hearing and deafness": ermen (TB-21), fengchi (GB-20), xiaxi (GB-43), yifeng (TB-17), tinghui (GB-2), tinggong (SI-19).

This treatment may be retained in cases of retrocochlear deafness due to meningoneuritis, shingles or mumps, and may be attempted when we desire to restore audition in toxic or even traumatic cases, if we catch the problem early enough.

169

In cases of sudden deafness of infectious or vascular origin (cochlear circulatory disorders), the ting points on the opposite side are indicated: guanchong (TB-1) and zuqiaoyin (GB-44), as we have seen above. This is nothing more than first aid treatment, which is, nonetheless, worthwhile associating with a specialist's treatment (perfusion of vasodilators, oxygen therapy, hyperbare, etc.), in an effort to restore audition.

In cases of deafness whose origin is central and vascular, we may needle the "window to the sky points." Tianyou (TB-16) is indicated in the *Ling Shu:* "Tianyou {TB-16} is to be needled in cases of sudden deafness or of loss of visual acuity."[227]

This rapid view of the etiologies of deafness allows us to show that Shao Yang is often involved. We will go into the other etiologies of deafness in the chapter devoted to Shao Yin.

Once again, we notice that the choice of points to needle in a given disorder varies with the different etiologies. The most common etiology of deafness among Shao Yang patients is presbycusis, secondary to arteriosclerosis, which occurs in old age. It is rather common.

The main Shao Yang points indicated to treat deafness are: GB-20, TB-17, TB-20, GB-43, GB-44, TB-1 and GB-2. To this we may also add SI-19.

Dental Arthritis and Occlusion, Facial Neuralgia

There is good reason to examine the relationships between the temporomaxillary articulation and the meridians Yang Ming and Shao Yang. In the *Ling Shu,* we read:

> Jiaosun {TB-20} is the jing point at which the energy of shou shao yang passes into zu shao yang. In disorders of the maxilla, we must needle the capillaries located between the nose and the ear.[228]

This means that the capillaries of this region are in the territory of Shao Yang.

From jiaosun (TB-20; tip of the ear), one branch of shou shao yang ascends to touwei (ST-8), descends to hanyan (GB-4) and to xiaguan (ST-7), makes a "U" on the cheek and the two maxillaries as far as quanliao (SI-18), before arriving at jingming (BL-1).

Zu shao yang begins at the external orbital edge, passes over the temporomaxillary articulation at tinghui (GB-2) and also at xiaguan (ST-7) by way of a distinct branch. Another distinct branch descends from tongziliao (GB-1), forms a "U" at the mandible, and climbs back up to jingming (BL-1). The energy flowing through these meridians and passing from one to another explains the role of Shao Yang in dental arthritis and dental occlusion.

The specific Shao Yang imbalance consists of a neuromuscular hyperexcitability (see Neurology, Shao Yang), with spasms and contractures, and more than accounts for these disorders. Shao Yang individuals are often people with square jaws who clench their teeth so much of the time that their masseter muscle is mobile and bulging. In this they distinguish themselves from hyposthenic individuals (Yang Ming-Metal), who tend towards ligamentary flaccidity.

170

Perhaps this temporo-maxillary contracture explains Qi Bo's strange observation:

> When the energy of the gallbladder is troubled, one bites one's cheeks; when it is the energy of the stomach that is troubled, one bites one's lips.[229]

Dental occlusion yields stress through the feedback from periodontal receptors and trigeminal nuclei.[230] Based on this research, we are able to understand trigeminal neuralgia secondary to malocclusion, which may involve all the branches of the trigeminal nerve, notably the superior branch with pain in the forehead, the temples and eyes, as well as the inferior branch, with pain in the cheek and the mandible. However, as Legrand comments, "Not all occlusions engender feedback."[231]

We can propose three ways of breaking the old pathogenic vicious circle. The first is technical and mechanical, involving the dental arch (occlusion, prosthesis, surgery, kinesiotherapy). The second is acupuncture and the third is trace element therapy.

Acupuncture therapy most often involves Shao Yang. The symptomology of shou shao yang is "pain in the external corner of the eye, swelling of the cheeks, pain in front of the ear."[232] That of zu shao yang is "pain in the head and the chin, and in the external angle of the eye."[233]

The *Ling Shu* indicates, "In cases of pain in the chin, needle the points of shou yang ming {large intestine} and bleed the points located at the angle of the forehead."[234] According to Chamfrault, the point in question is qubin (GB-7). Its semiology, described in the tenth chapter of the *Ling Shu* is, "chin and cheeks swollen and painful."

Practically all the local points are recommended and Zu Lien, quoted by Chamfrault, has meticulously codified the treatment of facial neuralgia.[235] We may add that almost all the points chosen for the treatment of opthalmic migraines are effective here. On the painful side, we treat the local points, as well as fengchi (GB-20) or yifeng (TB-17), and yanglingquan (GB-34), xiaxi (GB-43), taichong (LV-3), ququan (LV-8) and on the opposite side, ting points dadun (LV-1) and zuqiaoyin (GB-44).

Numerous doctoral theses have shown the efficacy of acupuncture treatment in cases of facial neuralgia. It goes without saying that the earlier the treatment is undertaken, the better, before starting chemotherapy.[236]

The trace elements prescribed in association with this pathology are manganese, magnesium and manganese-copper. The latter corresponds to the Yang Ming-Metal profile, where the articulation disorder is one of flaccidity.

The treatment of the meridians shou yang ming (large intestine) and shou tai yin (lung), or of the meridians zu yang ming (stomach) and zu tai yin (spleen), is theoretically identical to the one we have described and corresponds to the treatment of the divergent channels.

171

It is important here to determine the temperament of the patient in order to define the afflicted meridians. The nature of the malocclusion and the topography of the pain are precious aids, but are not always verifiable. It follows that the success of the therapy depends on the definition of the temperament of the patient. We can treat Yang Ming time and again, with no improvement at all, and then in a single session treat Shao Yang, with immediate and spectacular results, or vice versa, of course.

Ophthalmological Pathology

Presbyopia and Xerophthalmia

The element Wood corresponds to the eye and to vision. Its organ, the liver, and its bowel, the gallbladder, are both involved with the sensorial function we know as vision:

> The energy of the liver is linked to the eyes; it governs visual acuity.
> When the liver is healthy, the eyes see normally.[237]

The gallbladder is involved as well and ophthalmic indications are attributed to many points on its meridian, zu shao yang. The most obvious correspondence with Western physiology is that with vitamin A, which still goes by the name of retinol.

The liver is capable of transforming provitamin A, or carotene, found in our food, into active vitamin A, which is stored in the tissues. However, one function of the bile is to facilitate the absorption of the liposoluble vitamins, among them vitamin A. This vitamin A goes into the composition of the visual purple of the retina cells and enables us to see shapes. Its deficiency leads to hemeralopia, or loss of night vision. A vitamin A deficiency also leads to xerophthalmia, with swelling of the eyelids and corneal lesions. We see that vitamin A does not only concern the visual function. The poor absorption of fatty matters, common among hepatobiliary disorders, for example, hinders the absorption of vitamin A, which is liposoluble.

In practice, we notice that Shao Yang patients generally have good eyesight and rarely wear glasses. The opposite is true of Jue Yin individuals, who often have poor eyesight early in childhood, specifically shortsightedness (see Jue Yin).

There may be an intimate connection between visual acuity and the state of health of the liver and gallbladder.[238] In his treatise, *The Manner of Treatment of Renowned Doctors,* Tong Fun writes:

> As the meridian of Yang Ming (Stomach) has much blood and energy, and as the bladder meridian has more blood than energy, each time there is congestion of blood in the eyes, we must bleed the points of these two meridians. As the liver has more energy than blood, it will be preferable to needle rather than to bleed. Also, Shao Yang types having less blood should not be bled. Consequently, the more we bleed the points of Tai Yang and Yang Ming, the better the

172

visual acuity will be; but the more we bleed the meridian of Shao Yang or of the liver, the poorer the eyesight will be.[239]

Zusanli (ST-36) is the tonification point for the stomach meridian. Wang Tao writes, "After the age of thirty, apply moxas to zusanli, otherwise the energy will assail the eyes."[240] This means that moxibustion of zusanli (ST-36) is a form of preventive therapy against presbyopia of old age.

Among the points of Shao Yang, there are three points that deserve attention: fengchi (GB-20), to treat ocular hypertension, risks of hemorrhage, as well as acute or infectious pathology; linqi (GB-15), which is indicated as specific for all eye disorders by the *Da Cheng;* and most important, guangming (GB-37). The translation of guangming is "light", or better still, "clearness."[241] This point is indicated in the *Da Cheng* for "itching of the eyes and pain in the eyes."[242] Tong Fun indicates guangming for "ulcerations all around the eyes."[243] For this point the modern Shanghai authors indicate, "Hemeralopia, atrophy of the optic nerve, cataract, ophthalmic migraine."[244] We may conclude that guangming is the ophthalmological point par excellence, which would explain its name.

This point, located on the gallbladder meridian, is even indicated in vitamin A deficiency, if we interpret the associated ocular symptomology given by the *Da Cheng* as xerophthalmia: "Eye disease in children who show signs of malnutrition (swollen and hard belly, emaciation, yellow skin)."[245]

Other ophthalmic affections are studied in Jue Yin.

Infectious Pathology

Shao Yang plays an essential role in the traditional physiopathology of the penetration, meridian by meridian,[246] of perverse energy, in that it is the "axis" meridian. This is stated clearly by Qi Bo in the first chapter of the *Ling Shu:*

> If disorders dwell in the upper and external part of the body, we must needle the point yanglingquan (GB-34), as the perverse energy wants to penetrate into the body. We must chase it away before it manages to get within.[247]

Zona

This is a disorder that specifically affects the anatomical territory of the meridian Shao Yang. Geniculate zona, with auricular and bucco-pharyngial pain, involves shou shao yang more than zu shao yang, which is confirmed by its complications that include peripheral facial paralysis, hearing problems and equilibrium disturbances. Intercostal zona corresponds to the zu shao yang territory.

Opthalmic zona, due to its ocular pathology (conjunctivitis, cornea, iridocyclitis, paralysis of the third cranial nerve), is related to zu shao yang (gallbladder). This pathology is facilitated by various morbid processes that weaken the terrain (aging, hemopathies, neoplasia, immunosuppressor treatments, etc.).

173

This brings to mind disorders of Shao Yin (Kidney).[248] Here the perverse energy is "wind heat" or "wind dryness," which occurs when the weather is abnormally warm for the season. If we accept that perverse energy penetrates into the body only when the terrain is weak and that the virus enters through the upper part of the body (nasal cavities), the statement in the first chapter of the *Ling Shu*, quoted above, still applies.

It is thus Shao Yang that is the victim and yanglingquan (GB-34) which is to be needled, in association with zhigou (TB-6), with electric stimulation. This is the modern Chinese anesthesia protocol in surgery involving intercostal incisions. It is especially effective in intercostal zona pain.

In the *Da Cheng*, zhigou (TB-6) is indicated for "pain under the arm and at the sides of the chest, wounds, skin disease, dartre, eczema, etc."[249] It is thus an intercostal and brachial neurological point, and is also an important dermatological point of Shao Yang.

In addition to these points, we may needle the ting points on the opposite side, guanchong (TB-1) and zuqiaoyin (GB-44), as well as the local points, and plum blossom needle the lesions and local cephalic points. Yifeng (TB-17) is a particularly effective point to needle in cases of geniculate zona, along with fengchi (GB-20), yangbai (GB-14), tongziliao (GB-1), jingming (BL-1), etc.

Our experience with acupuncture treatment in cases of zona is extensive and we find that it is particularly effective in procuring rapid sedation of the pains, as it accelerates healing, prevents superinfection and subsequent pain. It dissipates or diminishes post herpes zoster pain by more than fifty percent. Of course, the earlier acupuncture is undertaken, the more effective it is, especially if undertaken in the days following the vesicular eruption.

The main points recommended for treating zona are: GB-34, TB-6, TB-17, GB-20, GB-14, BL-1, TB-1 and GB-44 on the opposite side.

In trace element therapy, copper-gold-silver is indicated in the acute phases,[250] and corresponds to anergia from deficiency of Shao Yin. It is useful to repeat here that manganese is effective against neuralgia.[251]

Traditional Chronobiology of Shao Yang

Diurnal Rhythm

The hour of shou shao yang is hai, from 9 to 11 p.m. The animal is the boar. The hour of zu shao yang, zi, is from 11 p.m to 1 a.m. The animal is the rat.[252]

Annual Rhythm

Regarding Shao Yang pains in the heart and in the thorax, the Shao Yang is in abundance which manifests in the heart. (Shao Yang = Fire Minister, heart = Imperial Fire.) By the ninth month, Yang is exhausted and Yin is in full blossom, whence comes pain in the heart and thorax; it becomes impossible to turn over when lying down: the

174

Yin stores things, immobilizing them. In severe cases, there are palpitations. The beings are enfeebled; the vegetative growth period has ended; the qi leaves Yang for Yin. If a superabundance of Yang persists in the lower part of the body, there will be tremblings in the legs.[253]

Duodecimal Terrestrial Rhythm

"The third and the ninth years correspond with Shao Yang."[254]

Monthly Rhythm

"Shou shao yang corresponds to the first month of winter, zu shao yang to the second month of winter."[255]

Rhythmic Cycles in the Lower Limbs

"The upper part of the body represents the heavens, the lower part, the earth."[256] In other words, the former evolves according to a $6x2=12$ cycle, the latter to a $5x2=10$ cycle.

The six meridians of the lower extremity correspond to the twelve months; although in the upper limb the energy evolves according to ten day cycles.[257]

"The first month is the birth of Yang. It corresponds to the gallbladder in the lower left extremity."[258] This is why it is called the first Yang, or lesser Yang. The second month is the bladder, the second Yang. The third month is the stomach, third Yang. In the succession of the limbs, the left (Yang) precedes the right (Yin).

Rhythmic Cycles of Shao Yang in the Upper Limb

"The first day represents the triple burner, on the left. The second day represents the triple burner on the right."[259]

Summary of the Shao Yang Temperament

Shao Yang individuals correspond to the coleric temperament defined by Gaston Berger, and are also known for being exuberant. Fond of action and enthusiastic, they are active, authoritarian, and they are moved by different moods, which often makes them angry, or sometimes violent.

Pathologically speaking, these types are given to disorders of cardiac rhythm, to high blood pressure or to arteriosclerosis in old age, which exposes them to circulatory problems that affect the veins more than the arteries, to presbycusis, and to cerebrovascular accidents. They are subject to biliary dyskinesia and are prime targets for cholelithiasis and even renal lithiasis (most often urinary calculi).

When they suffer from colonopathy, the pain is most often in the right side, with a possibility of diarrhea and hemorrhoids. The pain is violent and intermittent. Gastralgia and ulcers are not rare, unlike asthma, which takes on dramatic

175

proportions among Shao Yang patients. Regarding osteoarticular pathology, the Shao Yang patients are exposed to gout and to erratic arthralgia, more than to bone mineralization problems, which arrive with old age. The symptoms commonly grouped under allergies (urticaria, pruritis, allergies, migraines) are frequently found, as is dysmenorrhea among women. Hyperthyroidism is the major endocrine pathology found among these individuals. Tics, spasms, muscular contractures and temporo-maxillary contractures are typical of these agitated individuals, who are also victims of insomnia, anxiety and relational neurosis.

Thus we may summarize the pathology of Shao Yang patients, who may otherwise be optimistic people, as those who enjoy sports, enjoy good health and who don't at all enjoy having their momentum stopped by ill health.

We have shown that the miscellaneous meridians dai mai and yang wei mai, which shunt into shou shao yang and zu shao yang, are frequently involved in many of the energy imbalances and deserve to be opened by needling the points zulinqi (GB-41) and waiguan (TB-5).

A close inspection of the texts shows a good correlation between this temperament and the psychological and morbid behavior of Diathesis I and Diathesis III as defined by Menetrier, particularly in their Yang modalities, as they are linked to the bowel gallbladder (Wood) and the triple burner function (Fire). These correlations allow us to indicate the prescription of several trace elements: manganese, sulfur, iodine; and among elderly patients: manganese-cobalt, in treating subjects classified as belonging to the temperament Shao Yang.

Notes

[1] The nasal jia yi point corresponds to the gallbladder in nasal reflexotherapy. This point is needled when patients wish to stop smoking. See Requena *et.al.* (93), pp. 193-202 and Michel (49), pp. 50-52.

[2] Requena (93), pp. 193-194.

[3] Zhang Zhi Cong, quoted by Nguyen Van Nghi (66), p. 60.

[4] *Su Wen* (28), Chapter 8, p. 95.

[5] *Su Wen* (8), Chapter 44.

[6] *Ibid.*, Chapter 9, p. 48.

[7] *Su Wen* (28), Chapter 11, p. 103.

[8] Nervous tissue is also considered as one of the curious bowels in acupuncture (brain, marrow).

[9] Kaplan, referenced in Harrison (26), p. 452.

[10] See the relationships between the gallbladder and the uterus, menstruation, pregnancy and gynecological pathology, further on in this work.

[11] Robert *et.al.* (97).

[12] Quoted by Malmejac (42), p. 341.

[13] See Hamburger *et.al.* (24).

[14] *Ling Shu* (8), Chapter 12, p. 382.

[15] *Nan Jing* (64), p. 271.

[16] *Ling Shu* (8), Chapter 2, p. 315.

[17] *Su Wen* (8), Chapter 58, p. 204.

[18] *Su Wen* (28), Chapter 49, p. 214.

[19] *Ling Shu* (8), Chapter 10, p. 369.

[20] *Ibid.*, Chapter 16, p. 390.

[21] Shanzhong (CV-17) is the point of origin of the meridian shou jue yin (pericardium) and is of considerable importance in the thoracic physiology, in cardiac rhythm, etc.

[22] *Su Wen* (8), Chapter 18, p. 78.

[23] *Ibid.*, Chapter 21, p. 97.

[24] Quoted by Chamfrault (7), p. 912.

[25] *Ibid.*

[26] *Da Cheng* (7), pp. 564-916.

[27] *Su Wen* (8), Chapter 59, p. 206.

[28] Menetrier (46), pp. 75-76.

[29] For more information on the concept of jue, or energy blockage, see cardiovascular pathology, Yang Ming.

[30] *Su Wen* (28), Chapter 5, p. 84.

[31] *Su Wen* (8), Chapter 5, p. 32.

[32] Shanghai (105).

[33] Nguyen Van Nghi (67). See also, Nguyen Van Nghi, ''Hypertension arterielle,'' Le mensuel du medecin acupuncteur, No. 4, p. 20.

[34] *Ling Shu* (8), Chapter 21, p. 406.

[35] Shanghai (105).

[36] It is important here to refer to the discussion of cerebrovascular accidents in the chapter devoted to Yang Ming, in which we describe the concept of external feng and internal feng which corresponds to the surge of compressed energy (jue).

[37] Chamfrault (8) p. 523.

[38] *Ibid.*

[39] It is precisely advised that to needle this point, we must first needle yixi (BL-45), tianrong (SI-17) and tianzhu (BL-10).

[40] In Chinese, *Xue ya gang xin,* or ''excessive increase in blood pressure.''

[41] Menetrier (47), p. 46.

[42] *Ling Shu* (8), Chapter 60, p. 501.

[43] *Ibid.,* Chapter 10, p. 375.

[44] *Da Cheng* (7), pp. 563 and 578.

[45] Menetrier (46), p. 76.

[46] Nguyen Van Nghi (67), p. 677.

[47] *Ling Shu* (8), Chapter 2, p. 315.

[48] Ren ying represents the three levels of the left wrist pulse (Yang), and qi hao the right wrist (Yin).

[49] *Su Wen* (8), Chapter 79, p. 299.

[50] *Nan Jing* (64), p. 272.

[51] Requena (78).

[52] *Su Wen* (28), Chapter 7, p. 92.

[53] Quoted by Chamfrault (7), p. 567.

[54] Soulie de Morant (107), p. 569.

55 *Ibid.*, p. 536.

56 *Ibid.*, p. 567.

57 Quoted by Chamfrault (7), p. 519.

58 Zuqiaoyin (GB-44): fits of coughing, pressure in the chest and sides making it difficult to breathe, dyspnea.

59 Picard (75), p. 96-97.

60 Here, physical and emotional excess exhaust the energy of the organ, creating illness. Biliary dyskinesia represents the beginning and excess stages. A lithiasis is a sign of exhaustion and of deficiency.

61 *Ling Shu* (8), Chapter 10, pp. 368-369.

62 As a result of the impingement of the gallbladder upon the stomach.

63 Shangjuxu (ST-37) and xiajuxu (ST-39).

64 *Ling Shu* (8), Chapter 19, p. 402.

65 *Ibid.*, pp. 331-332. In this case we may be faced with cholangitis.

66 *Su Wen* (28), Chapter 45, p. 206.

67 *Ibid.*, Chapter 46, p. 214.

68 *Ibid.*, Chapter 38, pp. 183-184.

69 Nothing, however, enabled us to exclude any other infectious etiology, such as a hydatid cyst.

70 We can speak personally of one case, a patient suffering from hemochromatosis who complained of a bad pulmonary cough when he slept on his right side.

71 The bowel is deficient, but there is perverse heat energy.

72 *Su Wen* (28), Chapter 47, p. 210.

73 Quoted by Chamfrault (7), p. 880.

74 See Viral Hepatitis, Jue Yin.

75 Menetrier (46), p. 46.

76 See Requena (92).

77 Translated from the Vietnamese by Nguyen Van Nghi and published in my article on ulcers: Requena (90), pp. 389-396.

78 Chinese Medical Journal, Peking, No. 1, January 1974. See Requena (79), pp. 164-165, for detail.

79 From the research group at the Hospital of Tientzin. Traditional Western combined treatment of acute perforation of peptic ulcer.

80 Requena (86), pp. 40-60.

81 Menetrier (46), pp. 46-52.

[82] *Ibid.*

[83] The baliao are the points shangliao (BL-31), ciliao (BL-32), zhongliao (BL-33), xialiao (BL-34), in the sacred holes.

[84] Venal pathology is strongly related to the element Wood, as we explain in detail in Jue Yin in our discussion of varicose veins and phlebitis.

[85] *Ling Shu* (8), Chapter 10, p. 369.

[86] *Su Wen* (28), Chapter 8, p. 95.

[87] Gourion (21), p. 51.

[88] *Ibid.*

[89] *Nan Jing* (64), p. 268.

[90] *Ling Shu* (8), Chapter 30, p. 438. See also *Nan Jing* (64).

[91] *Ibid.*

[92] Chamfrault translates the passage as follows: "Shao Yang is a mobile, floating energy like the shuttle of a loom." We can add the commentary by Zhang Jing Yao, "Shao Yang is the axis {or hinge}, because the Yang energy is between the interior and the exterior, and at any moment it may open as well as shut" Nguyen Van Nghi (66).

[93] *Su Wen* (8), Chapter 62, p. 228. We may add that yangjiao is a meeting point with yang wei mai.

[94] One western equivalent of the term bi is rheumatism.

[95] *Su Wen* (8), Chapter 43, pp. 162-163.

[96] *Ibid.* Recall that the essence of wind is essentially mobile.

[97] *Ling Shu* (8), Chapter 17, p. 394.

[98] *Ibid.*, Chapter 73, p. 533.

[99] *Ibid.*, Chapter 10, p. 369.

[100] *Ibid.*, Chapter 28, p. 433.

[101] Quoted by Chamfrault (7), pp. 513 and 570.

[102] *Ibid.*

[103] The ahshi points are the points located in painful regions, or simply the cutaneous territory where the pain is the sharpest.

[104] Menetrier (46), pp. 45-46.

[105] *Su Wen* (8), Chapter 41, p. 156.

[106] Husson (28), p. 193, translated as the "chain of the Yang."

[107] *Su Wen* (8), Chapter 41, p. 157.

[108] Menetrier (46), p. 97.

[109] *Su Wen* (8), Chapter 60, p. 212. This first paragraph is obviously related to Shao Yang (Wood corresponds to the muscles), as can be seen in the Husson translation that follows.

[110] *Su Wen* (28), Chapter 60, p. 235.

[111] *Ibid.*

[112] *Da Cheng* (7), p. 347, for the point biguan (ST-31).

[113] *Da Cheng* (7), p. 561.

[114] Husson (28), p. 235.

[115] *Da Cheng* (7), p. 561.

[116] Husson (28), p. 235.

[117] *Da Cheng* (7), p. 451; *Da Cheng* (107), p. 599.

[118] *Ling Shu* (8), Chapter 10, p. 375.

[119] Pernice (71).

[120] *Su Wen* (8), Chapter 63, p. 233.

[121] *Da Cheng* (7), p. 561.

[122] For complementary treatments, see Pernice (71).

[123] Picard (75), p. 153. See also, Picard and Antonini, A., *Traitement medical etiologique de la coxarthrose.* Maloine, 1971.

[124] *Su Wen* (28), Chapter 8, p. 95.

[125] *Su Wen* (8), Chapter 8, p. 46.

[126] *Ling Shu* (8), Chapter 2, p. 315.

[127] *Su Wen* (28), Chapter 6, p. 90.

[128] See the corresponding chapter of Shao Yin concerning physiopathology and treatment of renal colic attack.

[129] *Ling Shu* (8), Chapter 35, p. 448.

[130] Zhang Zhi Cong, quoted by Gourion (21), p. 51.

[131] *Su Wen* (8), Chapter 35.

[132] See Renal Lithiasis, Shao Yin.

[133] *Ling Shu* (8), Chapter 4, p. 331.

[134] *Ibid.*, Chapter 35, p. 448.

[135] *Su Wen* (66), Chapter 23, p. 420.

[136] *Ibid.*

[137] Menetrier (46), p. 46.

[138] *Ibid.*

[139] Picard (75), p. 136.

[140] Serane and Pean, "Etudes psychosomatiques des lithiases renales," Maladies de la nutrition, vol. V, p. 1063.

[141] There's a common French expression to designate a well preserved old man: "He's still green."

[142] This specific etiology counts among the "emotional causes" of illness in Chinese medicine.

[143] This is a general term that includes all the psycho-affective troubles (the equivalent of the seven passions), not only sadness or fear.

[144] Shanghai (105).

[145] *Su Wen* (8), Chapter 7, p. 45. "Larynx" is an arbitrary term, chosen by the translator. Husson translates the term as angina. Further on, we will expand upon the ambiguity of this translation.

[146] Loss of weight and anorexia is associated with Tai Yin.

[147] *Ling Shu* (8), Chapter 10, p. 369.

[148] Pathology of pericardium includes all the disorders involving the arteries and the veins.

[149] *Da Cheng* (7), p. 566.

[150] Renying (ST-9) is the arterial point of the upper part of Yang Ming (see Yang Ming).

[151] Shanghai (105).

[152] Soulie de Morant (107), p. 725.

[153] The *Da Cheng* mentions "weakness of the arms and legs" for this point.

[154] Dazhu (BL-11) is the he point of the bones.

[155] We personally add xuanzhong (GB-39) to this list, when the myasthenia is severe.

[156] *Da Cheng* (7), p. 628.

[157] Chamfrault (7), p. 555.

[158] See Endocrinology and Gynecology in Jue Yin.

[159] Menetrier (46), pp. 90-97.

[160] *Su Wen* (28), Chapter 44, p. 202. Note that jin means muscles.

[161] *Ibid.*, Chapter 46, p. 214.

[162] Qiuxu (GB-40), indicated in the *Da Cheng* for "muscular spasms," is especially effective in treating nocturnal cramps in the lower limbs.

[163] The flapping tremor of the portocaval encephalopathies is a specific form of neurological affliction (of Wood origin) that causes the particular abnormal movements displayed by pre-coma cases (see also Viral Hepatitis, Jue Yin).

[164] See Schizophrenia (Tai Yin) to understand the concept of "ancestor."

[165] *Da Cheng* (7), pp. 517-8 etc.

[166] *Su Wen* (8), Chapter 28, p. 116. The Husson translation gives "convulsions" instead of epilepsy and lists five points that are different from those indicated by Wang Bing, which are those indicated by the modern commentaries Bai Hua Jie.

[167] *Ling Shu* (8), Chapter 10, p. 369.

[168] This is Shao Yang territory.

[169] *Ling Shu* (8), Chapter 24, pp. 420-421.

[170] Within the meridians flow blood and energy. There may be an excess of one and a relative deficiency of the other.

[171] Examined above.

[172] This is the hypochondriacal pain.

[173] This bears witness to the link between Shao Yang and the liver.

[174] These terms correspond to cardiovascular accidents and are developed in Yang Ming.

[175] *Su Wen* (8), Chapter 64, pp. 237-238. For the sake of comparison, we here give Husson's translation: "In Shao Yang, excess: bi of the muscles; insufficiency: bi of the liver. Too much fluidity: shan of the wind of the liver; lack of fluidity: gathering of qi, pulling in the muscles and episodic ocular pains" (28), p. 254.

[176] This disregulation of "blood and energy" in the meridians may involve the "fluidity" as well as its distribution (vasomotricity, circulation) by the shou jue yin (pericardium), which is considered equal to the sympathetic nervous system, and by shou shao yang (triple burner), corresponding to the parasympathetic. These imbalances account for acrocyanosis, for Raynaud's disease in these terrains (Jue Yin). We must admire the multiple physiological implications contained in a single Chinese system, *i.e.,* the relationship between blood and energy in a meridian.

[177] *Su Wen* (8), Chapter 60, p. 210.

[178] Taichong means "the supreme assault" and is the shu point of this meridian. It launches the energy in the meridian all the way to the top of the head. This point is indicated by Bian Que as one of the three points ruling over the superior part of the body. In his treatise *Elements of Chinese Medicine,* he recommends needling this point for all the nasal affections (along with hegu, LI-4).

[179] See also Blood Pathology, Psychiatry and ququan (LV-8), in the chapter devoted to Tai Yang.

[180] Other points such as guanchong (TB-1), a ting point, yemen (TB-2), the triple burner water point, yangfu (GB-38), the gallbladder dispersion point, are indicated in the *Da Cheng* with the symptomology "pain in the eyes."

[181] Same as xuanzhong (GB-39) in hyperthyroidism.

[182] Soulie de Morant (107), p. 564.

[183] *Ibid.*

[184] This is the qi of neuromuscular activity, movement from the interior towards the exterior.

[185] Soulie de Morant (107), p. 570.

[186] *Da Cheng* (107), p. 567. Quoted by Soulie de Morant for the point yangfu (GB-38), dispersion point of zu shao yang, indicated also for "cholecystitis, gall sand and stones."

[187] *Ling Shu* (8), Chapter 8, p. 347.

[188] Chamfrault (7), p. 563.

[189] Let us quote once more the semiology of tianjing (TB-10), the dispersion point of shou shao yang. "Soothes nerves, clattering teeth, hyperexcitations and delirium. Among very nervous women, sudden relaxation may bring on an attack of tears" Soulie de Morant (107), p. 539.

[190] *Su Wen* (28), Chapter 8, p. 95.

[191] *Ibid.*, Chapter 9, page 100.

[192] Is this the thyroid, or the vocal chords and the voice?

[193] *Su Wen* (28), Chapter 47, p. 219.

[194] *Ling Shu* (8), Chapter 19, p. 402.

[195] *Ibid.*, Chapter 43, p. 465.

[196] *Encyclopedia Universalis* (113), p. 767.

[197] See Hysteria in Jue Yin.

[198] Menetrier (46), pp. 45-109.

[199] *Ibid.*

[200] Nguyen Van Nghi, "Les insomnies" (61), p. 187.

[201] Menetrier (46), p. 109.

[202] This pathology is not related to hyperhidrosis.

[203] *Ling Shu* (8), Chapter 10, pp. 367-369.

[204] In Western physiology this is the case of bile, for example, which eliminates the waste products and the hormonal catabolites excreted by the liver, by reabsorbing water.

[205] *Ling Shu* (8), Chapter 12, p. 382.

[206] Chamfrault (7), pp. 519, 564, 568.

[207] *Ibid.*

[208] *Ibid.*, p. 543.

[209] This is by way of comparison with non-conjugate yellow or red bilirubin jaundice, which signals a disorder of the spleen, the circulatory system, transfusion, etc.

[210] We exclude primitive and secondary cancers of the liver, sclerosing cholangitis, cirrhosis and hereditary illnesses (Dubin-Johnson, Rotor), whose diagnosis must be made differentially.

[211] Which must be diagnosed differentially from cancer of the head of the pancreas.

[212] Viral hepatitis is treated in Jue Yin.

[213] Chamfrault (7), p. 559.

[214] In the patient standing at attention, this point is located at the extremity of the middle finger flat against the thigh, between the anterior edge of the musculus tensor fasciae latae and the musculus vastus lateralis.

[215] *Ling Shu* (8), Chapter 9, p. 355.

[216] *Ibid.*, Chapter 47, p. 474.

[217] Soulie de Morant (107), p. 760. Conscience implies shen, indicating Shao Yin.

[218] One famous example of Shao Yang deafness is Beethoven.

[219] *Ling Shu* (8), Chapter 10, p. 367.

[220] *Ibid.*, Chapter 26, p. 427.

[221] See Zona, further on in the same chapter. Let us point out that mumps treated by the cauterization of jiaosun (TB-20) are, in fact, a Tai Yin disease. Shanghai (105).

[222] See also Shao Yin.

[223] *Su Wen* (8), Chapter 45, p. 170. Husson translates, ''Sudden deafness, swelling and heat in the cheeks, thoracic pain, impossibility to move the legs '' (28), p. 206.

[224] This point is tinggong (SI-19).

[225] This does not mean that moxas on the opposite side are forbidden.

[226] *Ling Shu* (8), Chapter 24, p. 423.

[227] *Ibid.*, Chapter 21, page 406. (See Yang Ming, Cerebrovascular Accidents.)

[228] *Ibid.*, p. 407.

[229] *Ibid.*, Chapter 28, p. 434.

[230] Kroch and Poulsen in Legrand (37).

[231] *Ibid.*

[232] *Ling Shu* (8), Chapter 10, pp. 367-369.

[233] *Ibid.*

[234] *Ibid.*, Chapter 26, p. 428.

[235] Chamfrault (7), page 745.

[236] Facial neuralgia is the subject of a study done by the G.E.R.A.. See Trinh (111). See also, Le Grand (37).

[237] *Ling Shu* (8), Chapter 17, p. 392.

[238] This term, ''big gallbladder,'' given to the audacious by the ancient Chinese, may be viewed with a different eye. We find it worthwhile to pass on the anecdote told by Debeaux in his *Essay on Pharmaceutics and the Medical Manner of the Chinese:* ''Chinese warriors had so much respect for their dead that they dared not remove the slightest part of a body, soft or solid, in order to make medicine. The one and only exception to this respect of the dead involved the body of a dead enemy, which belonged to the warrior who had killed him, and who had the right to remove the gallbladder, by making an incision in the right side of the body with a knife.'' Debeaux bases his conclusion on the studies of Lariviere and comments, ''The human gallbladder is considered a potent remedy in eye disease.'' We might come to the conclusion that the victorious warrior intended to appropriate the belligerent virtues of his opponent, in consuming his gallbladder, and to strengthen his visual acuity at the same time. (9) and (14).

[239] Chamfrault (7) p. 804.

[240] *Ibid.*, p. 352.

[241] Shanghai (105).

[242] *Da Cheng* (7), p. 563.

[243] Chamfrault (7), p. 805.

[244] Shanghai (105).

[245] Chamfrault, (7), p. 802.

[246] Tai Yang, Shao Yang, Yang Ming, etc.

[247] *Ling Shu* (8), Chapter 11, p. 310.

[248] See Shao Yin and the concept of decrepitude, of defect, of immune weakness.

[249] *Da Cheng* (7) p. 517.

[250] Sal (102), p. 137.

[251] Menetrier (46), p. 46.

[252] The traditional time corresponds to the time of the time zone. In France today, 9 to 11 p.m. corresponds to the official time, 10 p.m. to 12 in the winter, and 11 p.m. to 1 a.m. in the summer.

[253] *Su Wen* (28), Chapter 49, p. 214.

[254] *Su Wen* (8), Chapter 66, p. 250.

[255] *Su Wen* (28), Chapter 7, p. 91.

[256] *Ling Shu* (8), Chapter 41, pp. 459-460.

[257] *Ibid.* Shou jue yin, which is not an organ, doesn't count in this cycle.

[258] *Ibid.,* Chapter 41.

[259] *Ibid.*

Jue Yin

Physiology of the Liver and the Meridian Zu Jue Yin

Before discussing the pathology of the Jue Yin temperament, it is important to consider the energetic and metabolic functions of the liver. Qi Bo defines the liver in the eighth chapter of the *Su Wen,* "The liver is the general who makes the plans."[1] The same statement, translated by Husson, reads, "The liver acts as the head of state, calculating and reflecting."[2] These two translations, together with the following passage from the *Su Wen,* bear witness to the importance of the liver and its metabolic role.

> When food is absorbed into the body, it is transformed into energy that penetrates into the liver. From there the energy spreads into the muscles, then into the heart and thence to the meridians and the arteries.[3]

The Role of the Liver in the Synthesis of Proteins

The liver synthesizes various proteins, the most abundant being albumin. When the liver fails to synthesize enough albumin, hypoalbuminemia results, causing edema and serous effusions, such as ascites, due to a drop in osmotic pressure. The ancient Chinese also made this observation:

> If the pulse of the liver is somewhat slow, there are troubles with the fluids (edemas, etc.).[4]

The liver is the main site of amino acid metabolism. Amino acids undergo various catabolic and anabolic processes within the liver. There are two important stages of catabolism: the oxidative deamination (LADH) and the transamination (SGOT, SGPT). The amino acid may subsequently enter the citric acid cycle, intermediary between the metabolism of lipids and glucides. We read in the *Ling Shu:*

> The East represents the celestial mysteries;[5] it is the symbol of the Tao that exists within man;[6] for it represents the transformation of nutrients that themselves engender intelligence. In the body it represents the liver.[7]

Other authors, such as Schatz, tried to establish correlations between DNA and the anterior heaven. These comparisons also attempt to justify a relationship between the liver, the celestial mysteries and the Tao.

Role of the Liver in Coagulation

The liver synthesizes coagulating factors: prothrombin, fibrinogen, factors V, VII and X. In the *Su Wen* we read, "The liver produces the qi of the blood."[8] In the *Ling Shu,* "The meridian Jue Yin contains more blood than energy."[9] In the Chinese theoretical framework, the organ gan (liver) and its meridian zu jue yin (in relationship with shou jue yin), play such a considerable part in the energetic physiology of the blood that we must go beyond the Western concept of the liver and superimpose several Western correspondences to account for the Chinese theory of the action of this organ.

The production of the qi of the blood attributed to the liver is one of the hardest of the syncretistic concepts in Chinese medicine to explain. Throughout the chapters devoted to the pathology of Jue Yin — cardiology, gynecology, endocrinology and neurology — we will meet with these correspondences.

Role of the Liver in Protein Catabolism

The synthesis of urea begins in the liver. This activity, along with that of the kidney, is part of the lower burner. It corresponds to san jiao and to the triple burner meridian shou shao yang (see Shao Yang).

Role of the Liver in Nutrition and in Absorption and Synthesis of Lipids

The liver synthesizes lipids, especially triglycerides. Along with the intestines, it synthesizes practically all cholesterol. The plasma and the liver contain an enzyme needed to convert free cholesterol to ester cholesterol.[10] Remember that the liver "corresponds to the muscles and the nerves" (phospholipids). Glucose is stored in the liver in the form of glycogen. Classically, this function has been related to muscular activity: "The liver nourishes the muscles."[11] This is not exclusive. When we fast, the liver must provide the tissues, especially the brain, with the glucose they need, as well as supplying the marrow, the peripheral nerves and the medulla renis. This is done by lipolysis and gluconeogenesis of amino acids liberated in the muscles.[12]

Role of the Liver in Eliminatory Functions

The liver is the main site of detoxification of exogenous substances (drugs) as well as endogenous substances (hormones). This is accomplished by conjugation and excretion by the bile and the urine, or by inactivation (reduction, oxidation, hydroxylation).[13] In Chinese medicine, the role attributed to the liver and to Jue Yin implies a close relationship between the liver, triple burner and gallbladder. The *Su Wen* relates the following discussion:

> "I believe the liver to be the most important[14] of the five organs," declared Lei Gong.

> "No," replied Huang Di, "it is the least important {noble} of the organs. Jue Yin is the last link of the Yin, it is the end of Yin."[15]

Thus, the liver is at once the general, and by virtue of its location at the end of the energy circulation, the end of Yin, it is also the least noble of the organs. At the end of the ying qi cycle, in the twelve meridians, "the energy is dirty." A part of it passes to the liver, then to the lungs and leaves the body through the nose upon exhalation.[16] This seems to correspond to the emunctory role of the lung, especially in regard to the metabolism of cholesterol, which is coupled with the liver and precedes the lungs in the circulation of the energy within the body.

Cardiovascular Pathology

Tachycardia, Auricular Fibrillations and Cardiac Instability

These are among the "excess of Wood energy" syndromes typified by the surge of the fire of the liver and of the gallbladder, previously described as a pathology of Shao Yang. They are representative of the cardiac erethism that is characteristic of those neurotonic subjects who become aggressive and hyperactive when the gallbladder meridian (zu shao yang) is in excess, and anxious and fearful when the imbalance is in the liver meridian (zu jue yin). The participation of the triple burner (shou shao yang) and the pericardium (shou jue yin) is certain in both cases, as is a direct link with the heart and the cardiac plexus.

Shanzhong (CV-17) is the point of origin of both the heart and pericardium meridians. It is also a Shao Yang passage. Disturbances may lead to rhythm irregularities:

> When the pulse of the first Yin and that of the first Yang slow down and come to a stop, it points to the Yin energy[17] reaching the heart {due to the inability of the liver and the gallbladder to start the fire of the heart}. The vicious energy may move up and down without regular patterns {because a disorder of the liver and the gallbladder will generate wind that moves around constantly}.[18]

Some thinkers, among them Nguyen Van Nghi, discriminate between the Yin and Yang of the liver. This distinction does help us to understand the mechanics of liver syndromes. If the liver is insufficient in its qi or jing, its Yin aspect, this insufficiency will cause the surging of its Yang. These minor and strictly functional symptoms can sometimes take on a more organic and serious aspect, as in the case of the prolapse of the mitral valve.

Prolapse of the mitral valve, or Barlow's disease, defined by the work of Reid in 1961, Barlow in 1963, and Criley in 1966, provides an interesting comparison with the concepts of Chinese medicine. Clinically, it is defined by functional symptoms that are present in at least 80 percent of all cases,[19] including atypical precordialgia, palpitations, neuro-dystonic disorders, dizziness and even fainting spells, intense asthenia and slight dyspnea after effort.[20]

Atypical precordialgia, which dominates on the left with needle pain, responds well to betablocking agents, but not to nitroglycerin. Palpitations correspond to the cardiac rhythm problems spoken of as part of the Shao Yang terrain. When we examine such a patient by auscultation, we hear a click that sounds like the opening of a valvular prosthesis. It may be proto-, tele- or mesosystolic and corresponds to the prolapse of the mitral valve. It is followed by a systolic murmur, which is often musical (like the cry of a goose) and signals regurgitation into the auricle through the deficient valve:

> The mitral valve is at first tight, then unfolds, goes beyond its goal, stretches, snaps, leaks and murmurs.[21]

The evolution of this syndrome, which we may no longer consider benign, involves three dangers. The first is mitral insufficiency, whose complications are rare but possible.[22] The second is bacterial endocarditis and the third is the danger of cardiac rhythm irregularities. There is a risk of sudden death if the problem is due to the desynchronization of repolarization. The family case history is of the utmost importance in these cases. As indicated, classical treatment involves the prescription of betablocking agents. In Chinese medicine, the dystonic and neurotonic context immediately brings the Jue Yin temperament to mind[23] and signals common problems of liver and pericardium meridians. We read in the *Su Wen* that the ''liver nourishes the muscles sustaining the heart.''[24]

This relationship between the liver (zu jue yin) and the heart, in which the pericardium meridian (shou jue yin) is the link, is even more explicit and suggestive in the disturbances due to energy imbalance in the liver. In the nineteenth chapter of the *Su Wen,* ''On Life Principles and Pulse Manifestations of True Energy,'' we find the following discussion:

> The Yellow Emperor asked, ''The pulse of spring is wiry. How can this be?''
>
> Qi Bo replied, ''The pulse of spring corresponds to the liver, the East, Wood. It is the birth of all creatures. Its qi is supple, light, smooth and stretches straight ahead like a young sprout. For this reason it is called wiry like a bowstring. If it is not so, it is pathological.''
>
> The Yellow Emperor asked, ''What type of pulse is contrary to the pulse just described?''
>
> Qi Bo replied, ''If the qi arrives full and violent, it is in excess, and the disease is external. When the qi arrives empty and tiny, this is a deficiency, and the disease indicated is internal.''[25]
>
> The Yellow Emperor asked, ''What is this illness like?''
>
> Qi Bo replied, ''The deficiency illness causes chest pains radiating to the back and descending down the flanks to where the fullness will abide.''[26]

We notice a correspondence with cardiac symptomology on the one hand, and with genital pathology, dystonia and spasmophilia on the other. We may interpret these latter syndromes as deficiencies that are expressed energetically as the descent of blood, along with its concentration in the area of the pelvis and the surging of the energy upwards.

Understanding these physiological movements of blood and energy is essential to a full comprehension of Jue Yin. In Chapter 21 of the *Su Wen* we find precious information on this subject. The title of this chapter is translated by Chamfrault as ''Relationships Between the Meridians and the Arteries'' and by Nguyen Van Nghi as ''Special Study of the Jing Mo (Primary Channels).'' It discusses the relative values of blood and energy within the meridians (jing mai):

192

The Yellow Emperor asked, ''The conditions of life, activity and rest, health,[27] are subject to variation in a man. Do the energy and the blood in the jing mo undergo related modifications during these variations?''

Qi Bo answered, ''Fear, anger, fatigue, work and rest may influence the energy and the blood in the jing mo and modify them.''[28]

Qi Bo goes on to discriminate between the different origins of dyspnea and of perspiration. In his conclusion on dyspnea, Qi Bo says:

This is why we say that diagnosis is above all an examination of the emotional and physical states to find out whether the patient is strong or weak, courageous or fearful.[29]

Concerning perspiration:

When fear has taken away the jing,[30] the perspiration comes from the heart.

When fear makes the patient run away, the perspiration comes from the liver.

Following these general observations, there is a discussion of pulse readings, meridian by meridian[32] and of their clinical significance. Qi Bo says of Jue Yin:

When the energy of first Yin arrives all by itself it is a reflection on the conditions of decreasing Yin; with true energy in deficiency and heart pain, upsurging energy accumulates below the heart and presses upon the lungs in the upper region, causing white sweats, which should be treated by a proper diet and medicinal herbs and by needling the lower shu point {taichong, LV-3}.[34]

In conclusion, we may say that Barlow's disease or a severe cardiac erethism is caused by an internal liver disorder and not by perverse energy. It is determined either by the emotions, by the patient's living or working conditions, or inadequate rest. This disorder is signaled by a deficiency of the ''true'' or pure energy (jing qi) of the liver that Nguyen Van Nghi calls the Yin root. This deficiency causes the upsurging of the Yang root. This is generally expressed in the following terms: Wood is transformed into Fire and surges upwards. This disorder also affects the pericardium meridian.

In a way, Jue Yin dissociates with an excess of shou jue yin (pericardium) and a deficiency of zu jue yin (liver). This is why the pulse of the whole meridian is affected. We may express this in still another way: there is a deficiency of blood, which is concentrated in the lower part of the body, and a surge of energy towards the upper part of the body. The liver no longer nourishes the muscles sufficiently, which in turn fail to sustain the heart. Clinically we see this as precordialgia in a dystonic context; vain or white perspiration. The exact translation given by Nguyen Van Nghi, ''depressing pain in the heart,'' is a perfect image of the mitral valve that prolapses. As we have seen, the treatment is tripartite, involving medication, diet and acupuncture.

193

In acupuncture, taichong (LV-3) corresponds to the element Earth and to a mild flavor that balances the excess Yang of the liver (Earth insults Wood). The *Da Cheng* indicates this point for "pale complexion and eyes, pain in the heart."[35] In cases of cardiac rhythm irregularities and disharmony of repolarization, with acute symptoms, fainting and danger of sudden death, I feel it is fundamentally necessary to needle the root and the knot of Jue Yin. This condition represents the separation, the rupture of Jue Yin with collapse of the Yin, which no longer sustains the heart, and violent upsurging of the pericardium (Yang). This explains the severity of the arhythmia, which is sometimes fatal.

The semiology of Jue Yin is intimated by Chapter 5 of the *Ling Shu* which deals with the roots and the knots of the meridians.

> The root of Jue Yin is in the point dadun (LV-1). Its concentration, the knot of its energy, is located in the point yutang (CV-18).

> If the Jue Yin axis no longer functions, the Yin meridian is as if knotted.[36]

In the *Da Cheng,* the semiology of dadun (LV-1), the root point of Jue Yin, is "arterial spasm, excess of heart."[37] Soulie de Morant adds, "sudden death, use moxas."[38] Chamfrault quotes, "The body is icy like that of a dead man, cadaverous fainting spell."[39] Given the laterality of the symptoms, we must normally needle this point only on the opposite side — dadun (LV-1) on the right toe — or apply moxas directly, especially if the patient has lost consciousness.

Yutang (CV-18), located on the midline at the level of the third intercostal space, is indicated in case of "malaise in the heart, fullness of the heart that impairs breathing, dyspnea."[40] This point means "jade palace." Chamfrault mentions its other name, juying, which means jade jing, or essence of jade. It is considered by all authors to be the point of concentration of the energy of the liver. The term jade signifies the precious value attached to the concept of jing, or essential energy. The message is clear: this point is able to revive the deficient jing of the liver and reestablish the internal balance of energy.[41]

Treatment of Cardiac Erethism

Apart from mitral valve prolapse, to treat a dystonic terrain and functional cardiac disorders (precordialgia, palpitations), I feel it useful to open the miscellaneous channels chong mai and yin wei mai by needling gongsun (SP-4) and neiguan (PC-6), starting with the couple on the right side. These remove the internal blockage. The same is true of tianchi (PC-1), which gives immediate and excellent results in neurotonic precordialgia. This point, a heavenly window point, enables us to exteriorize the energy blockage spoken of in Chapter 21 of the *Su Wen,* which is the cause of the depressing pain in the heart. It is also an important point in that it is the intersection of the liver and gallbladder meridians.[42] Tianchi (PC-1), "heavenly pond" according to the *Da Cheng,* is recommended in cases of thoracic obstruction of energy.

In treating cardiac rhythm irregularities and tachycardia, we must make mention of the classical indications of ximen (PC-4), neiguan (PC-6) and daling (PC-7). The latter is the dispersion point for excess in the pericardium meridian (shou jue yin). It is also advised in treating fright. Neiguan (PC-6), "internal

194

gate," opens yin wei mai and unblocks the energy of the thorax. In the *Da Cheng* (see Ophthalmology), it is particularly indicated in cardiac problems associated with ophthalmic allergy symptoms. We must also include jianshi (PC-5), a group luo point, when the renal pelvis is congested, which is often the case, or when there are functional ears-nose-throat symptoms such as aphonia or laryngitis.

As far as diet is concerned, the golden rule is to advise the patient to center his diet around cereal grains, which are mild flavored and correspond to Earth, like the point taichong (LV-3).

The third therapeutic aspect, medication, is handled with a prescription of *equisetum arvense* (horse tie).[43]

To recapitulate, the following points are recommended for treatment of this condition: LV-3, BL-18, LV-1, CV-18, PC-1, PC-4, PC-5, PC-6 and PC-7.

Diathesis I and manganese are the corresponding trace element coordinates for this whole cardiac terrain pathology. In functional cardiac disorders, such as "the periodic apparition of palpitations," tachycardia, precordialgia and cardiac instability — which are exaggerated by the patients' emotivity and nervousness — manganese, iodine and cobalt are the trace elements usually prescribed.[44] These "allergic" behaviors are common.

High Blood Pressure and Low Blood Pressure

The dystonic behavior common among Jue Yin subjects is often related to the instability of their blood pressure. This is especially the case among younger subjects who generally have low blood pressure that may alternate with periodically high blood pressure. Around the age of fifty, this situation is reversed and the basic clinical picture becomes high blood pressure. There is an undeniable influence exerted by the pericardium along with the liver, the mechanism of which is the same as that which causes cardiac instability and rhythm irregularities. The therapeutic role of zhongchong (PC-9) is well known. It is the tonification point of the pericardium, to be needled in cases of low blood pressure with fainting or lipothymia. This is one of the reanimation points. Soulie de Morant mentions zhongchong (PC-9) for "high or low blood pressure."[45] In both cases, the liver is involved. The symptoms that define dystony may be just as well applied to instability of the blood pressure: "forgetfulness, panic, confusion, dizziness."[46]

High blood pressure is defined in Chinese medicine as an excess of the liver, or of the Yang of the liver which is upsurgent.[47] This excess of Yang implies, again, an insufficiency of the Yin root of the organ, which is to say the failure of the Yin function, or jing qi, of the liver. This physiopathology may be compared to the Western definition of the physiological mechanism involved in some cases of high blood pressure, those in which the catabolic function of the hormonal steroids is troubled. This is what may occur when some Jue Yin women take birth control pills.

> The estrogen component in oral contraceptives may cause secondary high blood pressure among certain women, by stimulating the hepatic synthesis of the substrate of renin, angiotensinogen, which in turn activates the synthesis of increased quantities of angiotensin, and secondarily, of aldosterone.[48]

The synthesis of angiotensinogen in the liver constitutes the Yang root of the organ, which may be compared to the hepatobiliary function. In this mechanism, cholesterol represents the basis for the synthesis of various adrenal steroids, among which is aldosterone.

Besides interrupting the use of the contraceptive, the Chinese treatment (acupuncture, diet and medication) is, in this case, identical to that recommended for cardiac instability. I add to this prescription the trace element manganese. To quote Menetrier:

> Low blood pressure, which may be accompanied by symptoms associated with poor tolerance, and especially high blood pressure, which causes discomfort, are a part of Diathesis I.

> In this diathesis, and later in life, high blood pressure follows migraines[49] and is accompanied by symptoms of poor tolerance.[50]

> Manganese and iodine are almost always effective in improving the tolerance to high blood pressure.[51]

Venous Pathology of the Lower Limbs

Jue Yin is certainly related to the venous circulation and particularly to the lower limbs and the pelvic region where the circulation drains towards the heart through the vena cava system. It is as if there were a balance between the cavular and portal circulations that was maintained by the liver. This relationship between the lower limbs, the pelvic region and the liver makes women patients particularly vulnerable to this pathology, to varicosity and to acute phlebitis — conditions that are directly related to the episodes of genital life and to surgery of the pelvic region.

• Varicosity and Phlebitis

In the *Ling Shu,* we are told that "the liver produces the blood," and that "the pericardium governs all the vessels."[52] In clinical practice, we find that Jue Yin subjects (women more often than men) have particularly sensitive venous systems. This is particularly notable in the lower limbs in the region of the saphenous veins. Venous ectasia corresponds, in Chinese medicine, to an insufficiency of energy in the liver and in its meridian zu jue yin, which is sometimes accompanied by portal congestion. There is also a possibility of hemorrhoids or of pelvic congestion. In Chinese medicine, a deficiency of Yin of the liver causes a "concentration of blood downwards," and a surging of energy upwards. This is why the ancient texts quoted by Soulie de Morant state, "The liver is generally deficient in cases of jinmo chong chang {varicose veins}. Tonify ququan {LV-8}."[53] Ququan is the tonification point of the liver. It corresponds to the element Water.

Blood and energy blockage, with a deficiency of Yin energy in the lower limbs because of the liver, creates warmth in the feet. This is because of the insufficiency of Yin energy (cold) and the relative excess of Yang energy (warm) that descends through the Yang meridians. In the *Su Wen* chapter devoted to jue, energy blockage, the Yellow Emperor asked,

"How can energy blockages be warm or cold?"

Qi Bo replied, "Deficiency of qi in the three Yang channels of the leg causes a cold jue,[54] in the three Yin channels it causes a warm jue."[55]

"Why, then," asked Huang Di, "in the warm jue, does the heat begin in the soles of the feet?"

"In the Yin channels," replied Qi Bo, "the qi meets under the foot and concentrates in the hollow."[56]

This hollow is yongquan (KI-1), whose name means "gushing fountain."

Other lower limb points are indicated in the ancient texts; among them are zhubin (KI-9) for zu shao yin, shanggiu (SP-5) for zu tai yin and futu (ST-32). Zhubin, located on the inside of the calf, is the terminal point of yin wei mai, a Yin shunt miscellaneous channel linked to Jue Yin. Its symptomology is "shan: pain in the calf."[57] Shanggiu (SP-5), the jing point of zu tai yin, is mentioned for "edema, pain inside the thigh;[58] shan."[59] As for futu (ST-32), located on a bulge on the musculus rectus femoris, it is considered by the *Da Cheng* to be the "meeting point of the arteries and the veins."[60] Its semiology is "edema in the legs because of humidity," but also "all gynecological problems, in any region."[61] Soulie de Morant indicates this point for "varicosity, phlebitis, paraphlebitis and the venous return circulation."[62]

In circulatory problems in which the legs are numb or go to sleep, we are almost always able to find an imbalance in the transverse luo of the liver with a gallbladder deficiency. These symptoms correspond to the indications for ligou (LV-5), a luo point, and qiuxu (GB-40), a yuan point.[63]

The points indicated for the venous pathologies of the lower limbs are: LV-8, KI-9, SP-5, ST-32, LV-5 and GB-40.

Menetrier classifies varicose veins, as well as acrocyanotic circulatory disorders, in the dystonic diathesis (manganese-cobalt).[64] According to his experience, cases treated from the beginning and cases of dysesthesia in the hands and feet[65] improve "all of the functional symptoms" through the action of manganese-cobalt, sulfur, cobalt and magnesium.

Arteriole Pathology of the Skin

To demonstrate the role of the liver and of its jing function in relation to the blood vessels, it is useful to describe telangiectasia. Its classification is, according to Fitzpatrick:

A particular form of telangiectasia is known by the name of spider angioma. In liver disorders, a rare lesion, to which are associated vascular stars, makes up the telangiectatic "net" or "web," a little red spot formed by a lacing of fine veins that disappears under vitropression. We sometimes find spider angiomas in children and adults, often no more than three at a time, which have no pathological meaning. But there may be a great many of them during pregnancy, after taking contraceptive pills or in cases of thyrotoxicosis.[66] The presence of spider angiomas in great numbers or in a bulging form

197

indicates the possibility of a subjacent liver problem, an alcoholic cirrhosis, for example. The multiplication of these spider angiomas often indicates the evolution of a hepatic process, one that is true in more than half of atrophic micronodular cirrhoses, or toxic cirrhoses. We do not yet understand the mechanism that is responsible for the development of spider angiomas in hepatic affections and the role that the metabolism of estrogens in the liver may play is not clear.[67]

The whole range of cardiovascular pathologies associated with Jue Yin, which includes tachycardia, cardiac rhythm irregularities, high and low blood pressure, fainting, mitral prolapse, varicosity and telangiectasia, indicates the clear relationships that exist between the metabolic functions of the liver, vasomotricity, cardiac conduction and vascular endothelium.

In Chinese medicine, these relationships are grouped in a single meridian (Jue Yin) and in terms of qualitative Yin-Yang, blood-energy, jing qi-rong qi and qi disturbances. These relationships also demonstrate indirectly, by way of energetic logic, the incidents and accidents that may occur in emotional or stressful situations, or those due to overwork, nutritional errors or iatrogenic medication errors.

In a study of 23,000 women, C.R. Kay has shown that cardiovascular accidents were *five times as common* among women taking oral contraceptives as among women practicing other contraceptive techniques.[68] Use of a contraceptive pill is formally contraindicated for women who are deficient in antithrombin III.[69] In anatomopathological disorders of the blood vessels and in patients under the influence of synthetic estrogens, we find a thickening of the intima (muscular and fibrous dysplasia) and, less commonly, arteriosclerotic lesions. As for the well known cases of dyslipidosis among women taking pregestational estrogens, it is now considered that there is a predisposition in certain women that is revealed when the contraceptive is taken, and that, when the medication is stopped, regresses in only one third of all cases.

All these concepts may be grouped under the notion of temperament, or of predisposed terrains. It is not surprising to find that it is Jue Yin women who run the greatest risks and are simultaneously likely to have trouble tolerating oral contraceptives or have periodic high blood pressure problems, anxiety attacks, tachycardia, lipothymia, paresthesia, insomnia, heaviness in the lower limbs, pelvic pain or dyspareunia. All these are symptoms that are not as solely "psychological" as we are so often told.

Cardiac Liver

The hepatomegalia of right-sided or global cardiac insufficiency is not, of course, the illness of a specific temperament, but rather the logical outcome of the evolution of cardiomegaly. This was known by the ancient Chinese. In Chapter 21 of the *Ling Shu,* "Perturbation of the Energy Circulation," we read:

> When a patient has pain in the heart and his face is pale, he hasn't even the time to sigh during the day because he suffers so much; this is the symptom of liver disorder and, in this case, we must needle xingjian {LV-2} and taichong {LV-3}.[70]

According to the law of the five elements, when the son is ill, the illness spreads to the mother. This evolution is classic, although infrequent, and explains the title of the chapter quoted above. Xingjian (LV-2) and taichong (LV-3) are the rong and shu points of the liver. These points are to be needled when the organ and the meridian are diseased. The gravity of the explicit symptoms is great: precordialgia, severe dyspnea (even at rest) and pallor.

The *Da Cheng* confirms these symptoms. For example, for taichong, we read, "Pain in the heart and in the liver, with a tight pulse stretched like the string of a violin,[71] the complexion is as pale as a condemned person.[72] In cases of hepatomegalia and cardiac hepatalgia, the mu point of the liver, qimen (LV-14), is to be needled: "Intense dyspnea that prevents the patient from going to bed and sleeping, unbearable pain in the chest; energy that accumulates in the flank."[73]

Respiratory Pathology: Asthma and Allergic Rhinitis

These disorders are studied in further detail in the Shao Yang and Tai Yin chapters.

One specific form of excess asthma is that which is due to an excess of the lung and a deficiency of energy in the liver. The original imbalance may be in the lung. The temperament in this case is Tai Yin-Metal with a clear hyposthenic profile. However, this profile corresponds more often to deficiency of the lung (see Tai Yin). The deficiency may also be in the liver; in this case, the subject is Jue Yin.

There are numerous liver-lung relationships in Chinese medicine. "The production and transformation of the energy of the liver depends on the energy of the lungs," said Zhang Zhi Cong.[74] The controlling cycle influences this relationship — Metal saws Wood. On the other hand, according to the energy cycle, zu jue yin, the liver meridian, is last in the order of the twelve meridians and passes its spent energy to the lung. These two connections explain the intricate ties between the lungs and the liver and the difficulty we have therapeutically ameliorating this vicious cycle.[75] This is why the diathetic theorists developed a mixed diathesis — the arthroinfectious diathesis. In this diathesis we find a mixture of asthmas, rhinitis and eczemas.

The excess asthma etiology of Jue Yin patients is thus complexly combined with a deficiency of the Yin root of the liver, which is accompanied by the upsurging of the Yang root and abnormal production and circulation of wei energy. This excess production explains the amount of histamine that is produced in the liver, in the skin and in the lungs of such patients.[76] Allergic asthma also involves an abnormal synthesis of E-immunoglobulins in response to allergens that are not normally allergens. This, too, may be linked to a disturbance of wei qi (defensive energy) which is related to the liver. The allergen is nothing; the liver is everything. This explains the frequently seasonal rhythm of this type of asthma, with outbreaks in the spring.

The perverse energy at work is the wind.[77] Our treatment will therefore focus on the prevention of penetration by perverse wind, and thus on strengthening the

199

organ. The term "perverse wind" represents the allergen in the Chinese dialectic. Its point of penetration is fengmen (BL-12), "the door of the wind," indicated in the *Da Cheng* for "frequent sneezing, epistaxis, all the nasal disorders, abundant rhinorrhea, dyspnea, bronchitis and even whooping cough."[78] The terminal cephalic pathway of the liver meridian that leads to baihui (GB-20) and comes back down to energize the eye, the sinus, the nose and the lips is the means of explaining the frequent association of rhinitis and conjunctivitis and symptoms such as sneezing, stuffed nose and rhinorrhea. From fengmen (BL-12) on, Tai Yang involuntarily carries the perverse wind energy into the region of the head, to the nose and to the respiratory system where the insufficiency of liver meridian energy allows it to enter. This point must therefore be needled, or rather cauterized, as must feishu (BL-13), the shu point of the lung, "dispersion point for lung disorders; pain in the flesh with pruritis and abundant perspiration,"[79] and ganshu (BL-18), the shu point of the liver.

In addition to cauterizing BL-12, BL-13 and BL-18, we must needle taichong (LV-3), the "supreme assault," which gets the energy in the liver meridian moving and which is recommended by Bian Que in all the affections of the nose as well as for "fullness in the chest and sides." It may be necessary to disperse the lung more directly and to tonify the liver by needling chize (LU-5), the dispersion point of the lung, as well as ququan (LV-8), the tonification point of the liver.

To recapitulate, the points recommended are: BL-12, BL-13, LV-3, LV-8, LU-5; also GV-20, LI-20, GB-20 and LI-4.

According to practitioners of diathetic medicine, this form of asthma and exogenous allergic rhinitis (caused by pollen, dust, animal hair and other exogenous factors) is best treated with manganese in association with sulfur and, symptomatically, phosphorus. This treatment must be given with care and according to a subtle protocol[80] as reoccurrences are common and sometimes serious.

Acupuncture treatment and the association of acupuncture with trace element therapy give positive, consistent and long lasting results. Some cases can be totally cured. In all cases, we can avoid symptomatic treatments and desensitization. Acupuncture in these cases is spectacular in its results and the symptomatic effects are immediate.[81]

Gastroenterological Pathology

It may be interesting to take a closer look at the symbolism of the liver and its qi within the ancient Chinese writings. Remember, the liver is related to the element Wood and to the celestial energy of the East:

> The wind is a mysterious heavenly phenomenon.[82] For man, there is Tao. On earth, it is the transformation, source of the five flavors. The heavenly phenomenon engenders the spirit, the mutations of which are the energies. The spirit is the wind of heaven that is wood on earth and muscles. Among the forms of qi, it is that which softens. Among the viscera, it is the liver.[83]

This passage indicates many of the physiological and metabolic connotations of the liver — regulation, participation in thermo-regulation, circulation and muscular activity. This text does not distinguish between the physiological functions of the liver and the metaphysical aspect, Tao, the individual path that man must follow, and the mystery of heaven, which is the program written before his birth.[84]

According to the various translators, the mu point of the liver is called the "door of the times," "the door of the period," or "the door of hope." This is qimen (LV-14).[85] Speaking strictly medically, the observations made by the ancient Chinese concerning the volume and position of the organ lead us directly to gastroenterology:

> If one's liver is small and firm, one has no pain in the sides of the chest; if it is big, one often has pains in the diaphragm, and in the sides of the chest.

> If it is positioned higher than usual, one often has malaise in the chest.[86] If it is positioned lower than normal, one is uncomfortable in the stomach. If one has a delicate liver, there are frequent digestive problems.[87]

Gastritis, Ulcers

The element Wood in general and the liver in particular are frequently implicated in cases of stomach inflammation (gastritis and ulcers), as we may conclude from the above passage, as well as from the etiologies of gastritis presented in the *Trung Y Hoc* from Hanoi.[88] Of six etiologies mentioned in the text, three concern the liver:

- Concentration of the energy of the liver;

- Concentration of the energy of the liver with deficiency of the spleen;

- Excess heat of the liver and stomach.

The mechanism is not complicated: excess of the liver subdues the spleen and the stomach (Wood controls Earth).

The psychosomatic origin of the disorder is a significant part of the mechanism:

> When the pain is of psychosomatic origin, as is the case especially in inorganic gastralgia, needle ganshu (BL-18), the shu point of the liver, and taichong (LV-3).[89]

This tells us something about the frequency of this physiopathology that is clearly psychosomatic, especially among Jue Yin patients.[90] The choice of taichong (LV-3), the shu point corresponding to the element Earth, enables us to balance the excess of the liver by stimulating Earth. It is said of this point that it disperses, or harmonizes, the energy of the liver. This point also corresponds to the sweet (or mild) flavor that insults acidic or acrid flavors. These are particularly aggressive to the gastric mucus and should be avoided. We read in Chapter 22 of the *Su Wen:*

On jai yi days, fir and bamboo 1-2, the liver suffers from excess, it is contracted. One can relax it with sweet foods.[91]

Apart from ganshu (BL-18) and taichong (LV-3), it is useful to use pishu (BL-20), weishu (BL-21) and yanglingquan (GB-34) in association; and locally, zhongwan (CV-12) and qimen (LV-14), the mu point of the liver.

According to Menetrier:

Functional stomach problems, such as acidity, heartburn, pain and discomfort after meals, are part of the allergic behavior, although the lesions may be impossible to treat.[92]

Manganese is therefore the Wood trace element to prescribe. It must be said here that unlike treatment with trace elements, which is not effective in cases of severe inflammation (ulcers), acupuncture is particularly effective against ulcers and all other gastralgia, even in the most acute attacks. In my experience, I have been able to calm the most severe inflammations primarily through the use of hydro-puncture with injections of vitamin C, or better yet, using bilateral injections of redistilled water. A single point is treated at each session, for example, GB-34 or BL-18, or locally zhongwan (CV-12), or at the most painful points of ren mai (often xiawan, CV-10) "the lower door of the stomach," which corresponds to the duodenum and the duodenal bulb. This is continued for from two to five sessions with a one or two day interval between each. Needling a total of 12 to 15 of the other points in following sessions consolidates the treatment and delays or avoids recurrence.[93]

Minor Hepatic Insufficiency

Minor hepatic insufficiency is the daily bread of French doctors, and is a cultural trait specific to France as well as a subject of mockery at the hands of Anglo-Saxon hepatologists.

If a patient complains of eczema,[94] of a tenacious sinusitis, of "liver attacks" with vomiting, of headache, or of a mere migraine, the liver becomes the scapegoat for all these disorders, especially if the vomiting is bilious and if there is pain in the right side of the trunk. Clinical and biochemical investigations are nonetheless negative. If gallbladder x-rays happen to show an anomaly of form or of function, these patients are in danger of being told they must undergo an operation.

Often, after all, choleretics or repeated duodenal intubations bring such relief that we are obliged to admit the existence of a certain link between these disorders and the hepatobiliary function. For, although the hepatic cell itself is still normal in these conditions, it seems probable that the patients fail to properly excrete bile, and their digestion suffers.

It has been shown that their synthesis of endogenous cholecystokinin is insufficient. The inappropriate secretion of other digestive hormones — secretin, pancreozymin, gastrin, etc. — may play a certain part.[95]

This functional symptomology, although it may spare the British Isles, nonetheless seems universal and was known in ancient China and attributed to the same source. In the *Ling Shu* we read, "If the pulse of the liver is very slow, vomiting is frequent."[96] Qi Bo states, in the chapter devoted to jue, "Jue of the liver: abdominal swelling with trouble excreting, sleepiness."[97] These symptoms are in line with the enzyme deficits previously mentioned and the semiology may represent a sort of lingering dyspepsia associated with aerophagia, constipation, postprandial sleepiness and headache. It is halfway between the etiologies of gallbladder excess and spleen deficiency described among the causes of functional colonopathies.

Functional Colonopathies

In this case, the insufficiency of energy of the liver with a blockage of the blood represents a form of transition, rarely isolated, of certain functional right-predominant colonopathies. Nonetheless, the pathologies of an insufficient spleen will finally dominate the clinical picture:

> If the cause of the illness is a chronic wind, the illness will be *xan tiet*,[98] diarrhea with undigested debris.[99]

Zhang Zhi Cong made the following commentary on this passage:

> Wind corresponds to perverse Wood. If it remains within the organism for long, it will offend the spleen-Earth {through the inhibiting cycle, liver-spleen} and will bring on the illness *xian tiet*.[100]

This disorder begins with constipation that soon becomes diarrhea. The two alternate thereafter. There may also be hemorrhoids:

> When the feng {wind} triumphs over man's energy, the energy of the five senses is exhausted.[101]

> If one eats in excess, the circulation of the blood increases and the liver becomes congested, which affects the intestines and causes hemorrhoids.[102]

This remarkable passage shows once again the subtlety and precision of the ancients' powers of observation. However, the original text is not quite as clear as the Chamfrault translation would have us believe. Nguyen Van Nghi translates the same passage as follows:

> The invited wind infiltrates the energy. . . if at the same time there is nutrition in excess, the muscles and the blood vessels will be stretched out of shape, causing dysentery and hemorrhoids.[103]

Husson's version is just about the same:

> When the illness is caused by overeating, the muscles and the blood vessels are stretched, we notice a chang bi {bloody foam in the stools} and hemorrhoids.[104]

Nguyen Van Nghi comments, "The text is speaking of the muscles and blood vessels of the stomach and intestines."

The anatomical imprecision of the ancient Chinese allows us to make all sorts of interpretations regarding abdominal muscles, the portal system, the arterial system of the celiac trunk, smooth muscles and digestive tract mucous membranes and those of the rectum. One observation is certain: there is a distention of "muscles and blood vessels" due to overeating, and the pathology of the abdominal muscles is related to the liver. The same is true of the blood vessel pathology due to plethora and logically involving the portal system. This in no way diminishes the value of the ancient Chinese observations that include notions of cyclic rhythms never studied here in the West.

The treatment of all these functional disorders — dyspepsia, drowsiness, vomiting, constipation, diarrhea, flatulence, and hemorrhoids — is the same. We must therefore assure the opening of the key point of chong mai, gongsun (SP-4) and of yin wei mai, neiguan (PC-6). The first of these points corresponds to the luo point of zu tai yin (the spleen meridian) whose symptomology, whether in excess or deficient, is flatulence. The second, neiguan (PC-6), which means "internal gate," is indicated in all symptoms of thoracic blockage or blockage of the transdiaphragm abdominothoracic passage. Their action is remarkable and rapid. Ganshu (BL-18) is useful, but pishu (BL-20) is more highly recommended for dyspepsia.[105]

The mu points of the liver and spleen are also needled. Zhangmen (LV-13), the mu point of the spleen, is indicated for these symptoms:

> The patient eats but doesn't digest. Little piglet runs around in the belly {the image of colic pain}, belly swollen like a drum.[106]

Qimen (LV-14), the mu point of the liver, is also indicated when "little piglet runs up and down in the belly, and diarrhea."[107] In association, we may needle yanglingquan (GB-34), taichong (LV-3), zusanli (ST-36) or sanyinjiao (SP-6), according to whether the symptomology is hepatobiliary or gastropancreatic. Taichong (LV-3) is indicated for "constipation with blood in the stools, diarrhea." This means it is useful in cases of hemorrhoids and for the symptoms of alternating constipation and diarrhea. Zhongfeng (LV-4) is the jing point of the meridian, corresponding to the element Metal and inhibiting the wind with dryness and the acrid with the hot and spicy. It enables us to protect the colon against the aggressivity of the liver, just as taichong (LV-3) protects the stomach and the pancreas, as we have seen in gastralgia. Its semiology is "Malaise after eating, pain and swelling in the belly (or groin)."[108]

Last, but far from least, ququan (LV-8) is an essential point for treating deficiencies in the liver.[109] It is the tonification point. Its semiology includes "fullness in the belly and the flanks, diarrhea, dysentery with pus and blood, intestinal hemorrhage." It is therefore indicated when diarrhea prevails over constipation. It is also effective against acute dysenteriform syndromes and seasonal diarrhea that is not related to functional colonopathy.[110] Rectal hemorrhage with stools that are more or less foamy (with mucus) is also treated by this point. This etiology may correspond, among other dysenteric syndromes, to the onset of an ulcerative rectocolitis where the first manifestation was uveitis or some isolated disorder of the liver. In this case, the perverse energy is wind cold (see ulcerative rectocolitis in the chapter devoted to Shao Yin).

In summary, functional hepatic disorders, whether or not they are associated with colonopathy or hemorrhoids, are to be treated with the following points: BL-18, BL-20, LV-13, LV-14, LV-3, GB-34, ST-36, SP-6, LV-4, LV-8, SP-4 and PC-6. Acupuncture treatment of these disorders is remarkably effective and is enhanced when associated with trace element therapy.

There is a consistent correlation with diathetic medicine, as Menetrier classifies digestive disorders, with morning nausea, painful digestion, biliary vomiting, right-sided colitic type intestinal problems under Diathesis I (manganese).[111]

Hepatic Colic

These disorders are studied in detail in the chapter devoted to the pathology of Shao Yang and involve the gallbladder as much as the liver.

Viral Hepatitis

More often than not, viral hepatitis is a benign disorder and cures itself in 80 to 85 percent of all cases. The remaining 15 to 20 percent of the cases present complications that are multiple, sometimes serious and even fatal. For this reason, the pathology deserves close attention. In the benign cases, as no specific treatment has been developed outside of acupuncture, we believe that it is worth considering the contribution made by acupuncture treatment.

Once again we may note that knowledge of the patient's temperament is of considerable significance and importance. Among patients who suffer or have previously suffered from viral hepatitis there is a clear correlation with temperament. 65 to 70 percent of these patients are Jue Yin. In decreasing order of frequency, the remaining 30 percent come from Shao Yang temperaments, then Tai Yin, with a small percentage of occurrences among the other temperaments.

What is more important is that in the vast majority of these cases, those patients who have had viral hepatitis in the past show a much higher incidence of the symptoms and disorders associated with the Jue Yin temperament. Typically, this is the case *since the time of their hepatitis,* no matter that their symptoms are non-hepatobiliary digestive, emotional, gynecological, neurological or allergic. It goes without saying that the studies made of the after effects of this pathology have concentrated exclusively on the clinical and biological aspects of the hepatobiliary sphere, with the exception of asthenia. Personally, I feel that the aftereffects of viral hepatitis are more varied and more numerous than those commonly studied. This is why it is essential to understand the physiopathology of this affection according to the precepts of Chinese medicine and to develop a systematic treatment with acupuncture. The modern Shanghai authors confirm the importance of this idea.[112]

Acute viral hepatitis is a generalized infection that electively attacks the liver. There exist two forms that are clinically identical but immunologically different: hepatitis A and hepatitis B. Both forms may be transmitted orally or parenterally. Hepatitis A is known as infectious hepatitis, short incubation hepatitis and MS1 hepatitis. Hepatitis B goes by the name of serum hepatitis,[113] long incubation hepatitis, MS2 hepatitis and hepatitis with an antigen associated with hepatitis or the Australia antigen.[114] The modern authors in Shanghai refer to the chapters of the *Su Wen* concerning "pain in the sides" and consider viral hepatitis a disorder of the liver and the spleen, due to a heat-humidity perverse energy that is more or less associated with the wind (feng).[115] The wind is certainly involved here, given the target, the liver, the organ associated with the element Wood.[116]

I refer to several chapters of the *Su Wen* and *Ling Shu* to define this affection. Chapter 19 of the *Su Wen,* "The Perfect Mechanism of the Pure Energy of the Organs," in the seventh paragraph dealing with the feng and with its various manifestations, is particularly important. The whole passage is as follows:

> The feng {wind} is the first cause of all illnesses. When the feng han {cold wind} attacks man, the hairs stand up, the pores close, giving fever. To disperse it, we must use sudorification.
>
> When it penetrates into the jing luo, it causes paresthesia or painful swelling. To disperse it, we must apply hot compresses and cupping glasses, or use moxas or needles.
>
> If there is no treatment, the wind gains the lungs, causing a fei qi {pulmonary obstruction} manifested by coughing and a rising of energy.
>
> If there is no treatment, it gains the liver, causing a gan qi {hepatic obstruction} manifested by pain in the flanks, vomiting of food. In this case we must use massages, moxas and needles.
>
> If there is no treatment it gains the spleen, causing a pi feng {splenic wind} manifested by dan {jaundice} with a sensation of frightening abdominal heat and dark yellow urine. We must use massages, herbs and baths.
>
> If there is no treatment, it passes to the kidneys and causes a san ha with cloudy white urine. This disease is also called co {affection that spreads in depth}. We must use massage and herbs.
>
> If there is no treatment, it passes to the heart and causes khe {painful muscular contractions}. We must use thermoacupuncture, in the absence of which, within ten days, death follows.
>
> If the perverse wind is transmitted directly from the kidneys to the heart, then immediately to the lungs, it causes han nue, the cold-heat disease, and death, according to the rule, after three years. This is the evolutive order of the illness, and our therapy should be appropriate.
>
> However, if the illness comes on like lightning, we cannot base our treatment on this order. The order can also be disturbed in cases where its appearance is facilitated by emotional problems.[117]

The above text calls for several comments. First, it shows the order of attack of the organs by the wind. The lung is first to be attacked, after the jing luo, with respiratory symptoms, then the liver, then the spleen and only then do we see jaundice, which signals the disorder as a problem related to Earth.[118] This would lead us to believe that the passage of the common bile duct through the pancreas and its entry into the duodenum in the oddi sphincter depends on the energy of the spleen-pancreas, and that obstructive jaundice is due to a disorder of this energy.

In the pre-jaundice phase of hepatitis, particularly in hepatitis A, we find a fever ranging between 102° and 104° with flu-like symptoms: cough, coryza and pharyngitis.[118] These symptoms are accompanied by, or preceded by, myalgia with stiffness in the muscles that does correspond to luo disorders: "paresthesia, painful swelling." This can tend to lead the diagnosis astray, since the symptoms are so much like those of the flu.

In the second stage, the liver is attacked. We note nausea, vomiting and hepatalgia. In the third stage we find jaundice with dark urine, something like dark beer. This signals retention and that the spleen is affected. More exactly, the pancreas and its head and the passage of the common bile duct are affected. At this stage the overall condition of the patient is affected by asthenia (to a greater or lesser degree), by anorexia and often a weight loss of from six to eleven pounds.[119] These three signs together are pathognomonic of Tai Yin disorders and especially concern the spleen (see Tai Yin). American authors have declared that "a distaste of tobacco is a common and curious symptom of this illness."[120] This same symptom is found in cases of gastric cancer and shows the relationship between different disorders associated with the element Earth.[121] Upon examination, we also notice a splenomegalia in 20 percent of these cases.[122]

Many Tai Yin symptoms are found in the pre-jaundice phase of hepatitis. This lasts from 2 to 14 days. However, the respiratory symptoms may be absent and the jaundice may be present from the first. This shows that it is possible, as was mentioned in the *Su Wen,* for the perverse energy to attain the organ directly without going through the whole cycle. Anicteric forms of hepatitis show that the disease may spare the spleen. The intensity of the affection will be determined by the patient's defense system and by the virulence of the perverse energy. In general, it is jaundice that signals the illness. The *Su Wen* and the *Ling Shu* state:

> If the epidermis, the teeth and the fingernails are yellow, this is jaundice; the patient likes to sleep, his urine is the color of mahogany, his pulse is rapid, rough, he loses his appetite.[123]

> If the pulse of the spleen is turbulent, hard and long, and the patient is yellow, the patient lacks energy.[124]

Nonetheless, the Chinese were conscious of the participation of the liver in jaundice and subicteric affections. We read in the chapter of the *Su Wen,* "Normal Pulses":

> A slow and rasping foot pulse[125] indicates that the patient is asthenic.
> ... If the conjunctive tissues are yellow there is a liver problem.[126]

"If the illness comes on like lightning," we read in the text at the beginning of this discussion, "we cannot base our treatment on this order." This is particularly true for cases of hepatitis B, often called "serum hepatitis," or "syringe hepatitis," because of the predominance of parenteral cases. We might say that the patient injects the "perverse energy" directly.[127]

The premonitory symptoms — urticaria, polyarthralgia and migraines — are more often typical of hepatitis B. These symptoms are allergic signals that alert us to the excess of gallbladder energy (see Rheumatology, Dermatology and

Neurology in Shao Yang). This is true even if the pruritis may be otherwise explained by bile salts. In these cases, we may say that the perverse energy has gained the bile ducts and the liver directly. Angioneurotic edema,[128] or measle-like rashes, are other signs of an attack on the gallbladder energy by perverse heat (erythema) with stagnation of the blood in the epidermis and connective tissues. This was the ancient expression indicating an imbalance between energy and blood at the origin of eczema and rashes. This engenders the observation that when there is a pronounced Tai Yin disorder, the perverse wind energy is more often associated with humidity than with heat. When the disorder is Shao Yang (urticaria, migraine, arthralgia), the perverse wind is more often associated with heat.

In the text quoted at the beginning of this discussion, we read, "The order can also be disturbed in cases whose apparition is facilitated by emotional factors." This would tend to explain why some people who are carriers of the Australian antigen don't get hepatitis, or do so only long after exposure.[129] The passage goes on to describe the role of emotional energies:

> Anger is harmful to the liver and determines a state of deficiency.
> The energy of the lungs takes advantage of this to subdue the liver.
> Worry is harmful to the spleen, and determines a state of deficiency.
> The energy of the liver takes advantage of this and subdues the spleen.[130]

According to this, if the illness continues its evolution through the controlling cycle, it will attain the kidney and cause what seems, by the description of the symptoms, to be a renal affection.[131] If it passes from the kidney to the heart, the perverse energy will have gone through the five organs, the full controlling cycle. Traditionally, this represents the exhaustion of the body energy and death. This is why we read that "painful muscular contractures" (*khe* in Vietnamese),[132] which Chamfrault translated as "muscular contractures and blood circulation problems"[133] are present when the wind gains the heart. This may correspond to the myocardias that rarely complicate viral hepatitis.[134] Most often, however, the evolution of common viral hepatitis runs the risk of active chronic hepatitis or of persistent viral hepatitis, which is, fortunately, very rare. Only five to ten percent of hepatitis cases become chronic P.C.H. (persistent chronic hepatitis). Active chronic hepatitis (A.C.H.) seems related to the presence of HB antigens and leads to post-necrotic cirrhosis.

Clinically severe hepatitis, the acute yellow atrophy of the liver, or Rokitansky-Frerichs' disease, was known in ancient medicine as "impetuous jaundice" or "horseback jaundice."[135] Heat perverse energy dominates this form; the nature of heat explains its virulence. It is the equivalent of fulminant purpura, icterohemorrhagic leptospirosis or aseptic meningitis complications that are sometimes associated with viral hepatitis.

> If the spleen is attacked by the Yang, the patient feels that his head is heavy, he has pain in the cheeks and malaise in the heart; his complexion is green;[136] he is nauseous with fever. Then, when the perverse Yang battles with the body, he has pains in the kidneys that make it difficult for him to bend over or to straighten up. There is swelling in the belly and diarrhea. He also has pain in the chin.[137] If the condition gets worse, he will have abundant perspiration, with the

impression that his energy is ascending to the upper part of his body.[138] Then he is in danger of death. In this affliction we must needle the meridians of zu tai yin (spleen) and zu yang ming (stomach).[139]

Treatment in common forms of hepatitis is lacking. There is no specific Western treatment for viral hepatitis in its most usual form. Bedrest and an hypercaloric diet have been commonly suggested, though the notion of a high calorie diet is actually contested.

The best prophylactic treatment, when we know there is contagion, is obviously the sudorification treatment noted in the first paragraph quoted at the beginning of the discussion. This concerns the wind. In this case, needle yuji (LU-10), shaoshang (LU-11), yinbai (SP-1) and dadu (SP-2)[140] as soon as the flu-like or digestive symptoms appear.

Treatment of the jaundice phase involves the perverse energy of wind heat. The Yin symptoms — asthenia, anorexia and loss of weight — tempt us to apply moxa to the points that disperse perverse Yang in the organs: ganshu (BL-18), danshu (BL-19) and pishu (BL-20).[141] The temptation to needle these points is to be avoided. It is likely to cause a loss of energy, which may cause fainting or lipothymia with a drop in blood pressure.[142] Rather, needle zhiyang (GV-9) and dazhui (GV-14), the points indicated by the Shanghai authors as a basic treatment. The importance of zhiyang, because of its physiological and anatomical properties related to the diaphragm and the spleen,[143] is frequently associated with stress. In the *Da Cheng,* zhiyang is indicated for ''loss of energy, the patient doesn't want to talk, jaundice, anemia.'' It is recommended by Bian Que for ''generalized jaundice, with dark urine.''[144] Although the Shanghai authors are not clear in their explanation, I prefer to apply moxa on zhiyang (GV-9) and to needle dazhui (GV-14). We must alternate also zusanli (ST-36), sanyinjiao (SP-6) and yanglingquan (GB-34), or dannangxue (M-LE-23)[145] and yinlingquan (SP-9).

In the acute phase, zhongfeng (LI-4) is highly recommended. It is the jing point that corresponds to metal and that enables us to control the wind and reduce the heat. This point, which is mentioned by Pien Cho for treating jaundice, is indicated in the *Da Cheng* for ''generalized jaundice and loss of appetite.''[146] In general, it is better to apply moxa on these points, using a few needles daily — or twice a day, if the general condition of the patient and the retention are serious. Alternate the points chosen. In cases of itching, fengshi (GB-31) is a good replacement for cholestyramine.[147] Most often, patients recuperate rapidly, polyuria is prevented and the asthenia is rapidly cured.

Treatment of aftereffects or complications (including persistent chronic hepatitis and active chronic hepatitis) should utilize all the points treated in the acute phase with the exception of dazhui (GV-14). As well, the rong and shu points of the liver and spleen, xingjian (LV-2), taichong (LV-3), dadu (SP-2) and taibai (SP-3), are used in alternation. I have seen persistent jaundices that had lasted for several months disappear following acupuncture treatment.

Treatment of the fulminant form of hepatitis utilizes renzhong (GV-26).[148] Some of the facial miscellaneous points located on the chin and around the mouth are also employed.[149] The symptomology of renzhong (GV-26), which is indicated in all reanimation circumstances, is mentioned in the *Da Cheng:* ''Epidemic jaundice; the whole body is yellow, the urine is dark.''[150] I feel that considering a mortality rate of 60 to 90 percent, such a specific treatment is worth trying, along with classical measures of reanimation, antibiotic and corticotherapy. It goes without saying that the equipment must be sterile, which is systematic in any case. However minimal the bleeding in acupuncture, we must remember that 0.00004 ml. of blood are sufficient to transmit the hepatitis virus. Caroli tells of long distance runners in Scandinavia having caught the disease simply because of the scratches of briars along the path. It is because of poor hygiene in certain Asian countries that the World Health Organization has classified acupuncture among factors transmitting viral hepatitis.[151] In recapitulation, the points used in the treatment of viral hepatitis are: GV-14, GV-9, BL-18, BL-20, GB-34, LV-2, LV-3, ST-36, SP-6, M-LE-23, LV-4, LU-10, LU-11, SP-1, SP-2, SP-3 and SP-9.

In trace element therapy, Menetrier indicates copper, which is anti-infectious and corresponds with the spleen.[152] This corroborates the ancient Chinese hypothesis that there is an imbalance of this organ in these cases. We may retain the use of this metallic ion in association with acupuncture.

Cirrhosis of the Liver

There are many etiologies of cirrhosis of the liver. Long ago, the Chinese developed the relationship between this degenerative pathology of the liver and body fluid troubles:

> Huang Di asked, ''Please tell me about the symptoms of swelling and distension according to the different organs and bowels.''
>
> Qi Bo replied, ''For the liver, the swelling is in the sides, with pain spreading to the groin.''

In Chapter 4 of the *Ling Shu,* the quality of the liver pulse is correlated with ''body fluid troubles'':

> If the pulse is slightly tense and rapid, energy is accumulated in the sides; one feels as if a cup were upside down on the sides.
>
> If the pulse is slightly slow, there is trouble with the fluids.
>
> If the pulse is slightly small, this is the sign of a degenerative affection. If the pulse is very raspy, there is edema, water overflows all over the body.[154]

We know that these disorders are linked to insufficient albumin synthesis in the liver and that the drop in the plasmatic concentration of this protein results in a loss of osmotic pressure, causing transcapillary exudate.

Corticotherapy is aimed at increasing synthesis of albumin in the liver. However, although this does occur, Alpers and Isselbacher point out, ''They do not significantly modify the plasmatic concentration, which is evidence of the complexity of the interrelationships between synthesis and degradation of plasmatic proteins.''[155] It may be a good idea to combine acupuncture treatment with the prescription of corticoids. The protocol would include moxibustion of ganshu (BL-18), the shu point of the liver, and needling of xingjian (LV-2) and taichong (LV-3), the rong and yu points. This accords to the ancient precept, ''When the organ is diseased, needle the rong and yu points.'' This is the same protocol as that for active chronic hepatitis. For reasons that will be noted in a discussion on ascites (Yang Ming), we also use zusanli (ST-36), xiawan (CV-10), zhongwan (CV-12) and shangwan (CV-13).

Hepatic Coma

The neurological complications associated with hepatic insufficiency and acute atrophy of the liver are described in the *Su Wen:*

> In the hot diseases of the liver the urine turns yellow to start with, then the belly becomes painful and the patient goes to bed with a fever. If the combat {between correct qi and perverse qi} is lively, he is delirious and has convulsions, painful thoracic plethora; his arms and legs are agitated [156] and it is impossible for him to rest calmly. [157]

There follows a discussion of chronobiology with indications of the moment at which the disorder is aggravated or attenuated and an idea of the best time to treat the condition. The chronobiology follows a ten-day cycle:

> The illness is at its worst on the 7th and 8th days; perspiration appears on the first and second days. A backwash of qi may result in death on the 7th and 8th days. We must needle the liver and gallbladder meridians. If there is a backwash of qi, there is headache and vertigo, as the meridian brings the qi to the head. [158]

Muscular Pathologies of the Abdominal Wall

In Chinese medicine inguinal and crural hernias represent a disturbance of blood and energy and an accumulation in the pelvic region known as shan. The term shan covers all accumulation pathologies of the pelvic region, not only hernias, but also certain anuria, pollakiurias, severe infections of the ureter, the penis and the exterior genital organs.

Leung Kwok Po[159] presents the classification of seven types of shan from the work, *Zhu Bing Yuan Hou Lun (The Origin of Diseases)*, written in the year 610 AD: jue shan (stifled hernia), zhen shan (hernia of swelling), han shan (hernia of the liver), qi shan (hernia of the breath), pan shan (umbilical hernia), fu shan (hard hernia) and lang shan (hernia from a blow). The different shan are all related to a disturbance of ren mai (conception vessel) or du mai (governing vessel), which are associated with the liver meridian (zu jue yin). Thus, the liver is closely related to muscular disorders. It is also related because the liver meridian encircles the external genitals and the hernial orifices and follows the median line as far as the navel. The tendinomuscular channel is also concerned in this surface pathology. In addition to an etiological treatment of each shan, dadun (LV-1), taichong (LV-3), sanyinjiao (SP-6) and qihai (CV-6) are needled for this pathology, as well as for hernias.

Direct inguinal hernias, inguino-pubic or inguino-scrotal hernias involve the luo channel of the liver as well:

> The luo channel of the liver begins at ligou {LV-5}, and communicates with the gallbladder meridian.

> This secondary channel passes along the calf, up to the scrotum and to the penis.[160]

The symptomology of energy perturbation is here described as follows: "The scrotum is swollen; in case of excess, the scrotum and penis are elongated."[161] Imbalance in Jue Yin, in the primary channel and in the secondary luo and tendinomuscular channels is part of the pathology of the shan. The disorder is considered globally in terms of imbalance of blood and energy. Inguinal hernias correspond to the two final shan, tui shan and hu shan. Leung Kwok Po indicates their physiology and symptomology. Tui shan is "the attack of humidity against Jue Yin, and leads to a blockage of blood." The symptoms include "swelling in the scrotum for men; for women, swelling in the groin {labia majus pudendi}, but without pain and without itching." Hu shan is "an accumulation of cold, humidity or mucus in the scrotum caused by a deficiency of energy or to physical overwork." The symptoms are "swelling of the scrotum which disappears when the patient is lying down" (reducable hernia). In addition to the acupuncture points mentioned for tui shan, needle zhongfeng (LV-4), ligou (LV-5) and yinlingquan (SP-9); for hu shan, fenglong (ST-40) and jimai (LV-12).[162] It is interesting to note that these protocols are useful when surgery is contraindicated, particularly in the case of the enfeebled elderly.

Urinary Pathology

A disturbance of the energy in Jue Yin may lead to pelvic congestion and cause urinary difficulties as well as genital problems. No hard and fast distinction is made between the two in Chinese medicine. These disorders may be isolated, associated or may alternate, as they are considered in pulsology and semiology. One paragraph in Chapter 49 of the Su Wen[163] serves as the best introduction to this nosology:

> Regarding Jue Yin in orchitis and gynecologic tumors: Jue Yin is related to the number five {of the twelve terrestrial branches}. The third month is that of Yin within Yang. The xie {perverse energy} is in the interior, causing pain and swelling of the lower abdomen.

> The third month gives the impulse to the resplendency of the creatures, which bend like the branches under the weight of new vegetation: pain in the genitals and vesicles. The yin is still abundant, the dilated vessels are no longer permeable. This is what is called tui long shan.[164]

Other passages in the Su Wen show that it is the liver meridian, zu jue yin, which is involved in this pathology. The distinction between urinary and genital disorders is as much a question of symptoms as of physiology. The physiological mechanisms are subtle and relate to Yin-Yang theory in its correspondence with cold and heat, blood and energy and with organ and bowel, in their biao-li relationship (inner-outer lining).

Some light is shed on the urinary and genital physiopathology of Jue Yin in relationship with seasonal illnesses. In another chapter of the *Su Wen* we find:

> In Jue Yin, if the qi is in excess, yin bi {cold pain}. If it is deficient, re bi {hot pain}. If it is too fluid, wind of fox shan.[165] If there is not enough, accumulation of qi in the lower abdomen.[166]

The qi being too fluid corresponds to an insufficiency of blood and thus to excess of energy in Jue Yin. This points to pollakiuria. The opposite circumstances would lead to pelvic congestion with "accumulation." This may be translated as shan (orchitis, epididymitis, prostatitis or fibroma).

It is remarkable that in the case of a parallel variation of blood and energy in Shao Yang the symptoms are practically the same:

> In Shao Yang: excess = bi of the muscles. Insufficiency = bi of the liver. Excess fluidity = shan of liver wind.[167] Lack of fluidity = accumulation of qi, muscular strain and periodic ocular pains.[168]

Urinary Infections and Cystitis

Urinary infections related to Jue Yin may be caused by hot or cold perverse energies (yin bi or re bi).

• Heat Cystitis (Re Bi)

Re bi, cystitis caused by heat, involves problems of severe micturition. When Jue Yin or Shao Yang are deficient, heat may penetrate into the body, causing a re bi with hot pains. Qi Bo explains this mechanism:

> Xie {perverse energy} tends to fill a void of qi. If Yin is deficient, Yang goes there. This is why, when there is shao qi {lack of qi}, there is heat and perspiration. Dark urine is the result of heat in the belly.[169]

The term bi is a Chinese medical term that is difficult to translate. It has been translated as rheumatism, which is accurate to a certain extent. However, it may also refer to a disorder affecting an organ or its energy as well as another region, be it the corresponding tissue or the region energized by that organ. Bi of the liver may indicate either certain muscular atrophies (the muscles are related to the liver) associated with a liver disorder, or disorders affecting the liver and its energetic sector — the pelvic region, the lower urinary tract and the genitalia.

In cases of Jue Yin urinary infection, it is logical to expect the infection to strike the lower urinary tract, the bladder and the urethra, all located in the pelvic region which is energized by the liver. For the moment, we can eliminate the ureters, renal pelvis and renal calyces.

213

In cases of urinary infection due to perverse heat, there are certain accompanying signs that brand the disorder as being related to Jue Yin. Qi Bo states:

> The manifestations of the bi of the liver are: night frights, excessive thirst, frequent urination and upward strain, as during pregnancy.[170]

At a more advanced stage, the dysuria is more pronounced:

> The fever of jue yin of the leg {zu jue yin} causes lumbago with tension in the lower abdomen, dysuria that is not retention and mictions that are frequent but in small quantities and accompanied by apprehension. There is a lack of qi with malaise in the belly. We needle taichong {LV-3} on the liver meridian.[171]

At an even more advanced stage there may be retention. This is jue, which means serious energy imbalance and blockage:

> In cases of imbalance of Jue Yin, the lower abdomen is painful and swollen, the belly is swollen, the patient cannot urinate. He tends to sleep, and in sleeping he bends his legs.[172]

Following this retention stage, the kidneys may be affected, but only secondarily:

> In imbalance of Jue Yin with contractures, pain in the kidneys and swelling, and if it is impossible to urinate, with divigation, we must needle the points of the liver meridian.[173]

This is anuria and the point to needle is dadun (LV-1). This point is also indicated in cases of intestinal occlusion, which may be caused by blockage of the three Yin meridians of the foot, as the following passage indicates:

> In cases of imbalance in the three Yin meridians with anuria, intestinal occlusion and cold limbs, death will follow in three days.[174]

As we can see in these passages, the bi of the liver involves disturbances of the organ, of its meridian, of the territory it energizes and the related tissue. This is for Wood, the muscles, and is the case in the terminal stage of the disorder, which is accompanied by contractures and convulsions. Obviously, we must be careful in studying Chinese semiology that limits itself to the observed symptom. The bi of the muscles does not refer only to myopathy, but to all muscular symptoms associated with a pathology, ranging from convulsions to the myasthenia associated with hyperthyroidism, to spasmophilia and muscular hyperexcitability.

Xiao Yu states in the *Ling Shu* that food or medicine of a specific flavor, when absorbed in excessive quantities, becomes perverse:

> Sour flavor goes to the muscles {through the liver}. If we absorb too much sour food or drink we will have contractures and sometimes anuria.[175]

In cases of urinary blockage due to internal factors, wuli (LV-10) is indicated as well as dadun (LV-1).

In the *Da Cheng* the semiology of wuli is, "Anuria due to excess of Yang; tendency to sleep, the patient loves to sleep."[176] These specific symptoms refer to obnubilation, the first stage of a metabolic coma. Anuria, here, points to an organic disorder of the liver. Wuli (LV-10) is located over the internal pudendal artery, one osteo-unit below the inguinal fold in the pelvic region where the liver meridian begins encircling the genitals. Wuli means "five countries" which gives us some idea of the importance of this point in the balance of blood and energy within the body. This importance is shared by another wuli point in the arm, LI-13.[177]

- **Cold Cystitis (Yin Bi)**

Yin bi, cystitis caused by cold, is evident in cases of cystitis with clear urine, where cold is the perverse energy that is responsible. Pollakiuria of clear urine is one of the classical symptoms of aggression by cold.[178] In this etiological context the affliction is much less dramatic and potentially less tragic. As the *Su Wen* seems to indicate, this is one possible evolution of the dystonic terrain:

> Green cordal pulse,[179] stretched and vibrating everywhere, accumulation of breath in the heart, the sides are tensed, this is bi of the liver due to humid cold. As in shan, the loins are painful.[180]

This is the "cold pain," or yin bi. If there is a combination of cold and wind the illness takes on a capricious, intermittent aspect, as in chronic cystitis with clear urine, which we might call the "shan fox wind."

To treat these forms of cystitis, we must balance zu jue yin to prevent the penetration of the perverse energy by needling xingjian (LV-2), the heat point, and taichong (LV-3), the shu point. It is sometimes also useful to needle ganshu (BL-18) and qimen (LV-14). Menetrier's analysis of Diathesis I includes "primitive urinary disorders" and links these disorders to manganese.[181] He notes that cystitis is frequent among allergic subjects or among those patients who are anergic[182] and who suffer from severe infectious or chronic cystitis (see Tai Yang and Shao Yin).

Genital and Gynecological Pathology

Anatomy and Physiology of the False Pelvis

To understand this pathology, it is essential to have a clear picture of the energization of the external genitals, the gonads and the adnexa, located in the pelvic region. This area involves an intricate network of meridians among which are the spleen (zu tai yin), the kidney (zu shao yin)[183] and the liver (zu jue yin), as well as the miscellaneous channels ren mai, chong mai and du mai that envelop the uterus. The liver meridian (zu jue yin) is essential to the energization of the false pelvis, as we have seen in the pathologies of the stomach wall and the lower urinary tract. Not only the primary channel but also its extensions — the tendinomuscular and luo channels — are involved. In Chinese medicine, the role of the liver in the synthesis and circulation of the blood, in the venal circulation of the lower limbs and the false pelvis relates to the whole range of pelvic pathology of

215

women, from menstruation to pregnancy. The equilibrium of blood and energy in the miscellaneous channels is determined by the activity of chong mai (the blood) and ren mai (energy). As Zhang Zhi Cong comments in his discussion of complexion and pulse when referring to the tenth chapter of the *Su Wen:*

> The "curious" pulses refer to the pulses and complexions of the curious channels chong mai and ren mai that are the "seas of energy and blood."

> The blood of the five organs flows into the liver, which may be seen in the eyes; as the eyes govern the blood and the complexion, the face governs the energy and complexion.[184]

There is every reason to believe that chong mai is closely linked to zu jue yin and its role in the physiology of the blood. Recent biorhythm studies have shown a correlation between lunar and menstrual cycles and have enabled researchers to develop a contraceptive method based on the lunar cycle.[185]

These correlations were elementary for the ancient Chinese who had ways of calculating the appropriate phases conducive to the conception of male or female children.[186] These methods are not presented globally in the *Su Wen,* but Huang Di does mention:

> Jue Yin is the last link of Yin. This is the end of Yin and the beginning of Yang; in the cosmos, the moon is its symbol. When the moon begins to grow, the blood and energy in the body of a man begin also to take action. At the full moon, the blood and energy are at the height of their strength; they weaken thereafter.[187]

Because of its correlation with the lunar cycle and to the physiological cycle of blood and energy, Jue Yin is an important meridian for women. Its permanent mobilization makes it vulnerable, which explains the frequency of pelvic disorders and emotional problems among women who are of the Jue Yin temperament. There is still another relationship between Jue Yin, the blood and the uterus, which is based upon the energetic envelopes described by acupuncture theory, specifically the heart and pelvic envelopes. The pericardium meridian begins in the thorax, at shanzhong (CV-17). It describes a centrifugal radicular pathway into the upper limbs. At the thoracic level there is an extremely dense network of secondary channels (luo),[188] the "heart envelope," or xin bao luo, which literally means "channels enveloping the heart," and which is the actual name of the pericardium, shou jue yin. The role of this network is protection of the heart.

The envelope of the uterus is located in the pelvis and is known as bao luo gong, meaning "channels enveloping the uterus," or "envelope of the menstrual blood and the sperm." According to Nguyen Van Nghi, this envelope communicates with ren mai through the points zhongji (CV-3),[189] guanyuan (CV-4) and qihai (CV-6) and, by an internal channel to the kidney, the dwelling place of jing qi.[190] The bao luo gong protects the uterus. There is reason to believe that the bao luo gong is linked not only to the kidney, but also to the liver and the spleen, via the insertion points. It is also linked to chong mai and du mai through the internal channel connecting the kidneys that is common to the three miscellaneous channels stemming from them.

216

The link with chong mai supports the relationship with the liver and the blood. The bao luo gong seems to correspond anatomically with the sacral and pudendal plexi.[191] One very important point supports this idea: baohuang (BL-48) is called "envelope of the bao" or "envelope of life." Located on the external sacral loin branch of the bladder meridian, it is found bilaterally three units on the horizontal line of the second sacral foramen. In fact, the two envelopes are related. As we see throughout the text, this relationship operates through Jue Yin. Zu jue yin is directly linked to bao luo gong (uterus); shou jue yin is linked to xin bao luo (heart envelope). The interrelationships between zu jue yin and shou jue yin serve to explain certain genital and sexual indications of the points of the pericardium meridian. This is why shou jue yin was translated by the earliest Western authors as "envelope of the heart-sexuality meridian."[192] These relationships enable us to explain not only the functional thoracic symptomology related to gynecological problems, but also the associated vascular pathologies such as high blood pressure as well as the vagal reflex that is so easily triggered by certain gynecological maneuvers.

To complete our discussion of the energetic relationships of the pelvic region with the element Wood, we must recall the fundamental role of the gallbladder, the noble curious bowel that stores the essence. Remember, too, its link with the miscellaneous meridian dai mai, the pelvic region and the uterus, through its meridian, the zu shao yang:[193]

> The liver is attuned to the gallbladder because the latter is a bowel
> that contains the vital essence of the middle of the body.[194]

Dai mai is the miscellaneous channel that connects the curious function of the gallbladder with the kidneys, mingmen (GV-4), the pelvic region and the bao luo gong. The whole of the Shao Yang meridian is involved and shou shao yang, the triple burner meridian, also emerges in the false pelvis and plays a specific role.

Dysmenorrhea, Genital Infections, Ovarian Cysts and Fibroma

In acupuncture, we distinguish between dysmenorrheas due to excesses and those due to deficiencies.[195] Those caused by deficiency are, more often than not, related to a kidney deficiency, which is studied in the chapter devoted to the pathology of Shao Yin.[196] The modern authors from Shanghai agree with the distinction between excess and deficiency syndromes and link the deficiency cases to the kidney, as did their predecessors.[197] Excess dysmenorrhea is linked to the liver and to excess or blockage of its energy.[198] This pathology is similar to shan, of which dysmenorrhea may be symptomatic, or to which it may lead. This pathology is found almost always among women subjects of Shao Yang or Jue Yin temperament.

• Dark Liver Etiology and Fibroma

For the most part, the fullness and the blockage of this affection correspond to what the Shanghai authors call "dark liver." This etiology is nothing more than the accumulation of qi, the mechanism of energy and blood disturbance in Jue Yin or in Shao Yang. This is the same mechanism that causes cystalgia. Let us recall:

In Jue Yin, too much fluid causes shan fox wind; not enough means accumulation of qi.

In Shao Yang, too much fluid causes shan of liver wind; not enough means accumulation of qi, muscular twinges and episodic ocular pain.[199]

It is not uncommon to find this sort of cystalgia in conjunction with dysmenorrhea. The Shanghai text defines the clinical picture of these dark liver dysmenorrheas very well. Pelvic pain is present either the day before or on the first day of the period, with abundant menses and blood clots from which is derived the name "dark liver" and painful swelling of the breasts. Not only is this clinical picture consistently present in this etiology, it is associated with such signs as headache and migraines located on the pathway of the gallbladder meridian and linked to the ocular globe. Nausea, lipothymia or dizziness may be present. This is the terrain of allergies, hemorrhoids, slight hepatic affections, alcohol intolerance and fat intolerance, among other syndromes associated with the element Wood, Shao Yang or Jue Yin.

The evolution of these functional dysmenorrheas is specific. They often appear with the patients first period and occur until menopause. Parallel to this pathology, fibromas develop easily on a uterus that is conducive to their formation from the beginning. It is as if the congestion of the blood, which causes the pain and difficulty, makes elimination partial and causes some blood to remain in the myometrium. This is really a case of shan and corresponds to qi shan in the classification of Dr. Zhang. Significantly, emotional factors are preponderant in the formation of qi shan. Leung Kwok Po states, "In qi shan, there is a blockage of energy resulting from emotional shock, or following great anger or physical exhaustion."[200] This is representative of the psychological profile of Jue Yin and Shao Yang subjects. It corresponds to the western correlation between dysmenorrhea and the psyche. According to H. Michel-Wolfromm, dysmenorrhea etiologies are 20 percent organic, 20 percent psychological and 60 percent psychosomatic.[201]

The Shanghai authors advise the systematic needling of guanyuan (CV-4), qihai (CV-6), sanyinjiao (SP-6) and guilai (ST-29) in treating excess dysmenorrhea. The first two points are the connections of the uterine envelope. Sanyinjiao (SP-6) is the luo point of the three Yin meridians that terminate in the pelvic region and acts as a general regulator.[202] Guilai (ST-29) means "return" in the periodic sense and corresponds to our common usage of the term "period." This point has always been considered as a "special point of the genitals"[203] and is indicated for "Any disorder affecting the genital apparatus, metritis, prolapsus, sterility, amenorrhea, condensation, organic tumors or blood clots."[204] Blood clots would obviously point to uterine fibroids. To the indications for this point, Soulie de Morant adds "lump in the throat caused by emotions,"[205] evidencing a correlation between dysmenorrhea and dystonia. ST-29 is located on the liver meridian belt pathway beyond the chongmen (SP-12) and fushe (SP-13) points and before its loop around the genital organs.[206]

The Shanghai authors recommend treating the points tongli (HT-5) and ligou (LV-5) in cases of dark liver dysmenorrhea. These are the luo points of the heart and the liver. The authors state:

When the heart and the liver, the Fire Minister, is disturbed,[207] we must needle the luo points to bring the Fire Minister into the organs through the longitudinal channels.[208]

The *Da Cheng* indicates, for tongli (HT-5), "Communication with the interior, abundant menses, uterine hemorrhage due to excess."[209] For ligou (LV-5), the *Da Cheng* indicates "metrorrhagia, irregular periods."[210]

Remember that the semiology of excess or deficiency of the longitudinal luo of the liver is specifically genital.[211] Aside from the classical indications, we must not omit the points jianshi (PC-5), taichong (LV-3), ququan (LV-8) and yinbao (LV-9). Jianshi (PC-5) is the luo point of the Yin meridians of the hand. It is linked to the heart envelope and the uterus envelope as well, as are tongli (HT-5) and neiguan (PC-6).[212] These, too, are luo points. Jianshi is indicated for "irregular periods, circulatory problems, uterine congestion."[213] Ququan (LV-8) is indicated for "menstrual troubles among young women." Yinbao (LV-9), "envelope of the Yin," which seems to represent the liver meridian loop around the genital organs (Yin), is indicated for "irregular periods."

For qi shan that involve not only dark liver dysmenorrhea but also the evolution towards fibroma, the physician Zhang indicates two specific points, xingjian (LV-2) and zulinqi (GB-41).[214] Xingjian is indicated for "swollen and distended lower abdomen."[215] Zulinqi (GB-41), the key point of dai mai, is indicated for "swelling and pain in the breasts (mastosis), difficult or insufficient periods."[216]

Swelling of the breasts during the period is related specifically to a point on the gallbladder meridian and is linked to a disturbance of that organ (Shao Yang) rather than the liver (Jue Yin). This aspect of hyperfolliculinism, related to the catabolic capacity of the hormonal steroids, seems to be linked to the biliary function of the liver, which is more often treated through the Shao Yang meridians than through those of Jue Yin.[217] For these reasons, daimai (GB-26) and weidao (GB-28) are indicated. The intersection point of dai mai and Shao Yang is one of the special gynecological points. According to the *Da Cheng*, this point is indicated for:

> Pain in the lower abdomen, pain in the loins that radiates to the back, metrorrhagia, leukorrhea, irregular periods, uterine spasms, convulsions,[218] erroneous desire to go to the bathroom and the sensation of pelvic heaviness.[219]

Weidao (GB-28) means "liaison road" or "united paths." Chamfrault describes this point as being the connection point of Shao Yang and dai mai. It is also a point that links zu shao yang and shou shao yang, the gall bladder and the triple burner. This point is indicated in all disorders linked to the triple burner, particularly as concerns the role of the triple burner and gallbladder in the physiology of the body fluids. This is why it is indicated in the *Da Cheng* for edema as described in the chapter devoted to Shao Yang, as well as for incoercible vomiting[220] and loss of appetite.[221]

The Shanghai treatise, on the other hand, lists quite different indications: "Anexitis, endometriosis, uterine prolapse, intestinal hernia and chronic constipation."[222] The last symptom indicated is proof of the connections between the triple burner, the gallbladder, the dai mai channel and the physiology of body fluids and constipation.[223]

To recapitulate the points indicated in "dark liver dysmenorrhea" and fibroma, we must note: CV-4, CV-6, SP-6, ST-29, HT-5, LV-5, PC-5, GB-41, LV-2, GB-26, GB-28 and BL-48.

• Perverse Cold Etiologies, Genital Infections, Ovarian Cysts and Leukorrhea

Another excess dysmenorrhea etiology that is mentioned by the Shanghai text is one caused by perverse cold energy. This disorder occurs when the patient takes a bath, swims or simply bathes her feet in cold water. The *Da Cheng* tells us that these patients are more vulnerable during their periods. I have noticed that women instinctively avoid cold water at these times. This is a classical etiology mentioned in the *Su Wen*. In a passage in Chapter 39 on "The Origin of Pain," the pelvis-thorax axis of Jue Yin is explicitly described.

> The cold may lodge in the Jue Yin channel. This channel is related to the genitals and linked to the liver. The cold freezes the blood, the channel contracts and the pain radiates from the thorax to the lower abdomen. The qi is pushed back, and is lodged in the perineum; the cold ascends to the lower abdomen and pulls on the congealed blood down below, which is why the pain radiates towards the perineum.[224]

This etiology is cystalgia with clear urine, with which it alternates frequently with or without the symptoms of bi of the liver from cold humidity, such as "night fears, polydipsia, frequent mictions, upward tuggings as during pregnancy."

It is easy to tell the difference between this etiology and that of dark liver. Whereas dark liver dysmenorrhea is primary and commences brutally, this etiology is secondary. Since it is perverse cold energy that affects the menses, the pain will be constant throughout the period. The flow of blood will be fluid, rather than coagulated (cold indicates Water) and abundant. We will find polymenorrhea and the period will last relatively longer. It is not exceptional to see metrorrhagia during the cycle. In the presence of this perverse cold energy we find infections of the ovaries and the adnexa such as metritis, salpingitis, ovaritis and even ovarian cysts. These correspondences are even more likely when there is cold wind.

Let us recall the paragraph from the *Su Wen* concerning the pathology of the wind:

> The wind (feng) is the first cause of all illness. In absence of treatment, the illness passes to the kidneys and causes a shan jia accompanied by cloudy white urine. This illness is also known as gu, "affection that goes deeper." We must treat with massotherapy and phytotherapy.[225]

Husson translated this difficult passage as follows:

> If there is no treatment, the illness passes to the kidneys and causes a shan jia with sharp pain in the lower abdomen and whitish urine; this is also called gu {consumption}.[226]

220

The differences between these two translations point out how difficult it is to assimilate one interpretation of a text in regard to an etiology, particularly when we are dealing with wind.[227] The terms themselves are equivocal. Are we speaking of urinary infection, of cystitis or of genital infection with leukorrhea? The term consumption may refer to a much more serious, "deeper" as Nguyen Van Nghi would say, disorder that is a result of the same mechanism and to the same perverse energy, but occurs in the context of a more vulnerable terrain. This is how Chamfrault tends to see consumption as tuberculosis; here, genital tuberculosis. On the other hand, the term may be understood in the psychological sense which is closer to its popular usage, "to consume," such as being consumed by love or by passion.

Since we are dealing with shan, as the text explicitly states, and with perverse cold, there is a direct correlation with the han shan described by the physician Zhang:

> An internal accumulation of cold (predisposition) to which is added a new attack of cold causes a resulting blockage of blood and energy in the conception vessel (ren mai) and in the liver.[228]

Another interpretation of the shan that is of liver origin and causes leukorrhea is given by Qi Bo in Chapter 44 of the *Su Wen* that deals with the wei. Here, emotional factors are even more important:

> Countless preoccupations, deceptions, immoderate desires and carnal abuses tend to loosen the "chief muscle" (zong jin),[229] causing a muscular wei and also "white genital flow" (bai yin). According to the *Book of the Emperors,* the muscular wei comes from the liver through the action of the sex life.[230] This says a lot about the frequency of the psychosomatic etiologies of leukorrhea, in which an internal accumulation of cold,[231] along with the loosening of the abdominal and pelvic wall, eventually precipitates the constitution of hernias and uterine prolapse, or shan.

The Shanghai treatise advises treating xingjian (LV-2) and taichong (LV-3), "to provide heat and to fight the wind cold perverse energy in the uterus, in chong mai and in ren mai."[232] Xingjian is the heat point of the meridian. The *Da Cheng* indication for this point is as follows:

> Seven sorts of shan: swollen and distended lower abdomen, overlong periods, hemorrhages in the course of the period {which goes right along with the clinical context} and urinary incontinence.[233]

Taichong is the Earth point (sweet or mild flavor) that turns against the wind (Wood). The *Da Cheng* indicates, "Illness whose symptoms are Yin, pale complexion, painful shan, unending menstrual flow among young women." Apart from these two points, we may also needle the mu point of the liver, qimen (LV-14), which is not referred to by the Shanghai text, although the *Da Cheng* notes "trouble after having caught cold during the period."[234] The physician Zhang indicates guanyuan (CV-4) and zhaohai (KI-6) for han shan (cold hernia). Since zhaohai is the yin qiao mai opening point, it seems to indicate the kidney not only as a victim, as we have understood in the chapter devoted to the feng, but in a deeper sense indicates Shao Yin and its link with yin qiao mai.[235]

To recapitulate, the following are the main points to be needled in treating perverse cold dysmenorrhea: LV-2, LV-3, LV-14, CV-4, KI-6, with which we may associate GB-41[236] and BL-48. Let us not forget, however, that the *Su Wen* recommends massage and phytotherapy. Massage may no doubt assist in acupuncture therapy, especially the massage of the belt meridian dai mai. As for phytotherapy treatment, the Chinese pharmacopoeia includes a wide range of plants, among which we must select ti yu, the root of *Sanguisorba officinalis*. According to Chamfrault:

> This non-toxic, bitter plant refreshes the blood and stops hemorrhage. Used in the treatment of leukorrhea, it calms the pain, stops perspiration and is excellent in the treatment of Yang symptom diarrhea,[237] is used to treat abscesses,[238] blood vomiting and in all sorts of epistaxis,[239] overlong periods and hemorrhages of the genital organs.

According to Tong Fun, ti yu tonifies the energy of the gallbladder. Chamfrault says that this plant "acts upon the liver, kidney, large intestine, stomach and dai mai meridians."[240] In the West, this plant is recognized as acting upon all these conditions and is notably hemostatic, owing to the concentration of tannic acid. It is used for treating dysmenorrhea and leukorrhea. Freshly picked roots and leaves are gathered before the plant flowers and are used in decoction.

Commenting on dysmenorrhea, Menetrier says:

> Allergic subjects {manganese} will have abundant menses that are painful and close together, often with signs of hyperfolliculinism. Dystonic subjects {manganese-cobalt; pericardium, triple burner} will have irregular periods that are painful and preceded by folliculinic troubles.

The two clinical pictures overlap to define Jue Yin or Shao Yang dysmenorrhea. A rigorous examination of the diatheses, or as we say, the associated temperaments, allows us to make a more precise distinction. It is useful to combine manganese and copper for arthro-infectious patients who suffer often from cold wind dysmenorrhea and whose condition is improved by needling zulinqi (GB-41). It is common to find women patients who are at once Jue Yin and Shao Yang and for whom copper-gold-silver coincides with zhaohai (KI-6), which is also needled in the cold wind etiology. More often than not, Jue Yin and Shao Yang patients who suffer from dysmenorrhea correspond to the dark liver etiology. We then treat the Wood meridians in combination with manganese, sulfur and even iodine.

Acupuncture alone gives excellent results in these cases,[241] as does trace element therapy. The association of the two therapies seems useful, if not indispensable, especially in cases of fibroma. According to Menetrier, fibroma corresponds to the passage from the allergic diathesis to the dystonic diathesis.[242] I agree with Menetrier in saying that we must think twice before advising hysterectomies in these cases. It appears that an hysterectomy has a degenerative effect and brings on disorders that are usually post-menopause phenomena, including: spinal arthritis, especially arthritis of the cervical spine, generalized bone demineralization, presbyopia, hemeralopia and vein disorders in the lower limbs, as well as congestive vasomotor phenomena. All these syndromes are related in Chinese medicine to the energy of the liver and gallbladder, which are disturbed as much by hysterectomy as by cholecystectomy.[243]

Obstetric Accidents

Throughout pregnancy, it is important to be aware of the relationships between chong mai, the liver meridian, the blood and the uterine envelope. It is worth noting that Jue Yin women whose liver energy is constitutionally deficient have a higher risk of miscarriage due to the deficiency of the "uterine muscle" and a cerclage is more often necessary.

• Post-partum Hemorrhage

There is reason to believe that the liver meridian is directly linked to the placenta and to uterine contractility and that the xi point of the meridian (the point indicated in emergencies; here zhongdu, LV-6) may be useful in cases of uterine hemorrhage in general. Specifically, when the uterus does not retract sufficiently after delivery, zhongdu is indicated. This is indeed the case, as the *Da Cheng* indicates clearly for zhongdu (LV-6), "Uterine hemorrhage, after delivery the blood flows endlessly."[244]

• Retention of the Placenta

Jue Yin is mentioned in the *Da Cheng* in relation to placental retention but here it is shou jue yin that is involved. Neiguan (PC-6), "heart envelope" — the luo point of the meridian and also the opening point of yin wei mai, the curious meridian coupled with chong mai — is indicated: "Syncope after delivery, placenta that does not descend."

Bilateral electrical stimulation of yanglingquan (GB-34) and taichong (LV-3)[245] induce labor among women who are at full term and are properly dilated to such an extent that it would be dangerous to stimulate these points at an earlier stage. This has been described in modern Chinese literature and by Nguyen Van Nghi, whose fruitful observations I have confirmed in practice. This is not, however, new knowledge. The *Da Cheng* mentions that taichong (LV-3) and shanqiu (SP-5), if needled in the beginning of pregnancy, are likely to cause miscarriage.[246]

Puerperal Depression

The frequency of puerperal depression is explained by the fact that Jue Yin is a connective network between the envelopes of the heart and uterus, the liver, the heart, the psyche and the blood. These puerperal depressions are often without gravity, but may sometimes take on dramatic proportions. Jue Yin subjects are often victims of this depression. In Chinese medicine, puerperal depression corresponds to a deficiency of blood, here related to a loss of blood and to the exhaustion of the liver following delivery. Other blood deficiency syndromes, such as neurovegetative dystonia, spasmophilia, eczema and psoriasis of the scalp are often aggravated after delivery. The lipothymia and syncopes observed among spasmophilia patients, with a deficiency of blood in the upper part of the body and a concentration of blood in the pelvis, are the same symptoms as those observed in extra-uterine pregnancy. Clearly, for extra-uterine pregnancy, the deficiency in the upper part of the body and the concentration in the pelvis are more than just an image. Note also that lactation is closely related to Shao Yang and specifically to the gallbladder meridian.

Masculine Pathology

All comments concerning physiology made at the beginning of this discussion may also be applied to men. Male genital pathology obeys the same mechanism as does female pathology and accumulation of qi may also be observed among men. It corresponds to various specific etiologies of shan, such as prostatitis, impotence, orchitis, urinary infection, urethritis, scrotal eczema and inguino-scrotal hernia. The seven shan described by the physician Zhang concern the whole range of male pelvic pathology.[247] Erection disorders, genital eczema and genital infections correspond to a blood and liver meridian imbalance. It is especially the luo of the liver that is involved. Excess or deficiency may cause priapism, impotence or genital eczema.[248] In the tenth chapter of the *Ling Shu,* we may read:

> A secondary channel of the liver meridian (zu jue yin) begins at ligou {LV-5} and communicates with the gallbladder meridian (zu shao yang). This luo channel passes through the calf and the scrotum and arrives at the penis.
>
> If there is an imbalance of energy, the scrotum suddenly swells.
>
> If it is in excess, scrotum and penis are long; if it is deficient, there is violent itching in the scrotum.[249]

Among these pathologies we may mention tui shan, an attack of humidity against Jue Yin,[250] or jin shan (shan of the muscle),[251] that comes about "from the blockage of the blood or of the energy following trauma or excess of sexual intercourse."[252] The symptoms include "pain and swelling in the penis, purulent or nonpurulent lesion, spermatorrhea, lactescent urine."[253] This seems to be the case of the inflammation of the penis, infectious or not, in which we sometimes observe spermatorrhea. Jin shan, also translated as "muscular spasms,"[254] is described differently in the *Yi Xue Ru Men:*

> The penis is erect, stiff, and may not retract; sometimes it itches and is excessively painful. This is a result of an excess of coitus.[255]

This is a perfect description of priapism.

• Impotence, Eczema

Beyond these various symptoms, we observe among Jue Yin subjects (yet almost never among Shao Yang subjects) transitory sexual deficiencies, such as erection difficulty. This sometimes occurs the first time a man is about to have intercourse with a new partner. This may be what is referred to in a passage in the *Su Wen* concerning the pathology of the liver which mentions "periodic aversion to women." When this problem is transitory, it corresponds to what the *Da Cheng* calls "home fatigue." The zu jue yin points, zhongfeng (LV-4)[256] and ququan (LV-8) are the main treatment points. Ququan is to be treated with moxibustion. As many as 100 moxas may be used for deficiency after sexual excess.[257] These points are also useful in treating scrotal eczema. A deficiency of energy in the liver meridian and in the luo channel, as well as perverse cold, are accompanied by impotence and eczema. It is thus necessary to tonify ligou (LV-5).[258]

• **Priapism, Genital Infection, Orchitis**

At the other end of the energetic spectrum, an excess of the luo channel of the liver, or perverse heat, brings about balanitis, microbial infection of the genitals and priapism — in short, jin shan. To treat this, Dr. Zhang uses the points qichong (ST-30),[259] yanglingquan (GB-34) and taixi (KI-3).[260] Yanglingquan uses the Yang of the gallbladder to tonify the muscle of the pelvic band and to reduce the energy blockage. Taixi reinvigorates the jing qi that may have collapsed temporarily as a result of sexual overindulgence. The Japanese texts translated by Soulie de Morant demonstrate the principles in the opposite situation. In cases of overabundance of sexual energy, xingjian (LV-2) is needled.[261] This is the dispersion point of the liver. The message is clear: in case of deficiency, we must tonify and in cases of excess, we disperse. To treat impotence and eczema around the genitals among Jue Yin subjects, we needle LV-4, LV-5 and LV-8. To treat priapism, genital infection and balanitis, we needle ST-30, GB-34, KI-3, LV-2 and LV-5. In the context of diathetic medicine, we may quote Picard:

> Impotence and indifference among men are signs of a neuroarthritic terrain that tends towards anergy.[262] This coincides with the dystonic diathesis and indicates treatment with manganese-cobalt.

Bone, Ligament and Joint Pathology

The catabolic function of the liver may be compared to that of the lower burner (liver and kidney) and is partly dependent upon the Shao Yang energetic territory. The meridian Jue Yin is, nonetheless, also related to the purification function. Metabolic accidents are less frequent among Jue Yin patients than among Shao Yang subjects, as is the case of gout, or atypical arthropathy with hyperuricemia. As we have seen in the chapter devoted to the pathology of Shao Yang, the physiopathology of acute arthritis implies the concept of perverse wind. It is only logical that Shao Yang, triple burner and gallbladder, which is known as "wandering throughout the body," is more often exposed to this pathology than Jue Yin, which is Yin and therefore a deeper meridian and better protected against external aggression. When Jue Yin is attacked by perverse wind — with articular pain — the disturbance is much more serious. The liver organ itself is affected through the Yin meridian, or through a Yang meridian linked to Jue Yin.

Acute Dorsalgia

Dorsalgia due to aggression against Jue Yin and Yang Ming is known as feng jue (jue of the wind) which is described in the *Su Wen:*

> The disease of the secondary Yang {Yang Ming indicates stomach} and of the primary Yin {Jue Yin indicates liver} manifests itself through fear and pains in the back. The patients burp and yawn frequently. The name of the disease is *fong quyet* {feng jue}.[263]

Husson translates these symptoms as "fears, pain in the back and a tendency to whine and yawn."[264] Fear is a significant sign of aggression against the liver (Jue Yin), as is the case in the bi of the liver with cystitis. Burping and yawning are

225

clear signs of stomach trouble (Yang Ming), while whining (instead of yawning, according to the translation) is a typical Jue Yin symptom. According to Zhang Jing Yao, as quoted by Nguyen Van Nghi:

> There are several diseases called feng jue: in this paragraph it is secondary Yang and primary Yin; in Chapter 31 of the *Su Wen* and in Chapter 23 of the *Ling Shu,* feng jue refers to the disease of Tai Yang {bladder} and Shao Yin {kidney} meridians. In Chapter 46 of the *Ling Shu,* Qi Bo says, "the patient stricken with feng jue perspires because the flesh is undernourished in energy and because the pores remain partly open."[265]

The context of these chapters implies that we are dealing with an infection in which the perverse energy is cold wind that has congested and become warm (*i.e.,* cold-heat disease).

Articular Pains

An imbalance of Jue Yin, just as that of Shao Yang, can lead to articular pains. In an important chapter of the *Su Wen,* "Perturbations of the Energies and Their Influence on Man," describing the excesses and deficiencies of qi in the Wood, Earth, Fire, Metal and Water seasons, Qi Bo explains the variations of symptoms and pathologies of the heavenly variations:

> If there is a lack of Wood energy {spring} in the course of a year, the spring may kill instead of give birth[266] because Metal {autumn} triumphs over Wood. Fire avenges the aggression against Wood, and the summer is excessively hot and there are catastrophes in the east. In man, the liver is diseased within the body, on the outside it is the articulations that suffer.[267]

Although the factors responsible here are said to be cosmic and to reveal an abnormal perverse cold in the spring, there is an association of perverse wind and cold that deeply affects the liver and also the articulations of vulnerable patients (*i.e.,* Jue Yin subjects in poor health). The specifically osteoarticular etiologies covered by this physiopathology are not more or less than acute arthropathies, as are those of Shao Yang; in particular, gout and chondrocalcinosis. With the etiologies of chondrocalcinosis, we are met with the most fundamental failures, such as those found in the context of metabolic failure associated with gout or hemochromatosis.[268] In 10 to 50 percent of all cases of hemochromatosis, x-rays show subchondral lesions. Anatomopathology shows that these lesions are related to an infarction of ferric deposits in the synovial membrane. Among the etiologies of metabolic arthropathies that are directly linked to Jue Yin and to a liver deficiency, we find the osteoarticular manifestations of Wilson's disease, in which the bone demineralization is typically due to a kidney imbalance, showing that the illness has passed from the son to the mother. This is tubular nephropathy.

Lumbago

Lumbago is frequent among Jue Yin subjects. It would be wrong to conclude too quickly that lumbago is always a Shao Yin problem. Let us recall the comment in the *Su Wen* concerning the bi of the liver resulting from cold humidity:

"As in the shan, the loins are painful."[269] In other words, whether it is a bi of the liver or a shan, we find lumbago. The same is true of the jue of the liver.

• Lumbagos of Jue of the Liver

Apart from the dorsalgia mentioned previously, we are sometimes confronted with lumbago due to the jue of the liver. It is accompanied by "contracture, absolute deficiency, urine retention and delirium."[270] The absolute deficiency of the organ's energy is proportional to the general state of health of the subject. This may be seen in the description of the bi of the liver:

> The serenity of the Yin maintains the visceral spirits; its agitation ruins them. The misconduct of the qi, which tires and exhausts, is a concentration in the liver.[271]

Thus, the jue of the liver represents a picture of urgency and of decomposition of the organic function of the liver whatever the etiology. Here, contractures are not simple muscular spasms as was true in urinary pathology, but refer to abnormal movements, even convulsions. We find anuria, probably due to retention (this is liver territory), and absolute deficiency, which prefigures an abandonment of the viscera by the shen, the first sign of which is delirium. Even in a context of such gravity, the symptoms (including delirium) are nothing more than the exaggeration of the functional hepatic semiology. This is an exaggeration of the natural tendency of Jue Yin subjects. The same is true for lumbago, a secondary renal disorder leading to retention. This is another way for the son to pass the illness to the mother, as we have seen in tubular nephropathy.

• Shan Lumbagos

In a context of lesser gravity we find the shan lumbago. The *Su Wen* explains their mechanisms and treatment according to anatomical relationships:[272]

> Pain in the lower abdomen: there is accumulation (ji); we needle the infra-umbilical adipic fold without touching the lower abdomen, then on each side of the spine at the fourth intercostal space gaohuang {BL-43},[273] the iliac points juliao[274] and the points of the last rib, jingmen {GB-25}. We also induce the intro-abdominal qi to reduce the heat. If there are pains with dysuria and dyschezia, the name of the disease is shan, it is a result of the cold; we needle between the thighs and between the hips {territory of the liver, kidney and chong mai channels}, and we needle many times to make as much heat as possible and the disease ceases.[275]

• Acute Lumbagos

The best proof of the existence and specificity of the Jue Yin lumbagos is to be found in the discussion concerning Jue Yin in the chapter of the *Su Wen* that is devoted to the "Explanation of the Channels":

> It is impossible to bend or to straighten the loins as they are extremely painful: the third month awakens the growth of all creatures that bend like branches beneath the weight of new growth.[276]

This poetic passage refers to acute lumbago, comparable to that seen in the chapter devoted to Shao Yang. In a special chapter of the *Su Wen* devoted to lumbago, however, the paragraph that treats the gallbladder lumbago (Shao Yang) is quite different from the description of liver lumbago (Jue Yin).

> In cases of liver lumbago, there is tension in the loins that is comparable to that of a crossbow.[277] We needle outside the "fish belly" on a vascular network between the calf and the heel {ligou, LV-5}.

> In this disease, even the most talkative of patients becomes mute. We needle three times.[278]

Added to this information, we find, "lumbago with warmth in the upper part of the body: liver meridian."[279]

Notice once more that the loquacious aspect of these "liver" subjects is mentioned. It may be that this muteness from pain corresponds to the hepatic colic pathetism.

Acute lumbago is related to an excess of the luo channel of the liver that, according to the text, we must disperse by needling ligou (LV-5). The *Da Cheng* confirms this semiology: "Spasms in the back; the patient may bend neither forwards nor backwards."[280] To summarize, we may say that liver lumbago (zu jue yin) is a clinical reality that presents a number of aspects that vary according to the physiopathological mechanism: bi, shan, jue and acute lumbago. In trace element therapy, acute arthritic pain, as well as the corresponding terrain, is treated with manganese, as was mentioned in the discussion of this pathology in the chapter devoted to Shao Yang.

Endocrine Pathology

Hyperthyroidism

Hyperthyroidism coincides as perfectly with the Jue Yin temperament as it does with that of Shao Yang. Please refer to the discussion of endocrinology in the Shao Yang chapter.

Spasmophilia, Tetany and Neurovegetative Dystonia

These conditions also correspond to the Jue Yin terrain. Spasmophilia, "a tendency towards spasms," is an European clinical syndrome that as yet is neither defined nor delimited with any precision. It includes tetanic spasms and various other neurovegetative symptoms. Apart from its neuropsychiatric aspects, we may speak of either latent or active neuromuscular hyperexcitability, combined frequently with biological disorders.[281] Spasmophilia and tetany are inseparable from neurovegetative dystonia. They are more often than not exaggerated symptoms. The characteristic nervous behavior has been ascribed a handy name, "neurovegetative dystonia," that serves to hide our ignorance of its mechanisms or causes and, unfortunately, facilitate the systematic prescription of tranquilizers or of beta-blocking agents. Such prescriptions do little to re-establish an equilibrium and tend to prolong and perpetuate the malaise. This is all the more dramatic in

228

that the frequency of these syndromes, because of the stress inherent in modern ecology, is constantly on the rise. The "nervous" behavior associated with neurovegetative dystonia is close to the psychological profile of the Jue Yin subject.

In the discussion of gynecology, the direct relationship between the pericardium meridian (the envelope of the heart — shou jue yin) and the neurovegetative nervous system was noted. This correspondence allows us to state that neurovegetative dystonia is clearly an imbalance of this function, an imbalance of the Fire Minister. The Fire Minister (pericardium and triple burner) belongs to the element Fire, as does the Imperial Fire, heart and small intestine. The visceral qi, or vegetative soul of Fire, is shen. Shen, as we have seen, is the qi of the instincts and the emotions. It is particularly sensitive to emotional shocks, to emotive stress, be it affective, psychological or physical. It is only logical that Jue Yin subjects who are "nervous" by nature are prime targets of all these stresses, because of their characteristic instability. This is the terrain that is most often subject to spasmophilia and tetany. In cases of spasmophilia or of tetany, zu jue yin is also involved. Thus, the entire meridian is imbalanced. Remember that jue is variously translated by the following terms that speak for themselves: "exhausted, hidden, suffocated, breathless, weak."[282]

• **Physiopathology**

The liver is involved in the physiopathology of these disorders, because of its direct relationships with the muscles and with contractures:

> The east is represented on earth by the element Wood. Within the body, it represents the muscles; as an organ, it represents the liver. It corresponds to the color green. Its imbalance is contractures.[283]

The pulse of the liver varies with the symptoms:

> If the pulse of the liver is slightly raspy, there are contractures; the affection dwells in the muscles.[284]

However, an imbalance reflected in the pulse of the heart, the Fire organ, may give the same symptoms accompanied by precordialgia:

> If the pulse of the heart is frequent and tense, there are contractures. If the character of this tension is minimal, there will be pain radiating from the heart towards the back, and the patient is unable to swallow food.[285]

> The causes of these spasms are probably threefold: cosmic, alimentary and emotional.

> The cosmic etiology coincides with the periods when the cosmic Jue Yin (energy of the springtime, Wood) is deficient, which partly determines the times when the symptoms are aggravated or recede."[286]

The alimentary etiology concerns an excess of the corresponding flavor, here sour. "Sour food goes to the muscles {through the liver}. If one eats too much food or drinks too many sour beverages, there will be contractures and sometimes anuria."[287] In this affection, however, it seems that emotional energy is the predominant etiology. This is confirmed in the *Ling Shu* chapter on "The Role of the Mental":

> Troubles and affections affect the liver. The patient will have muscular contractures.[288]

• Clinical Observations

Clinically, latent spasmophilia frequently manifests itself subsequent to pregnancy, nursing, diarrhea, estroprogestative imbalance, corticotherapy, metabolic alkalosis (vomiting) and stress.[289] All these circumstances are harmful to Jue Yin in general and to the liver in particular, and tend to cause a deficiency of Yin of the liver (jing qi). There is a tendency to believe that spasmophilia predominates among women.[290] Due to the appearance of spasmophilia in the course of a woman's genital life, especially following pregnancy and delivery, this belief is easily justified by the specific sensitivity of the Jue Yin meridian in women. The classic terrain is "young women who are anxious, often insomniac, with antecedents, frequently, of depression."[291]

The clinical symptoms that bring patients to seek medical assistance include, in decreasing order of frequency: asthenia, which we may interpret as a deficiency of the liver ("fatigue and exhaustion" according to the *Su Wen,* Chapter 43); paresthesia of the extremities, predominantly of the upper limbs, because of abnormal energy circulation in the shou jue yin meridian (pericardium); cramps, with or without the tetanoid attack, a sign not only of imbalance in the liver and in the heart envelope, but in Jue Yin as a whole. There are also neurotonic manifestations, "fits of crying with uncontrollable sobbing, panting, convulsive fits that are always quite spectacular."[292] This behavior seems hysterical and corresponds to an excess of pericardium. We will discuss this further on in Jue Yin subjects. It is important to note that spasmophilia, hysteria, convulsions and epilepsy manifest themselves more or less indistinctly and often concommitantly in the same sort of terrain. Thus, it is hard to tell just where one starts and the other stops. This is particularly true for spasmophilia and makes a precise definition of the syndrome almost impossible. As the mechanisms of these different disorders are all the same, this is not particularly upsetting to the Chinese medical paradigm. The liver and its muscular sector are imbalances and the major factor of imbalance is a deficiency of blood — in other words, a deficiency of the essential energy (jing qi) of the organ.

The vomiting and the acute abdominal pain, when isolated, are difficult to distinguish from localized allergy attacks with intestinal edema. All these signs point clearly to a Jue Yin (liver) imbalance. There is mention of the possibility of an accompanying arthralgia occasionally coexisting with an allergic terrain (*sic*).[293] In short, all these symptoms, classically recognized by endocrinologists, were observed by Menetrier to correspond to the allergic behavior pattern, and fall under Diathesis I. The tetany attack corresponds to the paroxysmic manifestations of hypocalcemia. We find these attacks associated with spasmophilia, as we do with acute hypoparathyroidism.[294]

The tetany attack begins with paresthesia and formication in the extremities and in the peribuccal region. Then muscular fasciculations begin, followed by generalized contractures. In the upper limbs, these contractures manifest as carpal or metacarpal spasm; in the lower limbs the carpopedal spasm. In the face, the orbicular muscles of the lips upsurge and contract in opposite directions, giving the appearance of a fish face. This angular aspect represents a complete contracture of all of Jue Yin. As said, in the discussion of the prolapse of the mitral valve, "if the Jue Yin axis ceases to function, the Yin meridian is like a knot."[295] Peribuccal formication indicates contraction of the terminal meridian of the liver in its peribuccal cephalic branch. The accoucheur's hand is nothing more than convergence of the metacarpal and the carpal over the wrist, rolling up around the shou jue yin meridian, which is knotted. This is known as "Trousseau's Sign." In a description of the pathology of the secondary channel of shou jue yin, we may read:

> In case of imbalance, the patient feels heat in his heart; his arm and elbow are contracted, and there is swelling under his arm.[296]

In the lower limb, the contracture involves the pathway of zu jue yin as a whole (inside the calf and the thigh). This is why it takes on the aspect of a carpopedal extension.

In clinical practice the search for signs of hyperexcitability involves the Chvostek test (percussion on the peribuccal branch of the liver meridian) and, curiously enough, the less frequent Lust test (percussion of the head of the fibula among children). The fibula is located in the yanglingquan (GB-34) zone, the hui point of the muscles.

An electrocardiogram shows whether there are anomalies such as tachycardia, a shortening of the P-R segment, or a lengthening of the Q-T segment. These anomalies call to mind Barlow's disease. The Chinese physiopathology is strictly identical. We may quote Qi Bo once more:

> If the pulse of the first Yin {Jue Yin} arrives alone, we must treat the liver meridian. The exhaustion of the organ's pure energy {jing of the liver} causes depressing pains in the heart and a blockage of energy in the jing mai and is likely to cause white sweat.
>
> Diet and medication are necessary. We may also treat with acupuncture the lower shu point, taichong {LV-3}.[297]

This passage deals with the same neurotonic symptoms of the cardiac sphere found in Barlow's disease that represent a disturbance of the envelope of the heart resulting from a deficiency of the liver.[298] This may be compared to an energy blockage in Jue Yin with an excess of the pericardium luo channel:

> The shou jue yin meridian has a secondary channel that begins at the point neiguan {PC-6}, runs along the arm between two groups of muscles and enters the pericardium. If there is excess, there is pain in the heart.[299]

Jue Yin is like a rubber band. When the lower portion is deficient (deficiency of the jing qi of the liver), the blood may no longer circulate normally and settles at the bottom (accumulation of qi). It is as if the weight of the blood were stretching the rubber band downward. The tetany attack is analogous to what happens when the rubber band suddenly breaks. "The Yin meridian is like a knot." The liver shrinks into the lower portion (carpopedal spasm) and the pericardium shrinks and goes into excess. In the upper portion there are, then: accoucheur's hand, cardiac neurotonia, emotional symptoms and anxiety.

Other passages in the *Nei Jing Su Wen* also coincide with this dystonic symptomology:

> In liver affections, the patient suffers momentary blindness, and his sides are painful.[300]

Husson translates the passage, "Disease of the liver: dizziness and thoracic constriction."[301] According to modern authors, the disturbances of the electronystagmogram may explain these patients' dizziness. The frequent trophic disorders of the fingernails (brittleness, lines, white spots) are like a liver "signature" for this affection. These symptoms belong to the element Wood in Chinese medicine (see Table I and our discussion of dermatology in the chapter devoted to Shao Yang). Cataracts, specially among younger patients, are another such "liver" signature.[302]

Acupuncture treatment, particularly during the attack, will focus around the root and knot points of Jue Yin, dadun (LV-1) and yutang (CV-18). This is as if we were dealing with the cadaveric syncope of Barlow's disease, which is also a case of the rupture of the root and knot of Jue Yin. Apart from these points, the general balancing treatment will include taichong (LV-3), recommended by the texts and corresponding to the mild flavor; yanglingquan (GB-34), the special hui point of the muscles, indicated in all Wood muscular pathology; and neiguan (PC-6), the luo point of the shou jue yin. According to the circumstances we may treat ququan (LV-8) with moxibustion to tonify the liver, or needle the dispersion point of the pericardium, daling (PC-7), the indications of which are as follows:

> Pain or malaise in the heart, feeling that the heart is hanging with a hungry feeling at the same time; pain in the heart with the palms of the hands very warm; pain in the chest and in the heart with moaning and anxiety.[303]

We may also apply moxa to the beishu points of Jue Yin — jueyinshu (LV-14) for the pericardium, especially in cases of thoracic symptoms or vomiting, and ganshu (BL-18) for the liver, especially in cases of asthenia (See *Da Cheng*).

As far as diet is concerned, we may recommend whole grains (mild flavor), which are rich in magnesium, various vitamins and trace elements. Among the plants of the Chinese pharmacopoeia, mu ze cao is chosen preferentially. This is *Equisetum hiemale,* or shavegrass, a plant that is mild, slightly bitter and acts, according to Chamfrault, on the liver and gallbladder meridians. It influences the phosphorus-calcium metabolism because of its high concentration of silica. The ancient Chinese used it against all eye affections, especially for cataracts. It tonifies the liver and the gallbladder and is indicated in cases of overlong periods, of rectal prolapse and hemorrhoids.[304]

Massage is effective as well. According to the fifth aphorism concerning the five states of the body and mind (wu xing zhi):

> If the body is often frightened,[305] the liaison channels become congested and give rise to paresis, which we may treat with massages and alcoholized drugs {tinctures}.[306]

When we speak of massage, we mean energy massage along the Jue Yin meridian and the plexus points of ren mai, as well as along the internal and external spinal branches of zu tai yang (bladder meridian). These patients should be encouraged to practice energy exercises such as the Chinese taijiquan and/or Indian yoga or their modern derivatives (relaxation), or the martial arts, thus introducing into their stress-packed lives moments of decompression and of accumulation of qi.

To recapitulate the points indicated in cases of neurovegetative dystonia, of spasmophilia and of tetany: LV-1, CV-18, GB-34, LV-3, LV-8, PC-6, PC-7, BL-14, BL-18, associated with massage, whole grains, energy exercises and shavegrass.

Here again, there is a direct correlation with trace element therapy, since the dystonic behavior is responsible for the name of Diathesis III. Menetrier prescribes manganese-cobalt in cases of "dysparathyroidism," in association with phosphorus, which is related to muscle and cardiac tone as well as the calcium metabolism. He also prescribes magnesium. In most cases, the association of these various modes of therapy leads to a total relief of the symptoms and to an improvement in the patients' equilibrium, which is their fondest desire.

Neurological Pathology

The Jue Yin meridian plays an important role in neurology. It is involved in the encephalon, the cerebrospinal axis and in the motor nerves. A study of the classics shows that the neurological and psychiatric disorders associated with Jue Yin involve, more than anything else, an imbalance of blood and energy within the meridian. The flow of one of the two, upwards or downwards, creates a flow in the opposite direction of the other. We find the same mechanism as that found in the pelvic pathology (shan). As we are dealing with a global movement, the two are necessarily linked. This is obvious in gynecology in cases of "nervousness," neurovegetative dystonia associated with menstruation, pregnancy and post partum. This can progress as far as spasmophilia, tetany and even convulsions and hysteria.

The importance of the heart and uterine envelopes makes Jue Yin one of the fundamental axes of the balance of blood and energy in Chinese medicine. We have seen how the qi accumulates under the influence of emotional energy in the sperm and menstrual envelopes: "innumerable preoccupations, deceptions, immoderate desires and carnal abuses"[307] and causes dysmenorrhea and leukorrhea. The heart envelope is not excluded from these disorders and its meridian was even known as the "heart-sexuality envelope." In the realm of neurology, as elsewhere, the link between Jue Yin and the encephalon is established through the internal hepatoencephalic branch, which rises as high as the top of the head, baihui

233

(GV-20), and descends to the face. This shows the extent to which imbalances in cerebral physiology, either neurological or psychological, are linked in Chinese medicine to sexuality and the episodes of a subject's sex life. These concepts are astonishingly similar to modern physiology and psychiatric theory.

Acupuncture, which is by definition psychosomatic, represents an original and etiological therapeutic solution. Balancing Jue Yin, however, is not the only way to treat these disorders. (This is developed further in the chapter devoted to the Tai Yang temperament.) Once again, we come up against the necessity of determining the patient's temperament, and thus his vulnerable meridian. Otherwise, we need to be extremely gifted in sphygmology. As far as the neurological pathology of Jue Yin subjects is concerned, motor deficits are more central or proximal than peripheral. We may find other disorders such as epilepsy, convulsions and vestibular and cerebellar troubles[308] such as dizziness and memory loss. These disorders may be accompanied by headaches, a problem in and of themselves.

Headaches

Jue Yin headaches are often fronto-orbital and involve the eyeball, but they may also be occipital. They are discussed in the chapter devoted to Shao Yang and range from actual ophthalmic migraines to idiopathic or catamenial headaches.

• Warm Wind Headaches

As the links between Shao Yang and Jue Yin are very narrow, we may understand Qi Bo's comment:

> If the East wind blows in the spring, we will see the development of
> liver problems. These problems will be located in the neck.[309]

Husson translates this as the throat and the back of the neck. The back of the neck is certainly fengchi (GB-20), "the wind pond," but there are other "wind points" in this region including bingfeng (SI-12), fengfu (GV-16) and fengmen (BL-12), the "wind door." Their names imply an important role in the penetration of this perverse energy which takes place around the neck, the back of the neck and between the shoulder blades. Jianjing (GB-21), "the heavenly well," and tianliao (TB-15), "the heavenly bone," which comes before tianyou (TB-16), "the heavenly window," are points on Shao Yang that, as is clear from their names, are linked with the encephalon ("heaven").

This type of warm wind headache reminds us of the allergic etiology, as is often the case with perverse wind, whether the headaches be catamenial or essential, accompanied or not by edema (see asthma, rhinitis, conjunctivitis, hives and eczema). In Chapter 32 of the *Su Wen,* "Acupuncture of Heat," we find:

> In the heat disease of the liver. . . in case of backflow of qi, there is
> headache and dizziness, as the channel leads the qi to the head.[310]

Warm wind is the best definition of the allergenic perverse energy of the spring. When heat is associated with the wind, we may state that there is a plethora of blood. This is why, for a diseased liver, Qi Bo recommends, "Bleeding if there is a blockage of qi, headache, digestive problems or swelling of the cheeks."[311] The "swelling of the cheeks" seems to indicate an allergic edema.

234

• **Damp-Cold Headaches**

Damp cold headaches are quite different from warm wind headaches. Their context is defined by Nguyen Van Nghi in his discussion of the bi of the liver, gan bi:

> If the complexion is greenish, and if the pulse is slightly long and vibrating in both wrists, we may diagnose an accumulation of energy beneath the heart and in the flanks.[312] The illness is known as *can ty* {gan bi}, which is the same as *san khi* {shan qi}. accompanied by dorsalgia, cold feet and headache. It is caused by perverse damp cold.[313]

Zhang Zhi Cong adds:

> The damp cold always attacks the lower part of the body, through the feet. This perverse energy gains the liver meridian (zu jue yin), which brings it to the knees, to the genitals, to the flanks and then to the top of the head. This is why the patient has cold feet, dorsalgia and headaches.

> Qi Bo does not consider this phenomenon to be related to the spleen but to the liver, because the perverse energy does not follow zu tai yin (spleen) but rather zu jue yin (liver).[314]

This last comment is interesting. Since we are dealing with humidity, it would be logical to think that the perverse energy would tend to enter the spleen meridian (Earth involves humidity), as is classically indicated in Chapter 30 of the *Su Wen*. This happens in cases of leukorrhea (Tai Yin) or of peripheral neuropathy (see Tai Yin).[315]

Thus, the liver may be attacked by heat and wind, the penetration taking place through the throat and the back of the neck. The symptoms are by nature Yang — sudden violent headaches. The liver may be attacked, on the other hand, by the damp and the cold, and the penetration is located in the lower part of the body (through the shu point taichong; LV-3), and the symptoms are more Yin, more diffuse, more progressive and longer lasting, often nocturnal. We may also say, without much risk of error, that the warm wind headaches occur most often among women who suffer from "dark liver" dysmenorrhea or some other shan syndrome (fibroma, for example), or among men who are likely to suffer from genital infections, from priapism or from sexual overexcitation. Cold damp headaches, on the other hand, are secondary to leukorrhea and han shan (shan from the cold), or impotence, frigidity, pruritis vulvae or scrotal eczema. Treatment is studied in the corresponding sections of this book.

Dizziness

Our discussion of neurovegetative dystonia and headaches is based on the importance of the liver and of Shao Yang for the energization of the vestibular and cerebellar regions. This energization is also responsible for the phenomenon of dizziness. Once again, we must distinguish between excess and deficiency dizziness — between internal and external dizziness, since either excess or deficiency

235

of the liver meridian is likely to cause dizziness. This discrimination is made clearly in the *Su Wen,* first in Chapter 22:

> If the liver is diseased, there will be pain in the sides radiating towards the lower abdomen and a tendency to get angry.[316] If the disease is the result of a deficiency, the vision is troubled and hearing impaired;[317] there is a feeling of terror as if someone were grabbing at you. We take the points of the liver and gallbladder meridians. We bleed them, if there is a blockage of qi, headache, hearing problems and swelling of the cheeks.[318]

In Chapter 19, we find another passage:

> The pulse of spring {liver} is "like a cord."

> The qi arrives full and violent. It is in excess, and the illness is external. Or else it arrives empty and minimal, there is deficiency and the illness is internal. . .

> The excess makes the patient irritable,[319] uneasy, dizzy, confused, out of his head. The deficiency causes pains in the chest that spread to the back and down the sides, where the patient is fat.[320]

Notice a contradiction between the two texts concerning excess in the sides and vestibular disorders. The first text considers these to be due to an excess; the second, to a deficiency. This shows that there is a different reference, as an upsurge of energy can be caused by a deficiency of liver and an accumulation of blood in the lower part of the body.

In Chapter 69, Qi Bo discriminates between excess and deficiency of the element Wood, and thus of its viscera, the liver and the gall bladder:

> In the excess of the element Wood, the people suffer from diarrhea (sun xie), lack of appetite, heaviness of the body, malaise, borborygmus and abdominal tension[321] because of the exceptional shining of Jupiter.[322] In the extreme, there is obnubilation, anger, dizziness and cerebral trouble.[323]

Here we see an excess of blood an a deficiency of energy in the upper part of the body:

> In the failure of Wood, the people suffer from internal cold,[324] pain in the sides, in the lower abdomen, borborygmus and diarrhea. There are cold-hot illnesses, ulcers, dermatitis, abscesses and acne, coughing and colds under the sign of Mars[325] and Venus.[326]

Thus, excess dizziness is caused by an excess of liver energy, with a concentration of blood in the upper part of the body. Deficiency dizziness is a result of an insufficiency of energy of the liver, with a concentration of blood in the pelvic region and a concurrent upward surge of energy. The external (perverse energy) and internal (nutritional, emotional) etiologies follow this distinction to a greater or lesser degree.

In Western neurology, a discrimination is made between dizziness caused by central or peripheral factors. In dizziness due to central factors, the functional symptoms are limited to a drunken sensation and a non-systematized instability or imbalance.[327] Closer examination may reveal a spontaneous central nystagmus, asymmetric deviation of the indexes and associated neurological signs. We may mention Wallenberg's syndrome among these etiologies and a vertebrobasilar insufficiency. This is the excess Wood etiology in cerebrovascular accidents. There are also tumors of the posterior cavity and subjective syndromes subsequent to cranial trauma. In cases of tumor, we may make a comparison with the accumulation of qi associated with fibromas. Here, the accumulation of qi is located in the upper part of the body (encephalon) because of the excess of blood. In cases of cranial trauma, the dizziness is due to a blockage of energy within the meridians. There is concentration and excess. Acupuncture alone is capable of relieving the symptoms. We needle fengchi (GB-20).[328] Multiple sclerosis is another cause of central dizziness. All or almost all these syndromes stem from an excess.[329]

In cases of peripheral dizziness, all the subjective manifestations are due to a disorder of the membrane vestibule and of the eighth nerve pair.[330] These symptoms are comparable to those associated with dystonia, with the overwhelming dizziness associated with nausea and vomiting, or to a characteristic sensation of drunkenness, sometimes brought about by a sudden change in the posture of the head. There are associated cochlear symptoms including deafness and tinnitus. There may be a spontaneous nystagmus — in this case the deviation of the indexes is harmonious. Among these etiologies we find otospongiosis (degeneration, Yin indicating deficiency); infectious and inflammatory causes studied in the chapter devoted to Shao Yang, which are Yang; vascular and tumoral causes, particularly neurinoma of the eighth pair of nerves, and toxic causes, among which are streptomycin and ethylic intoxications.[331]

• **Meniere's Disease**

The origin of Meniere's disease is endolabyrinthine, defined as labyrinthine hydrops due to a hypertension of the endolabyrinthine fluids. It is manifested by dizziness with nausea and vomiting. The patient must lie on his side with his head turned towards the affected side. The dizziness is accompanied by a unilateral buzzing, such as that heard in a seashell, sometimes with a hissing, sometimes with unilateral surdity. There are bilateral forms as well. The condition occurs at regular intervals, from several weeks apart to several months or even years apart. Between attacks, there may be a persistent hypoacusis. In mild cases, the patient may complain more of headaches or of intellectual problems[332] than of dizziness. His problem may be thought of as being neurotic.[333]

The Chinese interpret this syndrome as a disorder of Jue Yin not only because of dizziness, which is considered to be the result of an excess of energy, but also because of the vomiting. This syndrome seems to be a perfect example of an external attack of perverse energy. We may compare the syndrome with the symptoms described by Qi Bo in cases of imbalance due to perverse energy: ''If the liver pulse is very slow, the vomiting is frequent.''[334] The association of vomiting and dizziness eliminates imbalance of the kidney meridian (the ears) as a potential cause.[335] The ancient physician makes another comment that directs our interest toward the endolabyrinthine fluids: ''If the liver pulse is slightly slow, there are problems with the fluids'' (edema, etc.). Thus, Meniere's vertigo seems to be the result of an external perverse energy disorder with complications related to the fluids. The capricious nature of the disease, which goes away and comes back like a fox — something like the repetitive "cold" cystitis — is a signature. We may read the signature as wind, and more precisely, cold wind.[336]

A stagnation of this perverse energy in the ear explains the physical sensation of pressure in the ear, as it does the necessity to put weight on the affected ear by sleeping on that side. Such an excess demands sleep and obscurity. The patient lies down and closes his eyes.

It is worth pointing out that this excess (whose origin is external, especially when cold is a factor), is likely to come about when there is a deficiency of liver, or rather a deficiency of the energy of the liver with a deficiency of blood in the upper part of the body and an accumulation of energy in the lower part. This explains the anxious or dystonic behavior of these patients, who tolerate their symptoms poorly and beg for prescriptions of tranquilizers. Acupuncture treatment of this disorder, which is more often than not unilateral and involves the Jue Yin meridian, is quite simple. It is the same as that indicated in the *Ling Shu* for tinnitus:

> When there is buzzing in the ears, we must needle zhongchong {PC-9}, then dadun {LV-1}, on the side opposite the ear in which the patient hears the buzzing.[337]

Nothing is more logical than needling the ting points. For zhongchong (PC-9) the *Da Cheng* indicates "chills with headaches"[338] which is the equivalent of dizziness, according to the American authors, Victor and Adams.

In conclusion, it is interesting to compare the Chinese physiopathological interpretation of neuritic dizziness with the "epidemic" dizziness described by Basser and Cogan. Cogan describes a syndrome specific to young adults, in which an interstitial keratitis (see Ophthalmology) is associated with dizziness, tinnitus, a nystagmus and a sudden deafness of uncertain cause.[339] In treating Meniere's disease we must treat PC-9 and LV-1, and we must balance Jue Yin between the attacks by needling the appropriate points and using moxibustion.

Trace elements indicated in treatment of "functional" dizziness are manganese, iodine, sulfur,[340] and, in short, all the trace elements associated with the element Wood (Diathesis I). Manganese-cobalt is also indicated in states of anxiety and for dystonic behavior.

Epilepsy

The Chinese etiologies of the epileptic syndromes are studied in the chapter devoted to Tai Yang. The Shao Yang etiology has already been mentioned. Jue Yin epilepsy does not exist.

There are, however, five epileptic organ etiologies that correspond to the disorders of each of the five organs: heart, spleen, lung, kidney and liver. The semiology of each one of these is different and the texts describe them by comparing the cries of the corresponding animals. The element Wood corresponds to the chicken. The description of the attack is as follows: "Liver epilepsy: the face is black and blue, the head wagging with fright or with joy, the cry of the rooster."[341] This description implies congestion of blood in the head, visible in the black and blue color of the face, and proves the etiology of excess of blood in the upper part of the body.[342] The wagging head (fear, stress, joy, emotion) is a typical Jue Yin symptom, and is evidence of the instability and the nervous and emotional sensitivity of these patients. Acupuncture treatment and correlations with the trace elements are described in the chapter devoted to Tai Yang.

Multiple Sclerosis

We will not attempt to explain precisely the origin of this disease, as any explanation is as yet hypothetical. However, it is interesting to apply the analogical reasoning that is specific to Chinese thought. Such reasoning is based on a semiological identity that corresponds with a strictly energetic physiopathology.

• Clinical Observation

The initial symptom in 40 percent of all cases of multiple sclerosis is an optical neuritis.[343] It appears suddenly and within a few days leads to a partial or total loss of sight in one eye (amaurosis), associated with oculomotor difficulties. In cases of partial loss of sight, there is a characteristic scotoma and a spontaneous nystagmus. This neuritis, when accompanied by inflammatory papillitis, regresses rapidly and totally in at least one third of all cases, or after several months of recuperation, or persists as an aftereffect. A brain stem lesion, involving the third, sixth or fourth nerves, can lead to diplopia or to intrinsic paralysis (myosis, accommodation troubles).

These clinical observations may be compared to the teachings of the ancient physician Qi Bo:

> Fainting and dizziness with sight and hearing problems[344] are caused by an excess in the lower part of the body and a deficiency in the upper part. The illness is in zu shao yang (gallbladder) and in zu jue yin (liver). If the case is severe, the disease passes to the liver.[345]

Other disorders of the brain stem or the medulla are responsible for the other 60 percent of these cases. The locations are varied, accounting for the multiplicity of symptoms and the presence of dysarthria, intentional trembling, ataxia, equilibrium disorders, troubles with vibratory sensitivity, motor deficits of one or more of the limbs (spastic or not), varied sensitivity disorders, facial anesthesia, dizziness and vomiting, according to whether the disorder involves the brain stem, the cerebellum, the vestibule or the medulla. It is particularly characteristic of this sort of pathology to begin with formication in the extremities, dizziness and temporary amblyopia.[346] In disorders involving the medulla, there are often bladder problems with dysuria, tenesmus, pollakiuria and urinary incontinence. Among male patients, these symptoms are often associated with impotence. About five percent of these patients suffer epileptic attacks.[347]

In Chinese medicine, the symptoms that characterize this pathology are as follows: eye problems, hearing difficulties, dizziness, vomiting, muscular paralysis, urinary incontinence, vesical pain, impotence, tenesmus and epilepsy.[348] Here once more, the common denominator of all these symptoms is none other than the liver (Jue Yin), with insufficiency of blood, and thus, a deficiency of liver. The muscular pathology is a result of "a severe disorder of the liver," that Qi Bo feared, faced with dizziness and amaurosis in the passage we quoted earlier. The diseased organ, along with its territory, represents the Chinese concepts of wei, of qi or of bi, implying severe deficiencies and chronic affections.

This is how we must interpret the astonishing passage in the *Su Wen:*

> All the channels[349] are attached to the eyes, all the marrows to the brain, all the muscles to the articulations, all the blood to the heart, all the murmurs to the lungs. In the morning and in the evening, the wind {breath} and the blood pass through the eight "valleys" {ba xi: elbows, knees, wrists and ankles} of the limbs. During sleep, the blood regains the liver, enabling us to see.[350] When they receive the blood, the legs may walk, the hands grasp and the fingers touch. If we are exposed to the wind upon rising, the blood is congealed in the skin and this is a bi,[351] or in the vessels {meridians} and it is a qi,[352] or in the legs and it is a jue. In all three cases, the blood cannot enter the cavities[353] and this is the cause of the bi and the jue.[354]

It is in this chapter that the symptoms we spoke of earlier are listed: fainting, dizziness, etc. Thus, in acupuncture, the symptoms of multiple sclerosis seem to be the result of a severe disorder of the liver and of its tissues (the muscles) — such as a bi, a qi or a jue — in which the physiology of the blood plays a fundamental part in the nutrition of the dependent cerebral structures: optic nerve, vestibule, brain stem, medulla.

• Examination

Patients who suffer from multiple sclerosis and who complain of functional symptoms involving a single limb show signs of disease. A good example of symptoms involving both limbs would be a bilateral Babinski. This means, in Chinese medicine, that the perverse energy and the "congealed blood" are blocked within the secondary channels, and especially in the luo channel of the liver meridian. This calls for needling on the opposite side. The study of the psychological behavior of the patient is especially enlightening; among multiple sclerosis patients, we sometimes notice a euphoria, a paradoxical gaiety that results from a disorder involving the white matter of the frontal lobes.[355] This is interpreted in acupuncture as an imbalance of the pericardium meridian shou jue yin ("the patient laughs all the time"). On the other hand, we also find patients who are depressed, irritated, moody and who have disorders such as memory loss as a result of disseminated lesions.[356] This behavior is typically zu jue yin. (See Psychiatric Pathology.)

The interrogation of a great many patients concerning their personality and behavior prior to the onset of the disease shows, without exception, that the Jue Yin profile is subjacent to the illness. We must note, however, that this psychological profile is more often than not combined with the Shao Yin profile. Personal history and associated morbidity among these patients include the whole range of Jue Yin symptoms, as is the case among Shao Yin patients. Among the former, we find we find signs of insufficiency of the blood of the liver, along with pre-existent myopia and gynecological problems. Among the latter, we find signs of insufficiency of the kidneys given the immunity role assigned to the kidneys in Chinese physiology, such as repeated sore throats during childhood, boils and superinfection.[357] All these observations point consistently to the importance of a patient's terrain in the onset of this disease.

• Weakening Factors

Certain factors that precede the onset of disease have been considered to weaken the patient and facilitate the disease. They include various infections, emotional shocks and wounds, as well as pregnancy, which seems to increase the frequency of the attacks among patients who are already diseased.[358] All these circumstances, including the wounds, aggress the Jue Yin meridian, particularly those concerning the state of the blood within the meridian of the liver.[359] The prevalence of women patients among those who suffer from this pathology accredits our insistence upon terrain, upon predisposition to illness, as well as our hypothesis involving insufficiency of blood of the liver in Jue Yin according to the energetic explanation of this disease in Chinese theory. We may thus easily include as a weakening factor the episodes of genital life among female patients.

• Biological Examination

Classically, we find hypergammaglobulinemia of the cerebral spinal fluid. Seric gammaglobulins are disturbed in 60 percent of all cases.[360] These disturbances are associated in a good many cases with a relatively low rate of cholesterol and with perturbations of the beta-lipoproteins and in their specific flocculation tests. This may indicate a profound disorder of the absorption or the metabolism of lipids in the small intestine (under the influence of the bile) and in the liver. One physiological manifestation of the liver blood deficiency might well be a disorder of lipid metabolism (here the cerebral lipids, phospholipids) and a subsequent alteration of the myelin sheaths that they constitute.[361]

• Etiology

The cause or causes of multiple sclerosis are still unknown today. Certain epidemiological factors, however, have been demonstrated. The affection appears to be rare between the equator and the 30th or 35th latitudes North or South. It is much more frequent in higher latitudes.[362] If an individual moves from a region of high risk to a region of lower risk before the age of fifteen, his chances of contracting the disease become those of the low risk region. Over the age of fifteen, there is no such change. In Chinese medicine this would be interpreted as a "latent perverse energy," that would be contracted at an early age but that would remain latent for a number of years. This hypothesis would tend to support the idea of a partly external origin (virus or allergy and autoimmunity).[364] It is curious to note, in passing, that there are analogies in Chinese and Western medicine: we speak here of latent infections, for example, or of cold auto-antibodies, in immunology.

• Anatomopathology

It is interesting to compare microscopic studies with the Chinese hypothesis of an insufficiency of liver blood (which covers, by the way, all the various venous circulatory disorders, from varicose veins to hemorrhoids, including the cardiac liver, which we have already studied). Histological examination of recent lesions notices perivenous demyelinization, sparing the cylinder, a neurological reaction and a mononuclear vascular infiltration.[365] This perivenous distribution of the lesions might well be the modern interpretation of the "congealed blood" in the vessels, or meridians, mentioned in the *Su Wen,* which hinders the normal action of the fingers, the hands and the legs.

In determining a differential diagnosis, there is a possibility of confusion between multiple sclerosis and certain forms of amyotrophic lateral sclerosis, or of combined degeneration of the marrow stemming from a vitamin B12 deficiency (presence of megaloblasts in the bone marrow, anemia and absence of gastric acid secretion). Amyotrophia and its fasciculations enable us to identify the former affection. Both, however, seem to be combined Tai Yin/Shao Yin affections. The former disease resembles specific peripheral polyneuritis, the second resembles anemia and an absence of gastric secretion.[366]

• Chinese Etiopathology

To summarize from a perspective of Chinese etiopathology, we may say that multiple sclerosis appears consistently within the framework of the predisposed terrain of the Jue Yin temperament, or more concisely, to the combined Jue Yin/Shao Yin temperament. We may speak of a constitutional predisposition to a deficiency of blood within the Jue Yin meridian that, along with Shao Yang, energizes the occipital region, the vestibule and the cerebellum, the eye, the optic nerve, the brain centers involved in vision, the motor nerves and muscles and the medulla. This deficiency facilitates the penetration of a latent perverse energy that involves the wind which, unlike the bi of the liver, penetrates through the cervical points and stays "hidden" until other circumstances (cosmic, emotional, gynecological) trigger the onset of the disease. In Chapter 80 of the *Ling Shu,* dealing with "The Concentration of the Energy of the Meridians in the Eyes," Qi Bo states:

> When the perverse energy attacks the back of the neck, it penetrates
> through to the eyes, then to the brain, which is why there may be diz-
> ziness.[367]

The capricious evolution of the illness, coming and going, is typical of perverse wind affections. The Chinese compared these to the fox, a clever animal that knows how to hide.

Whatever the Western etiology (virus, allergy, autoimmunity), the analysis of the features of this illness according to the traditional Chinese reasoning classifies it among combined organ-tissue disorders, such as the qi, the bi and the wei. There is probably association with the cold. This leaves us with a perverse cold wind, a symptomology that may be compared to the description of the bi of the liver: "pain in the back, headache, cold feet."[368] Along with rachialgia resembling "electrical discharges" described by Lhermitte, these are typical manifestations of multiple sclerosis. The absence of rachialgia, however, does not contradict the Chinese bi etiology. In the chapter of the *Su Wen* devoted to these pains, Huang Di asked:

> "What happens when the bi is without pain?"

> Qi Bo replied: "If the bi is in the bones, the body is heavy; if it is in
> the vessels, the blood is congealed.[369] In this way there are five bi
> without pain. In all forms of bi, cold causes formication, heat causes
> sedation."[370]

This last comment says something of the use of moxibustion in this sort of affection.

We must not forget the role played by Shao Yin in this pathology. Shao Yin, after all, is responsible for energizing the bones and the marrow. The kidney is the dwelling of jing qi, the essential energy related to the curious bowels: endocrine glands, nerves, vascular system, gallbladder and uterus. The heart is the dwelling of the shen. It is the organ of the blood and the blood vessels. Jing and shen are in balance.[371] An insufficiency of the former may cause signs of excess of the latter, as we learned in the chapter devoted to the wei. The illness leads to physical and psychological behavior that is Yin in nature and immediately visible.

It is not impossible that the cold-wind penetration enters through the zu jue yin and zu shao yin meridians, through the lower limbs. It is, however, the symptomology that will enable us to determine whether the perverse energy is located in the lower limbs, in the back of the neck or in both. There is a good chance that the initial penetration of the latent perverse energy is located in the upper part of the body where it remains hidden:

> All the meridians are concentrated in the eyes, and through the eyes,
> are linked to the brain and to the neck. When the perverse energy
> attacks the neck, it penetrates through to the eyes and then to the
> brain, which is why there is dizziness.[372]

Whether the triggering factor is internal, external or cosmic (perverse cold in the springtime), the imbalance will be discovered in the lower part of the body, within the meridians of the lower limbs. It will activate the latent perverse energy waiting in the upper part of the body. It is this combination and this alternative that enables acupuncture to explain the capricious nature of the illness with its moments of activity and its regressions.

If this traditional physiological interpretation is valid, our analysis is not without value. As there is a cosmic factor that is involved in predisposition and in triggering the internal pathology, the precepts of Chinese chronobiology enable us to predict the season, the month and also the years during which the condition is likely to be aggravated. The fact that the onset of symptoms typically occurs at the age of thirty, a time that is considered by the Chinese to be the "springtime of life" is one of the intriguing aspects of Chinese energetic epidemiology.

• Treatment of Multiple Sclerosis

In treating multiple sclerosis attacks, ACTH alone has proven effective in controlling the disease and in accelerating the recuperation.[373] A significant number of patients, however, fail to respond to this treatment.[374] It is well known that such treatment has no influence upon the evolution of the disease and shares the long term disadvantages common to the corticoids.[375] In light of this knowledge, it may be of value if we propose acupuncture treatment of multiple

243

sclerosis. This should be applied in association with adjuvant techniques such as re-education and symptomatic relaxation treatments, and in place of such treatments as tranquilizers and antidepressants.

● **Treatment During a Period of Attack**

During attacks, or if we are lucky enough to observe a patient who is undergoing an original manifestation, we must examine the little capillaries along the pathway of the liver meridian, and also in the cervical and neck regions. Needle and bleed the ones that appear dilated. Owing to the certainty of "blood congestion" in the secondary channels, we can probably observe the phenomenon in examination and apply the traditional *Su Wen* method, which "chases away the perverse energy."[376] This has always proven effective in practice. We must meticulously inspect the wind points and heat them with moxa when they are pathological. For all attacks, it is useful to needle taichong (LV-3), or treat this point with moxa.[377] This is the shu point of penetration of perverse energy in the lower limbs. The shu point is also the point of the Yin meridians indicated by Qi Bo in the treatment of the bi.[378] The *Da Cheng* indicates for taichong (LV-3), "Illness with Yin symptoms,"[379] as well as "Pain in the spine and insensitivity in the fingertips."[380] Soulie de Morant adds to these indications, "Trouble moving the lower limbs, walking; numbness in the lower limbs."[381]

● **General Treatment**

To effect treatment it is essential in all cases to needle the luo point of the liver meridian on the side opposite the functional deficit, or bilaterally, whether or not there are symptoms on both sides. Again, priority is given to the side opposite the one most affected. The *Da Cheng* indicates for ligou (LV-5), the luo point of the liver:

> To be dispersed when there is weakness and flaccidity in the lower limbs, when the legs and feet are cold, numb, difficult to bend or to straighten.[382]

Among the points of the liver meridian, we may choose to needle xingjian (LV-2), taichong (LV-3) and ququan (LV-8), but certainly not all at the same time. The illness is serious, "the organ" is affected, so we must treat xingjian (LV-2) and taichong (LV-3) regularly and in combination as these rong and shu points are the Yin meridian points to treat when the organ is affected. Qi Bo chose to needle these points in cases of wei pathology:

> "What is the treatment of the wei?" asked Huang Di.

> "We tonify the rong point, we liberate the shu point, we regulate the tonus and we re-establish the flow of qi in the meridians that correspond to the diseased tissues during their specific periods."[383]

One detail does not escape our attention: "during their specific periods."

We may prefer to treat ququan (LV-8) with moxa.[384] This is the tonification point that, when heated, strengthens the blood and energy of the liver. This point corresponds to distal and medullar neurological semiology (anal and vesical sphincters) according to the *Da Cheng*, and is particularly indicated.[385] Chamfrault transmits Doctor Zhang's advice in these cases:

> When the legs are paralyzed due to wei, we needle dazhu {BL-11} as well as ququan {LV-8}.[386]

Dazhu (BL-11) is the special he point for the bones and is located in the cervical region. This point links the cold wind, Jue Yin, the bones, the kidney, Shao Yin and the muscles. If the wei is complicated by a Shao Yin temperament, it must be treated by needling the rong and shu points of the kidney, rangu (KI-2) and taixi (KI-3), which are indicated for "fear, paralysis of the lower limb, atony of both legs, fatigue and insensitivity in the feet."[387] It seems that these two points are especially indicated in cases of paraparesis. We may also strengthen the Yin by cauterizing the beishu points on the back: ganshu (BL-18) (the liver shu), shenshu (BL-23) (the kidney shu) and mingmen (GV-4).

Three other points are fundamental in treating multiple sclerosis. Yanglingquan (GB-34), the special hui point for the muscles and for the gallbladder, is indicated in all muscular deficits, whatever the etiology (see Neurology, Shao Yang). Naohu (GV-17), special hui point for the marrows, is located on the occipital bone, over the cortical visual zone. Naokong (GB-19) on the Shao Yang meridian is on the same horizontal line as naohu (GV-17). The first two points are to be needled. The third, naokong (GB-19), "deficiency of brain," is located over the cortical visual zone and must be cauterized. It is indicated for "depressive states, shock causing diplopia, pain in the eyes, clouded vision and dizziness."[388] We may also mention the specific Jue Yin key points: gongsun (SP-4), the chong mai key point and neiguan (PC-6), the yin wei mai key point, as well as the points houxi (SI-3) and shenmai (BL-62), key points of miscellaneous channels more or less directly concerned with the energization of the neuraxis. The use of general points such as gaohuang (BL-38), baohuang (BL-48) and shenque (CV-8) depends on the individual case.

The length of insertion of the needles should be rather short. Few points should be needled in a given session, as the more points we needle and the longer we stimulate, the more we disperse the energy. We must remember the aphorism found in the *Su Wen:* "In needling Jue Yin, we release the blood, and not the qi."[389] We must be cautious about multiplying the number of insertions among patients who suffer from an insufficiency of blood in Jue Yin. "We must avoid wounding the energy in this case."[390] In any case, we should use moxa as much as possible in treating an illness that is as Yin as multiple sclerosis. The sessions should, for this reason, be repeated and closely spaced. The optimal number is three per week, or every day during the attacks, with periods of rest between each session.

In illness as profound, chronic and severe as the bi and the wei, to which we may compare multiple sclerosis, it is a good idea to accumulate as many success factors as possible, by choosing the time of the year and the time of the day that best serve our purposes. We must recall Qi Bo's recommendation of the "specific period." The specific period related to Wood is the spring. The specific days are jia and yi (pine-1 and bamboo-2). If we take the trouble to apply the laws of acupuncture according to the season and if we take multiple sclerosis as an example, in the spring of the year 1980, we would choose the days closest to the spring equinox, being careful to begin treatment as the moon waxes for the reasons developed in our discussion of gynecology.[391] In 1980, the new moon fell a few days before the 21st of March, so there was no problem. The jia and yi days that year were the 23rd and the 24th of March.[392] These will be the best days of the year on which to begin treatment. Next we must choose the best time, according to the rule of encounter and pursuit.[393] The hour of the liver is chou, from 1 am to 3 am. In this case the liver is deficient, so we have to go in pursuit of its energy when it weakens, which is the following hour, to strengthen it. The following hour is yin, from 3 am to 5 am. At that time, on jia day, the 23rd of March, the open miscellaneous channel that links man to the cosmos is dai mai, whose opening we may facilitate by needling zulinqi (GB-41).[394] In France, on daylight savings time, these hours correspond to those between 5 am and 7 am.[395] Zulinqi is not a bad choice, as it opens Shao Yang through dai mai. We must needle only the point opposite the diseased side, or begin with this point if we choose to needle bilaterally. Then, we needle ligou (LV-5) on the opposite side, or xingjian (LV-2) and taichong (LV-3) either on the opposite side or bilaterally. Afterwards, we will apply moxa, either to taichong (LV-3) or to dazhu (BL-11) and ququan (LV-8); or to ganshu (BL-18), shenshu (BL-23), mingmen (GV-4); or taixi (KI-3). The choice of points to treat will vary according to the other points treated according to the therapist.

The following day, the 24th of March, is the next most favorable day. At the same time, the yang qiao mai is opened by shenmai (BL-62), which is a neurological point of certain value and whose action is especially central and medullary.[396] This is particularly true for male patients. We may vary the choice of associated points to be needled or treated with moxa in the same manner of the previous day's treatment. Theoretically, the following two days should find an improvement, as we read in the *Su Wen:*

> Liver disease heals on the days bing (3) and ding (4), and gets worse
> on the days geng and xin. If it is not fatal, it is stationary on the days
> ren and gui, and begins on the days jia and yi. It awakens at dawn,
> attains its height in the evening, and calms down at midnight.[397]

The following days, bing and ding, corresponding to the 25th and 26th of March (1980) are equally favorable for continuing the treatment at the same time of the day. Between 3 a.m. and 5 a.m. on the 25th, the opening meridian will still be dai mai, through zulinqi (GB-41). That day we may add yanglingquan (GB-34). On the 26th, the opening meridian point is fortunately gongsun (SP-4), which is closely linked to Jue Yin, to the physiology of the blood and to the energy of the liver and the envelopes. We will needle this point contralaterally if the symptomology is asymmetrical, and couple it with neiguan (PC-6), which opens the associated meridian, yin wei mai.

This reasoning was used by the ancient Chinese therapists in their treatment of serious diseases. It merits at least one such digression to show how careful we should be in following systematic and standardized protocols in acupuncture, and in the interpretation of their results.[398] It would certainly be worthwhile to undertake serious methodical therapeutic experimentation, in view of establishing a treatment for this disease that makes invalids of so many young adults. Our analysis would lead us to examine the following points: the capillaries, LV-2,

LV-3, LV-5, BL-11, LV-8, KI-2, KI-3, GB-34, GV-17, GB-19, BL-18, BL-23, GV-4, SP-4, PC-6, SI-3, BL-62, BL-38, BL-48 and GB-41. As far as therapeutic associations go, we might prescribe Chinese massage, practiced by a qualified massotherapist, along with the classical techniques of re-education and, in general, any other adjuvant therapy that might be of value, including a careful study of the patient's diet and trace element therapy. Menetrier expresses his reservations about treating this illness with the trace elements, but speaks of a pertinent association with other, related pathologies. He speaks of manganese-cobalt and cobalt[399] associated with phosphorus.[400]

Psychiatric Pathology

Cerebral Physiology of Blood and Energy in Jue Yin

Common functional or psychiatric disorders such as insomnia, reactional neurosis, anxiety, neurovegetative dystonia and even spasmophilia are typical morbid states associated with the Shao Yang or Jue Yin temperaments. Described in various parts of this book,[401] these are typical of the symptoms a "psychosomatic" patient complains of when he consults an acupuncturist. The other mental disorders that result from aggression of the Jue Yin meridian may be considered as an excess or deficiency of blood in the upper part of the body or in the head. Strictly speaking, these are not symptoms that are specific to the Jue Yin temperament, but severe imbalances whose etiologies are varied. Drugs, stimulants or medication are important factors in acting upon the liver and upon its meridian. We cannot exclude the possibility that these disorders occur in relation to a predisposed terrain and are a compensation by the most vulnerable organ and meridian affected by a toxic agent. Since the same toxic agent may tend to affect a different organ or a different meridian among patients of a different constitution, this observation holds true for all the temperaments, not only Jue Yin.

It is as if a single perverse energy may choose among three different Yin meridians in the lower limbs, with penetration in each of the three causing a very different pathology.[402] It would be interesting to study how the aspects of tobacco intoxication vary according to the temperament of the smoker: one pathology determining a cancer of the lung, for example, rather than a cardiovascular disorder. Regarding the mental problems associated with Jue Yin, we may recall Qi Bo's remark, which applies as well to the biao-li meridian, Shao Yang:

> When there is an excess of blood, the patient is angry. If there is a deficiency of blood, he is anxious and fearful.[403]

A similar remark is to be found in the *Ling Shu:*

> The liver governs the blood, and within the blood dwells the soul {hun}.[404] When the energy of the liver is deficient, the patient becomes fearful, anxious. When it is in excess, the patient becomes irritable and is always angry.[405]

This passage shows us once again that it is indeed the liver that is so important in the physiology of the blood.

247

It is easy to understand that an excess of the liver, which goes along with the blood in its ascension within the body, will cause a concentration of blood in the upper part of the body and will give rise to Yang behavioral symptoms such as agitation, aggressivity, fury and delirium. A deficiency of blood causes a descending movement, a concentration in the lower part of the body, with deficiency in the upper part. This creates a Yin symptomology with an agitation, which is not at all aggressive but rather fearful, and delirium that is not furious but rather confused, and obnubilation. If we examine the patterns involved in alcohol intoxication, which is notoriously devastating to the liver, we may classify as excess of blood in the upper part of the body the pathological inebriety that gives rise to agitation (manic motor excitation) or to megalomanic delirium. This behavior may be complicated by the presence of another temperament, particularly Tai Yang or Yang Ming.[406] This inebriety results in a state of furor; the patient wreaks havoc all around him and can go so far as to kill. Afterwards, there is a tendency to sleep and to forget. This raises the problem of an epileptic complication,[407] which represents the most drastic behavior of Shao Yang[408] or even Jue Yin, with an excess of blood in the upper part of the body. Another form of this excess is known as the delirium tremens.

On the other hand, we have the mental disorders, a result of deficiency of blood in the upper part of the body, that are represented by a relative loss of memory accompanied by asthenia and psychasthenia, ranging from memory problems common to Jue Yin subjects to the typical Korsakoff's psychosis, another complication of alcohol intoxication. We also find hysterical behavior among these deficiency syndromes. We will develop a few of these syndromes.

Delirium Tremens

A brief description of the delirium tremens will serve to show to what extent this disorder is linked to an excess of blood in the upper part of the body within the Jue Yin meridian. There is an occasional prodromic phase that is marked by violent trembling and vesperal overexcitation. As seen in our discussion of multiple sclerosis, the evening is the time when liver disorders are aggravated. In the active stage, the patient is agitated and his incoherent behavior is full of fear and aggressivity.[409] In many ways, this behavior is illustrates the disorder. His face is red and puffy, his lips dry; there are signs of Fire in the head. He is mentally confused and is in a constant state of hallucinatory delirium that is often like a dream.[410] His hallucinations are primarily visual (the eye is the Wood organ, and the temporal lobe is energized by Shao Yang) and cenesthesic, gaining in intensity and precision at nightfall.[411] He has a fever that ranges from 100° to 104° Fahrenheit, with all the classical signs of an excess of Fire: "Great thirst, dryness of the mouth, oliguria, tachycardia," as was classically described for this syndrome.[412]

In Chapter 17 of the *Su Wen* we read, "When there is an excess of Yang, or of Yin, one dreams of massacres or calamities. . . excess of liver energy brings dreams of anger."[413] When it is not obvious that the patient is an alcoholic, we must make a diagnostic discrimination of delirium tremens, acute toxic delirium, acute epileptic psychosis, intracranial hematoma and acute azotemic encephalitis, whose description is to be found in the *Ling Shu*,[414] and meningeal hemorrhage, frequent among alcoholics.[415] These various etiologies are all forms of the same energetic mechanism — ''excess of blood in the upper part of the body'' — especially the intracranial hematoma, which represents the patent and substantial form of this energetic concept. This may be compared to cerebral tumors with vestibular symptoms and dizziness, which we have already mentioned.

Physiological and therapeutic confirmation of these various states is to be found in Chapter 22 of the *Ling Shu,* dealing with ''mental troubles'' or ''troubles of the consciousness''[416] and in which we find the main etiologies of comas and demential states. In this chapter, Qi Bo states:

> In treating such a patient, we must observe him meticulously and patiently, before deciding on which point to needle.

> When the patient is suffering an attack, certain meridians that show abnormal signs must be dispersed and bled. The blood that is gathered in a recipient should be agitated. If it is not agitated during the attack, we must apply moxas twenty times on the coccyx.[417]

Nguyen Van Nghi quotes this passage in his article devoted to ''the depressive states'' and translates the term ''agitated blood'' as coagulation.[418] This would tend to mean that rapidly coagulable blood corresponds to an excess of blood and thus to a movement towards the upper part of the body. Blood that coagulates slowly corresponds to a deficiency or deficit of blood in the upper part, with a concentration in the lower region.

This alternative of excess or deficiency among cases of mental agitation leads Qi Bo to make the following qualification:

> Always, at the beginning of the mental troubles, we first needle the point ququan {LV-8}, located over the artery. If need be, we may bleed it a bit, and the patient will calm down after a while, and if not, we apply moxa twenty times to the coccyx; the point changqiang {GV-1} is the liaison point between zu tai yang {bladder} and the miscellaneous channel du mai {governing vessel}.[419]

It is clear we are either dealing with an agitation due to an excess of blood in the head, where we would needle ququan (LV-8), or with an agitation that is a false Yang symptom. In this case it is a major deficiency and we heat changqiang (GV-1). This point activates all the Yang energy and mobilizes it towards the upper part of the body. This point name means ''always strong'' or ''long and powerful,'' depending on the translation.

Let us point out two things: first, ququan (LV-8) is chosen to disperse the excess, regardless of which meridian is imbalanced (the text refers to several). This tends to confirm the importance of zu jue yin (liver) in this specific physiology of the blood. Second, ququan (LV-8) is the tonification point of the meridian that corresponds to the element Water (cold) and that is indicated in cases of multiple sclerosis. The reasoning is exactly the opposite. For multiple sclerosis, the point was stimulated with moxa to bring heat to the blood, making the blood rise within the body. In this case, we needle and even bleed the point, causing an immediate and brutal dispersion of the excess; there is a decongestion of the blood and a downward movement. If indeed, agitation because of an excess of blood is synonymous with hypercoagulability, in the specific case of delirium tremens

249

(given the hepatic disorder), we are likely to find coagulation problems, a lowered rate of prothrombin and a delayed coagulation time, which is just the opposite. The etiological discrimination based on the blood taken from the patient is much more complex and involves cosmic[420] and energetic factors that we will see later in this work.[421] Ququan (LV-8) is also indicated in coagulation deficits.

Memory Deficits and Psychasthenia

• Serious Memory Problems

Serious memory deficits are the result of the inverse of the mechanism we have just described, as was indicated by Qi Bo in the *Su Wen:*

> If the blood descends toward the lower part of the body, and if the energy rises, the patient is delirious and has trouble remembering.[422]

This is a calm form of delirium, a type of obnubilation with dreamy confusion and temporospatial disorientation. The most characteristic type is Korsakoff's syndrome, which associates the two symptoms, since there is a fixated amnesia that is usually compensated for by fantasizing and "false recognition," characteristically accompanied by temporospatial disorientation.

• Slight Memory Problems and Psychasthenia

In everyday practice we frequently hear of slight memory problems. Here again, we might apply the principle of analogy that is specific to Chinese semiology. Accordingly, the intensity and the nature of the symptoms are proportional to the degree of "organicity" of the disorder. Among Shao Yang subjects, muscular hyperreflexia or effervescent nervousness in the coleric character may become epilepsy, manic homicidal fury or apoplexy. With Jue Yin subjects we find the Yin symptoms of the liver combining to form a more or less complete profile of psychasthenia or neurasthenia with physical disorder,[423] anxious and fearful personality ("fear that someone will jump him" says the text), volubility, slight disorientation, temporary obnubilation felt as a momentary confusion, and memory storage problems.[424]

This profile is polymorphously visible at all ages. It is often combined with one or more of the dystonic symptoms, signaling a deficiency of blood, or a deficiency of the liver with various spasms, thoracic or abdominal. Other symptoms include facial congestion, paresthesia, fits of tears and spasmophilia. These symptoms are sometimes, but not always, associated with dysmenorrhea, impotence, frigidity, allergies, migraines, angioneurotic edema, eczema, gynecomastia, depression or insomnia.

Menopause among female patients or andropause among the male patients is a special time at which physiological circumstances are associated with those more psychological in nature. The Chinese model enables us to understand why this moment is felt more dramatically and more intensely by women independently of any esthetic or superficial preoccupations, which are too often blamed as being responsible for the discomfort. Acupuncture treatment of slight memory disorders and of psychasthenia concentrates on the strengthening of the energy of the liver and of the blood and also on the balancing of Jue Yin. We must regularly disperse shou jue yin (pericardium), which is often in excess, with the accompanying psychological symptoms of the Fire Minister rising to the upper part of the body. Particularly during menopause, the shen itself will be affected and a combined treatment will be necessary.[425] We will again apply moxa to ququan (LV-8), but we must also treat certain points whose nature is more psychic, either on the median line of du mai or on either side of the spinal column on the branches of zu tai yang (bladder meridian).

In the space between D9 and D10 are located the points jinsuo (GV-8), "retracted muscle," (which is well named), on the D9 spinous process. On either side we find ganshu (BL-18), the shu point of the liver, and on the external branch, hunmen (BL-42), "the door of the soul" or "door of the hun," which is the shen of the liver. The *Da Cheng* indicates for jinsuo (GV-8), "Weakening of the nerves; the patient talks a lot, pain in the heart and dizziness."[426] Judging by its name, we may think that moxa applied to this point will be beneficial in treating spasmophilia. It is also indicated for epilepsy whose origin involves the liver (see Epilepsy, Tai Yang). We have already spoken of asthenia in relation to ganshu (BL-18). The indication for this point is "when the liver lacks blood."[427] The name of hunmen (BL-42), "door of the hun," means that we may reach the hun and act upon it. The hun, or the qi of neuromuscular activity, according to Needham, is considered in the *Su Wen* to be the advisor of the shen (conscious principle of the heart).[428]

Soulie de Morant considers the hun to be the hereditary or acquired mind, the dwelling place of conscious and unconscious memory, "the three memories," as he says. He translates it as "parrot memory," by which he means an automatic memory principle. The Chinese might, thus, learn "by liver" rather than "by heart," as we do. But as the hun is the advisor of the shen, it is all the same.

The three memories discussed by Soulie de Morant correspond to the conscious and subconscious memories on the one hand, and on the other to a physical or genetic memory. In light of this, let us recall a passage from the *Su Wen:*

> The East represents the celestial mysteries; it is the symbol of the Tao that exists within man; for it represents the transformations of nutrients that themselves engender intelligence.
>
> In the body it represents the liver.[429]

This might help us to understand from an energetic viewpoint the particular importance of hereditary defects among alcoholics, as well as their frequent neurological or psychiatric nature — epilepsy, behavioral problems, intelligence defects.[430]

We will give all the indications for hunmen (BL-42): "Pain in the heart that radiates to the back, muscular spasms, anorexia,[431] cadaveric syncope,[432] direct effects upon the hun {three memories}," according to Soulie de Morant, and "neurasthenia," according to the modern authors from Shanghai.[433] In the inferior intervertebral space between D10 and D11 are located two complementary points that correspond to the gallbladder, the Wood bowel, the bowel of the East. Zhongshu (GV-7), which means "central axis," roughly corresponds to the midpoint between C1 and the coccyx. Soulie de Morant, for reasons that are unknown, adds a question mark: "Heart: valves?"[434] Chamfrault notes that this is the point of departure of the energy of the meridian du mai.[435] This point, located horizontal to danshu (BL-19), the beishu point of the gallbladder, presiding bowel at the birth of Yang, corresponds to the beginning of the energy of du mai. Yang-gang (BL-48) is translated as the "precis of Yang" by Chamfrault and Nguyen Van Nghi; as the "firmness of Yang" by Soulie de Morant; and as the "principle of Yang" by the Shanghai Hospital Medical Group. The name probably stems from "essence of Yang,"[436] that represents the jing of the gallbladder.[437]

This point is mentioned in the context of "great asthenia, anorexia,"[438] whose semiological equivalent is to be found in viral hepatitis. It is indicated for treatment of hepatic symptoms: "red sclera, dark red urine, trouble urinating. . . "[439] Certain points of shou jue yin (pericardium) are also important in dealing with memory deficits, especially when the emotions flare up. Three of them are indicated by Soulie de Morant: ximen (PC-4), neiguan (PC-6), zhongchong (PC-9). The first two are involved with the global regulations of Jue Yin, liver insufficiency, thoracic blockage and the relative excess of the pericardium. The third serves to tonify Shao Yin (heart) in case of failure of the shen, depending on the age of the patient, or in circumstances that influence the emotions. This side of the question is dealt with not only in our chapter devoted to Shao Yin, but also to Tai Yin and Tai Yang, which are all involved in memory deficits.

We shall, however, consider the hun as being primary in these disorders, then the shen, which the hun advises, and to a lesser extent, the po. Psychasthenia and memory deficits caused by deficiency of the blood of the liver and by essential imbalance within Jue Yin are treated with the following points: LV-8, GV-8, BL-18, BL-42, BL-19, BL-43, PC-4, PC-6 and PC-9. As far as the correlation with the trace elements goes, Menetrier states:

> Memory deficits are linked to the allergic diathesis. They are improved with manganese. They can become aggravated to the point of total memory loss, during the evolution towards the dystonic diathesis, and are frequent during menopause. There is a possible action with manganese-cobalt.[440]

He goes on to mention the specific action of magnesium, of phosphorus and of aluminum.

Hysterical Neurosis

At the fringes of Jue Yin behavior, it is sometimes difficult to say where ends the boundary of neurovegetative dystonia, spasmophilia, psychasthenia, anxiety, emotional and affective hypersensitivity and where begins hysterical neurosis.[441] Beyond the clinical manifestations and their causes, the diagnosis depends on a thorough investigation of the personality of the patient. Still, there is no clear limit between personality factors and neurosis and, once again, we find a demonstration of the semiological analogy in Chinese medicine that enables us to better understand our patient beyond the strict discrimination between organic and psychiatric diagnosis. Chinese medicine tells us that all the manifestations of hysteria depend on the same mechanism that determines the functional or organic symptoms of a neurological disorder (epilepsy) or of an endocrine disorder (hypocalcemia). This knowledge allows us to speculate about an original therapeutic solution that will correct the common imbalance, thus going much further than the modern etiological sanctions for treatment of each of these disorders. In view of this speculation, a semiological analysis of the hysterical patient's symptoms deserves our undivided attention.

In secondary to hysterical neurosis, we find descriptions of asthenia, frequent headaches (which direct our thinking towards Jue Yin from the beginning), syncope, epileptic seizures, conversions with spasms or contractures. With sensorial manifestations we find amblyopia, diplopia, amaurosis; we also find the usual visceral manifestations including vomiting, digestive spasms, enuresis and dysuria, as well as dyspareunia and menstrual problems.[442] Apart from the depressive context,[443] as far as psychological symptoms go, we often note memory gaps when the patient is asked to give his own personal case history. These gaps correspond to episodes of his life that are of affective importance. The affective and emotional hypervulnerability of these subjects makes them extremely sensitive to the criticism of those around them. This instability visibly affects their moods; they have a spectacular tendency to change moods rapidly, going from bursts of laughter at one moment to fits of tears in the next. Sexually, the hysterical woman is classically frigid, in contrast with her seductive and provocative attitude. Male patients suffer from impotence or from premature ejaculation, although outwardly they act like Don Juans and are exaggeratedly virile. All these manifestations fit perfectly with the syndromes and illnesses associated with Jue Yin that we have studied, as well as with the personality profile of Jue Yin subjects defined in the beginning of this work. Everything points to a single mechanism of energy imbalance in Jue Yin, with a deficiency of the liver and of the blood contrasted with an excess of the pericardium.

This is confirmed by Soulie de Morant, who quotes from the dictionary *Zi Yuan,* which defines the disorder *xi si de li a,* or hysteria:

> Women who have a deficiency of blood {and therefore a predominance of Yang}, if they must bear worries or fear or overexcitation, suffer from this illness frequently. They have false ideas, their joy or discontent are extraordinarily exaggerated. If the illness is serious, there are contractures and speech difficulties, similar to depression caused by shock (feng tian).[444]

We may classify hysteria as a root and knot disorder. The classical description found in the *Su Wen* is that the whole meridian is knotted. This covers all the somatic symptoms, such as contractures and spasms, as well as spasmophilia. When there are psychological symptoms, it is the shen of Fire (heart), the qi of the emotions, which are also disturbed. The changes of mood bear witness to the inversion of Yin and Yang, excess and deficiency, within the element Fire and within its meridians, shou jue yin (pericardium), minister of the sovereign heart (xin), and shou shao yin (heart).

In Chapter 62 of the *Su Wen,* where we read, "If there is a deficiency of blood the patient is anxious and fearful," Qi Bo states:

> The heart governs the psyche; when there is an excess of psyche, the patient laughs to no end. When there is a deficiency, he can't stop moaning and groaning.[445]

In the discussion of the specific symptomology of shou jue yin in the tenth chapter of the Ling Shu, we read:

> If the trouble is serious, there is excess in the chest and in the sides,
> the heart is very agitated, the face is ruddy, the patient is very gay,
> and laughs.[446]

We can compare the migraines caused by perturbation of the circulation of energy to the headaches common to hysterical patients:

> In cases of migraine with crying and groaning, we needle the artery
> in excess and we bleed it, then we regularize the energy at the point
> of the liver meridian, zu jue yin.[447]

Acupuncture treatment of hysterical neurosis therefore involves the regulation of blood and of the liver meridian, as we have seen, notably through the treatment of ganshu (BL-18), as indicated in the *Da Cheng*.[448]

We must also balance the shen, the psychic energy of the heart, not only through the intermediary of its minister shou jue yin, but also by way of the points of the heart meridian itself. In ancient Japanese texts, as well as in the modern Shanghai texts, we find this protocol: lingdao (HT-4), tongli (HT-5), ximen (PC-4), daling (PC-7) and renzhong (GV-26). Lingdao (HT-4), the "road of the spirit" has a name that is close to lingtai (GV-10), "temple of the spirit," which is above xinshu (BL-15) the beishu point of the heart and on the same horizontal as dushu (BL-16), the shu point of du mai.[449] Tongli (HT-5), the luo point of shou shao yin, is indicated for "headaches, dizziness, groaning, the patient becomes suddenly mute, and does not want to speak."[450] Not that the patient does not *want* to speak, but is incapable of speech. Ximen (PC-4) is noted for "fear of those around, timidity, fear."[451] The name of this point means "door of the last point," "door of space"[452] or "door of the fissure."[453] It is the xi point to disobstruct shou jue yin.

The varying translations of the meaning of ximen give us the image of a door opening into a space, of an interval between two points. If we put these ideas together, we have the door of the last point in space, or the interval beyond. We have a fissure that represents a schism between two distinct modes of reference. Between these two modes of reference is the space of change of reference. There is also the idea of apparent manifestation. That is, the one hundred forms that constitute the manifestation, which we find in baihui (GV-20), located at the top of the skull, the "one hundred reunions." The fissure could be the interval between the one hundred aspects of the manifestation and the invisible coherence that creates that manifestation.

It is easy to see that hysterical neurosis is no small matter in that it results from the disorder of the shen, the great Fire that puts order into the great confusion. Proof of the dimensions of this disorder is to be found in the physiological properties and the names of the points we use to treat it.[454] Daling (PC-7), the dispersion point of the meridian, is classically indicated in cases of hysteria.[455] The *Da Cheng* indicates it for cases of "epilepsy or madness: the patient can't stop laughing, crying or groaning, his mind wanders."[456] Judging from the indications of the single point, the disorder is comparable to epilepsy. Daling is indicated by Soulie de Morant to "disperse the vessels and the sexual organs," which links hysteria to sexual disturbances with an excess of libido.

Zu Lien, in the *La nouvelle science d'acupuncture et des moxas,* prescribes the following treatment:

> If the patient alternates between laughing and crying, we will needle renzhong (GV-20), yangxi (LI-5), lieque (LU-7),[457] daling (PC-7) and shenmen (HT-7).

We will retain also the classical indications for baihui (GV-26) and xinshu (BL-15), the shu of the heart, in treating hysteria. These points are often cauterized. As we have said in the chapter devoted to Shao Yang discussing the correlations with the character types of Gaston Berger, the author himself linked the nervous temperament to nervous anxiety (Dupre's psychoneurosis) and to hysteria.[458] This confirms the close correspondence between the nervous character type, or the Jue Yin temperament, and the constitutional aptitude to become hysterical.

The relationship between the uterine envelope and that of the heart constitutes the anatomical and energetic basis according to which the ancient Chinese were able to establish a natural link between hysteria and sexuality. Such a link was made only during the eighteenth century in the West, when, in 1731, the name hysteria[459] was given to this aspect of mental illness. Two centuries later, Freud undertook the study of the relationship; the theories of psychoanalysis and the concept of libido stem directly from the interest of the young Viennese doctor in what is now known as hysterical neurosis.

Dermatological Pathology

Energetic Physiology of the Skin

The traditional analogy skin-Metal might lead us to believe that any cutaneous accident is simply nothing more than an imbalance of the element Metal and of its organ, the lung, or its bowel, the large intestine. The dialectic of the *Nei Jing Su Wen* is more subtle. The cutaneous surface is divided into four levels. There is a microcirculation of energy through the luo channels. To understand this Chinese concept of microcirculation, we need to distinguish between the primary luo channels and the secondary luo channels.[460]

According to their depth beneath the cutaneous surface and their diameter, we distinguish between the great luo and those meridians whose physiological role is superimposed upon the circulation of the blood. These constitute the secondary luo channels, luo mai, the transverse luo (capillary anastomoses). The sun luo are as intimately linked to the physiology of the luo mai (luo channels) as the arteries and veins are to the jing mai, the primary channels, and the great luo. The fu luo represent the ramifications of the sun luo toward the cutaneous surface. The xue luo, meaning "luo of the blood," are the endings of the fu luo.[461] The xue luo represent the microcirculation of the dermis and of the epidermis and may link with the jing ming, the tendinomuscular channels. Within this anatomical structure, rong and wei energies establish intimate relationships.

255

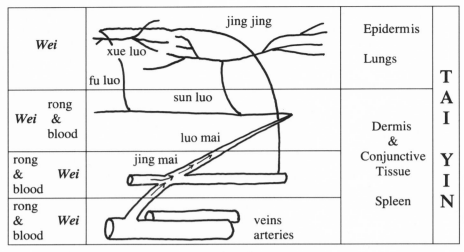

Figure 9

The relations between wei qi and the blood explain the repercussions of perverse energies (wind, heat, cold) upon any cutaneous lesions as well as the role of the blood and of the microcirculation in the defense of the organism. The physiology of the microcirculation is so closely linked to wei qi that any wei disorder will create a blood disorder. This is the case in cutaneous and respiratory allergies, and photosensitivity (solar erythema). In the same way, any blood disorder will affect the wei qi in the skin. This is the case in alimentary, chemical or medicinal allergies, or in idiopathic rashes.

When we study cutaneous pathology, we must take into account the physiology of wei qi and of xue. We have already seen the role of the inferior burner, the kidneys (adrenal glands) and the liver in the physiology of wei qi. For blood, xue, three organs are traditionally involved: the heart, liver and spleen. The heart is the "dwelling place of the blood." As it is the circulatory pump, we must interpret the term blood as meaning "greater circulation." A heart disorder will cause a circulatory disorder. "The liver produces the blood." Here we are dealing with the metabolic function, specifically albumin and the coagulation factors. "The spleen regulates the blood." This is at once the hematological and vasoregulatory function with the aid of the lung and of Yang Ming.[462] We might also say that the cutaneous territory is under the dependence of Metal, since the lung involves the epidermis, but also of the Earth, since the spleen affects the dermis and conjunctive tissue. In other words, the skin is governed by Tai Yin "which opens outwards."

This territory is the field of combat between the exterior and the interior. The external aggressor tries to outwit wei qi to penetrate xue. Xue attempts to push back the undesirable external agent with the assistance of wei. Accordingly, we may distinguish schematically between two sorts of illnesses. In the first, the external illness results from a superficial or metabolic disorder of the blood and of the defensive wei. In this case it begins in the xue luo, the most superficial of the luo channels. The illness is more Yang — violent and intense — but is of short duration and reversible. This is the case of disorders that occur among patients whose constitution is Wood and corresponds to Shao Yang and Jue Yin.

In the second case, the external illness results from a deeper disorder of the blood and of its autoregulation — more from the vasoregulatory aspect than the defensive aspect of wei. It is a Yin illness and dwells in the fu luo and sun luo. As it is Yin, it is insidious, dull and chronic. These are the skin problems that affect the Metal or Earth constitutions and the temperament Tai Yin or Yang Ming more often.

The first case results in all sorts of cutaneous manifestations of allergies, including urticaria, pruritis and contact eczema. The illnesses of the second case are much more serious and affect both the organ and its territory (epidermis or conjunctive tissue). These illnesses are the bi and the wei of the lung and the spleen. These constitutional disorders are represented by chronic eczema and psoriasis, as well as the cutaneous symptoms of the collagen affections (periarteritis, polyarteritis nodosa, scleroderma).[463] This may be understood when Qi Bo says, in his discussion of defensive energy in the *Ling Shu:*

> If there are no painful phenomena, the disease does not correspond to
> an energy disorder. The disease lies within the blood.[464]

Urticaria, Eczema, Angioneurotic Edema

The cutaneous manifestations of allergies are numerous: contact dermatitis, urticaria, angioneurotic edema (Quincke's edema), erythematous rash, eczema. These are tangible aspects of a Jue Yin disorder and coincide with the allergic temperament, or associated disturbances of the liver and cutaneous vasomotricity (pericardium). They may occur in isolation or accompany other Jue Yin disorders of the same nature: asthma, rhinitis (hay fever), dysmenorrhea, gynecomastia. Roughly, the manifestations linked to delayed hypersensitivity are contact dermatitis and eczema, whereas those linked to immediate hypersensitivity are rashes and edema. Urticaria and eczema of the genital region are classically linked to a deficiency of the longitudinal luo of the liver, which more or less proves the role of a deficit of the liver and of the blood in their occurrence.

However, the same deficiency of the blood allows the perverse energy, which is Yang, to penetrate into the body. Based on the visceral manifestations discussed above (*i.e.,* asthma, rhinitis), we may infer that the perverse energy that causes these is the same as that affecting the skin and enters into conflict with the wei qi on another level. That perverse energy is none other than the wind. Judging from the clinical symptoms, we are dealing with warm wind energy. We quote Qi Bo concerning the penetration of the wind into the epidermis:

> When the wind is retained in the skin, it may neither enter deeper into
> the body nor escape outside the body. The wind is mobile and chang-
> ing. . . If the cutaneous orifices close, there is warmth and
> languor.[465]

It is interesting to compare this text with all the aggravating circumstances classically indicated in relation to allergies. Emotional tension, a rise in temperature and physical exercise may aggravate urticaria.[466] Emotional tension as an aggravating circumstance is evidence of the psychosomatic role of the emotions and the incidence of shou jue yin (pericardium) on such a terrain. A rise in temperature and physical exercise are circumstances in which heat aggravates the symptoms that result from stagnant blood, captive beneath the skin, and from a deficiency of blood. Qi Bo says:

> Energy and blood like the heat and detest the cold; their circulation ceases when it is cold, and flows when it is warm. This is why, when the energy is enclosed within the Yang, there is a deficiency of blood.[467]

Allergic edema obeys the same mechanism. This is why the English use the term angioneurotic edema.

Acupuncture treatment of these cutaneous accidents focuses on points of the liver and gallbladder meridians. In the paragraphs concerning "swelling of the skin," we find:

> In all swelling, we must tonify taichong (LV-3), the yu point; for illness with swelling, dadun (LV-1), the ting point; for problems from swelling, zulinqi (GB-41).[468]

The *Da Cheng* tells us, in Chapter 6, "Pruritis is caused by a deficiency, it is Yang; we must not needle deeply."[469] Concerning allergic reactions from intoxication, In his *Yi Xue Ru Men* (c. 1575), Li Yan wrote, "Swelling due to poisoning: edema of the whole body: needle xingjian (LV-2)."[470] These indications were repeated in the modern texts. The *Yi Zhi,* a Chinese work published in 1919, mentions, "Angioneurotic edema indicates insufficiency of the liver and the need to tonify taichong (LV-3) and ququan (LV-8)."[471] Soulie de Morant relegates all these symptomatic aspects of the insufficiency of the liver to the tonification point ququan (LV-8):

> The direct effect of ququan {LV-8} is to tonify the liver, it is indicated in all deficiencies, yellow stools, constipation, migraines, asthma, skin problems, eczema, angioneurotic edema, etc.[472]

The stimulation of xingjian (LV-2) makes sense, since the role of the rong point is to get the blood flowing and unblock the stagnation.

Eczema is also treated through the action of the shou jue yin points, specifically daling (PC-7), the shu point and dispersion point of the meridian. Indicated by Zu Lien, in *La nouvelle science de l'acupuncture et des moxas* for the treatment of eczema,[473] daling is an important dermatological point. In the *Da Cheng,* its indication includes the following symptoms: wounds, abscess, eczema, dartre,[474] as well as "bubbles in the palms of the hands." Soulie de Morant compares this to dyshidrosis, a special form of eczema that is more often than not secondary to mycotic intertrigo.

To recapitulate the points indicated in treatment of allergic cutaneous accidents, we note LV-2, LV-3, LV-8, PC-7 and also GV-21, GV-23 and LI-11. There is, of course, a perfect correlation with trace element therapy.

> In cases of eczema, the allergic behavior is obvious, especially the psychosomatic manifestations and the equivalences."[476]

> The action of manganese and sulfur is incontestable, but often insufficient.[477]

There is every reason, then, to combine trace element and acupuncture therapies in these cases. In cases of urticaria, which corresponds to the same diathesis, manganese has a remarkable and long lasting effect. In rebellious cases of eczema, Menetrier advises treatment with manganese-cobalt (symmetrical eczema, neurovegetative participation, tendency to become chronic). As we say in Chinese medicine, the illness "settles in" and goes deeper.

We may mention, for example, the strange and unexplained manifestation of palmar erythema that accompanies cholestatic hepatitis, as it relates to the dermatological indications of the palmar point laogong (PC-8), located close to daling (PC-7), but that is also indicated in cases of jaundice: "Jaundice with yellow sclera."[478] This confirms the fact that shou jue yin and zu jue yin are inseparable, as are the liver and the pericardium, the liver and the skin. This is an example of the way a functional hepatic disorder, whose etiology is allergic, or due to an intolerance in the broader sense of the term, may influence the cutaneous vasomotricity within the territory of shou jue yin. We may also mention certain factors of "liver blood disorders," such as pregnancy and synthetic estroprogestins, which may cause cholestatic hepatitis.

Lichen Planus, Duhring's Disease and Herpes

These affections signal the passage from a functional state to one that is chronic, particularly lichen planus. According to Menetrier, this justifies a prescription of manganese-cobalt. In Chinese medicine, these illnesses represent a blockage and an aggravation of the stagnation of xue in the epidermis. It is remarkable to what extent the dystonic behavior of the patient becomes more predominant, the signature of a pericardium disorder. At the same time, the topography of the lesions is noteworthy. There is an eruption of purple, pruriginous wheals on the insides of the wrists, the arms, the elbows. This follows the pathway of shou jue yin (pericardium), as well as appearing in the loins and around the genitals, which is zu jue yin (liver) territory. It is not rare to find lesions over the jugal mucous membranes. Lesions around the fingernails makes them brittle to the point that they may disappear altogether. On the scalp the aspect is one of pseudopelade.

Lichen sclerosis et atrophicus represents an excess that has become organic. The Chinese called this a "retraction of the external genitals," a symptom of a major deficiency of the liver, especially of its longitudinal luo channel. Among women patients, we find kraurosis vulvae, characterized by a centrovulvar sclerosis and atrophy, causing stenotic atrophy of the labia minus and of the vaginal infundibulum. Among male patients we observe an atrophic balanitis with progressive sclerosis of the preputial ring. Acupuncture treatment of lichen planus is based on the protocol for eczema. It works well in synergy with the trace element therapy prescription of manganese-cobalt and sulfur indicated by Menetrier. We will apply moxa to ganshu (BL-18), jueyinshu (BL-14) and ququan (LV-8). This treatment is indicated in cases of Duhring's disease and for herpes as well.

The polymorphous bullous eruption of Duhring's disease, which is also very pruriginous, is accompanied by an alteration in the general state of the patient's health, especially in eosinophilia and its specific sensitivity to iodine. This is evocative of Jue Yin disorders. The same is true of gestational herpes that occurs

259

toward the sixth month of pregnancy, in which the bullous eruption is located on the abdomen and the extremities. According to Menetrier, there is an obvious dystonic behavior that is generally involved in cases of Duhring's disease.

Chronic edema, pruritis and urticaria are sensitive to the action of manganese and sulfur combined with manganese-cobalt. In cases of herpes, which Chinese medicine groups with eczema and lichen, the dystonic behavior requires manganese-cobalt, according to Menetrier.[479] Its buccal or genital location, its tendency toward recurrence and its catamenial rhythm are all signs of a Jue Yin disorder caused by dry wind or by warm wind and coincide perfectly with the Jue Yin behavior observed among these patients.[480] The herpes virus is the deeper equivalent of the exterior zona virus. The former attacks at the Yin energetic level, Jue Yin, the latter the Yang energetic level, Shao Yang.[481] The treatment is discussed with Ophthalmology, further on.

Pathology of the Scalp

The periodic loss of hair, which is physiological and which everyone notices in the springtime, is related to the liver, zu jue yin, which rises to the summit of the skull. The action of sulfur as a catalyst, recommended by Menetrier, is well known to Western empirical medicine; a good many balms and creams contain sulfur. Care for the scalp and the hair in the spring has always been part of eugenic preoccupations. The *Su Wen* makes a vague allusion to this in the second chapter:

> The three months of spring evoke a deployment (fa chen). The universe is waking, the creation is shining. We go to bed late, we get up early, we go outside, let down our hair, we are at ease and we get a taste of life. . .[482]

The lesions of lichen planus on the scalp are certainly not the only dermatological manifestation of a deficiency of blood in the liver. In practice, we often notice that psoriasis of the scalp coincides with the Jue Yin temperament. However, the lesions are generally isolated, sparing the rest of the cutaneous territory, and are anatomopathological in form, "eczematoid psoriasis."

More common and less severe are desquamations (dandruff) on a dry scalp, which is nonseborrheic. It is understandable that a precise diagnosis of these lesions is difficult. In Chinese, these dry desquamations are called bai xie, literally, "white parcels." One point indicated in their treatment is qianding (GV-21). We may ask ourselves if this point and shangxing (GV-23) are not meeting points with the cephalic branch of the liver meridian after its passage through baihui (GV-20). Qianding (GV-21) is not only indicated for bai xie, but also for "feng in the head," with the symptoms of a "ruddy and swollen face, edema in the face, swollen and painful back," according to the *Da Cheng*. This corresponds to urticaria and angioneurotic edema of the face. This point is included in *Da Cheng* protocol for "swelling in the head," next to daling (PC-7).[483] But qianding (GV-21) is also indicated in other wind disorders of Jue Yin:

> Dizziness, ocular inflammation, stuffy nose, abundant rhinorrhea, polyps in the nose, pediatric affections, convulsions, epilepsy with

frequent seizures, pain and swelling at the top of the head among children with clear rhinorrhea.[484]

If xinhui (GV-22) is indicated only for bai xie by Soulie de Morant, there is also an impressive Jue Yin symptomology noted for shangxing (GV-23):

> Swelling and pain in the forehead, the face and the head, coryza, stuffy nose, inflammation of the cornets, nasal polyp, dizziness, ocular pain, myopia, keratitis. . .[485]

Acne, Onychopathy

To conclude this discussion of dermatology, we will mention that the physiopathology of acne involves, of course, the liver and Jue Yin. The study of this affection is developed in detail in the chapter devoted to Tai Yin. Onychopathy is directly related to disturbances of the liver and the gallbladder. These have been discussed in the chapter devoted to Shao Yang. They are, however, often symptomatic of a liver disorder, as in the case of brittle nails secondary to lichen, or in leukonychia secondary to spasmophilia.

Infectious Pathology

Cold-Hot Diseases

The infectious pathology of Jue Yin is dominated by symptoms of the evolution of perverse wind within the organism. Throughout this chapter we have seen disorders caused by an excess of wind, warm wind, cold wind and humid wind. There is in Chinese medicine, however, a Yin modality of perverse energies; in other words, pathology due to insufficiency, here of wind energy, effecting a very different symptomology.

> "How do we name the transformations of diseases that have achieved their accomplishment?" asked Huang Di.
>
> "The winds become cold-hot," answered Qi Bo.[486]

In Chapter 69 of the *Su Wen,* Qi Bo's answer becomes clear. This chapter deals with cosmic influences in disease. An excess or deficiency of Jue Yin energy, for example, is easily determined by the two figures of the celestial stem and the terrestrial branch attributed to the year. Thus the fourth year of the decimal cycle of the stems, since four is an even number, is Yin. In the fourth years (such as 1977 or 1987) the wind is deficient. Qi Bo says:

> A failure of Wood gives free reign to a cold dryness. . . The reply of the fire {summer} gives free reign to torrid heat; the diseases are cold-hot: ulcers, dermatitis, abscess and acne.[487]

Facilitated by meteorological conditions, the cold-hot illnesses will strike those patients whose internal Wood energy is weak. These patients may, of course, contract such diseases otherwise, as a result of internal (psychic or alimentary) or external (perverse energy) circumstances, as is the case in epidemics, or in

261

endemics through direct contact, depending on the transmitting agent. The dermatological illnesses that are cold-hot as a result of cosmic or meteorological circumstances are marked, logically enough, by a cold and hot symptomology.

Abscesses (boils), pimples (acne), herpetic and other ulcers, and dermatitis (lichen, psoriasis, eczema, pruritis), are hot illnesses. There is stagnation and warming of the blood (see Dermatology), but the absence of fever or thirst, and cystitis or pollakiuria, symptoms that are sometimes associated with these illnesses, are cold symptoms. The cases just mentioned are studied in the discussion of dermatology. Their aspect is often functional; in other words, superficial and benign. They result from a conflict between the wind and wei qi, as explained by Qi Bo:

> Spreading through the intervals of the flesh, the wind attacks wei {the wei energy} whose channels become disturbed, which tumefies the tissues and ulcerates them.[488]

This stage may represent the evolution from functional to chronic.

Other illnesses, which present dermatological disorders, are much more serious and organic, possibly even fatal. These may be considered in our discussion of cold-hot affections.

> Transformations of the illnesses that have achieved their accomplishment are the winds of the meridians that become li, cold-hot affections {collapse of the nose and cutaneous ulcers — leprosy or syphilis}.[489] When a cold wind settles down in the meridians, this is a li feng, sometimes a cold-hot {the first being the conclusion of the second}.[490]

This is one degree further than a cold-hot illness, as far as the intensity of the conflict is concerned. The conflict is no longer between the wind and wei qi, but between the wind and rong qi. This is more serious. Qi Bo says, "In the li, the rong qi is attacked, the heat is spoiled and the blood is troubled."[491]

• Leprosy

It is important that we examine leprosy to show the specific aspects of one disorder of Jue Yin. Leprosy is the only disease that causes both cutaneous and neurological disturbances. The Chinese concept of "cold dryness" may be compared to Hansen's bacillus, which is responsible for the disease, and to acid-alcohol-fast bacillus, analogous to Koch's bacillus, that causes tuberculosis, and may also be classified as cold humid disease (see Tai Yin). In tuberculoid leprosy, it is interesting to note the hypertrophy and moniliform aspects of the external popliteal sciatic nerves at the head of the fibula that corresponds to yanglingquan (GB-34). We must remember what Qi Bo had to say of this point: "There is one point that is very important, it is yanglingquan {GB-34}. This point governs the cold and the warmth."[492] Husson's translation adds the following precision: "The cold-hot points are beneath the external condyles of the knees {yanglingquan of the gallbladder}."[493] Again, in neurological disorders, there is the "monkey hand," due to the atrophy of the intrinsic muscles of the hand that results from paralysis of the median nerve on the territory of the pericardium (shou jue yin). The cubital disorder on the shou shao yin meridian (Heart-Fire), at the elbow, at shaohai (HT-3) (he-cold point), is evocative of the mechanism "vengeance of Fire," and here, the Fire is imperial. The same is true of the atrophy of the foot muscles that results in what is known as *Talipes equinus*.

Monkey hand and *Talipes equinus* are the signs of an organic disorder of Jue Yin, which in functional pathology results in the carpal and the carpopedal spasm. In the same way, in lepromatous leprosy, the functional aspects of Jue Yin rhinitis are intensified as the disorder becomes organic. The classical initial symptoms of this form are a nasal catarrh, epistaxis and respiratory difficulty. Total nasal obstruction and laryngitis[494] are also possible. This rhinitis leads to the destruction of the nasal septum.[495] These clinical signs may be compared to the ancient Chinese observations found in the paragraph on wind, quoted above:

> In the li, the rong qi is aggressed, the heat is spoiled and the blood is troubled. There follows a collapse of the structure of the nose, an alteration of the complexion and ulcerations of the skin.

The frequent ganglial, splenic and hepatic localizations confirm once again that the meridians and organs deeply affected are those of Jue Yin, and also those of Tai Yin (see Infectious Pathology of Tai Yin).

Independent from the balancing of these organs and by use of the points geshu (BL-17),[496] ganshu (BL-18), pishu (BL-20) and gaohuang (BL-38), we should try to needle the meridians and especially the local points where the conflict is materialized — yanglingquan (GB-34), shaohai (HT-3), quze (PC-3), and laogong (PC-8). This treatment should be instituted at the beginning of the disease in association with modern chemotherapy. The *Da Cheng* indicates for shaohai (HT-3) cold point, "Scrofula, contracture in the elbow."[497] The physician Zhang indicates for quze (PC-3), "Epidermal affections."[498] Soulie de Morant recommends this point for median nerve disorders, indicating for laogong (PC-8), "Palmar aponeurosis retraction." Laogong (PC-8), the heat point of the meridian, is indicated in the *Da Cheng* for hot or cold abscess in general.[499] In conclusion, we notice that in this cold-hot disease the specific locations of the lesions are found at the cold and hot points of the meridians of the heart and the pericardium, inside the elbow (cold), and in the palm of the hand (hot). Symptoms are consequently treated by stimulating the same points. This is why, in the lower limb, apart from yanglingquan (GB-34), we must not forget to stimulate the hot and cold points of the liver meridian, xingjian (LV-2) and ququan (LV-8).

This examination of leprosy enables us to understand why we needle daling (PC-7), the shu point, and laogong (PC-8) in all forms of abscesses and why we treat with moxibustion, according to the ancient texts, in all dermatological problems.[500] Whether the disease comes from Jue Yin (because of a weakness of Wood) or is internally triggered or exaggerated by some cosmic (meteorological) failure of the same energy, the meridians of the Imperial Fire and the Fire Minister, along with the heart and the pericardium, are of major importance in the onset and the evolution of this disease through the mechanism of vengeance of Fire against Metal, as given in the *Su Wen*. This enables us to understand certain aspects of dermatology in general, and the mechanism and treatment of abscesses, boils and acne in particular. Aside from this logic, the use of the points of the pericardium in dermatology would appear to be only symptomatic.

• **Syphilis**

Syphilis, another infectious pathology of the Jue Yin, did not await the return of Christopher Columbus from Haiti to make itself known; even the writings of Hippocrates make allusion to it. As we will determine from a rapid and theoretical clinical review of syphilis, this li, affecting Jue Yin, displays the whole range of typical symptoms. In the primary stage the usual location of the lesion is the glans penis and the labia majus, *i.e.* on the external genitals, which are energized by the liver meridian. In the secondary stage, not only do the asthenia, the fever, the headaches and the articular pains follow a pattern of classical vesperal recrudescence (indicating the periodicity of aggravation proper to the liver),[501] but the concomitant polyadenopathy, with its preferential subepitrochlear and subtrapezial localization (heart and small intestine meridians, respectively), is in Fire territory.

The dermatological lesions are typically cold-hot, and include: roseola, opaline plaques on the labial commissures on the tongue (the cephalic pathway of the liver meridian, as with lichen planus) and on the genital mucous membranes (the liver meridian pathway) and alopecia areata, which is just as evocative of Jue Yin cutaneous lesions. The classic complications we may expect at this stage are jaundice and hepatitis, with a high alkaline phosphate level and a histological aspect very different from that of viral hepatitis, or arthritis, iridocyclitis and even uveitis. All these lesions are proof of the suffering of the liver (Jue Yin). Complications such as nephritis, periostitis and the meningeal syndrome show the suffering of the kidney and the heart (Shao Yin).

In the third stage, there are lesions of the subcutaneous tissue located on the genitals that are similar to those found in leprosy, and are accompanied by rawness, softness and ulcerations. However, these do heal. The visceral disorders include aortitis, tabes, general paralysis and, sometime later, ocular lesion. The aortitis, it is interesting to note, follows endarteritis obliterans in the vascularization of the vessels by the vasa vasorum. In Chinese medicine this endarteritis of the microcirculation is the equivalent of a Fire Minister (shou jue yin) disorder on the territory of the aorta/Imperial Fire (Shao Yin). The *Ling Shu* explains, "the pericardium meridian alone rules over only the blood that circulates in the vessels."[502]

The neurological and psychic symptoms, general paralysis and tabes are typically Jue Yin disorders: progressive dementia, with memory troubles (ancient, and then especially recent memories), disorientation, talking nonsense, illusions, false recognition, hallucinations, Argyll Robertson's pupil, dysarthria, labiolingual trembling and trembling of the limbs.[503]

Dorsal-lumbar tabes is the result of a demyelinization of the posterior colomnae, with shooting pain similar to Lhermitte's sign, as found in multiple sclerosis,[504] sensory troubles, static ataxia (different from cerebellar ataxia), trophic degeneration and arthropathy (Charcot) and an associated atrophy of the optic nerve. We find the same ocular lesions here as in the second stage: iritis, photophobia, ophthalmoplegia, chorioretinitis.

Syphilis represents a severe assault of perverse wind, li, upon the Jue Yin meridian. The nature of li is deficiency and this, along with the nature of the wind, explains the latencies of several months or years between the different periods. The onset of cold (neurological) symptoms similar to those of multiple sclerosis on Jue Yin/Shao Yin territory, as well as hot symptoms (aortitis) and syphilitic arteritis, reminds us of cardiovascular disorders on Shao Yin and Tai Yang[505] territory. An example is the megalomaniac form of the delirium (Tai Yang), which is observed along with general paralysis.

Serious Infectious Pathology of Jue Yin

In Chapter 49 of the *Su Wen,* "Explanations of the Channels," we may read:

> Dryness of the throat in severe cases, this is the consequence of the fight between Yin and Yang.[506]

At this stage, the weakened energy of the body has not been able to overcome the perverse energy. If the perverse energy triumphs, it means the exhaustion of Jue Yin. Qi Bo describes the "agony of Jue Yin":

> Central warming up, dryness of the throat, desire to urinate, upsetting sensation of warmth. In severe cases, the tongue rolls up,[507] the testicles retract.[508]

Apart from the retention of urine and the retraction of the external genitals, signs that are typically Jue Yin, it is interesting to note the two mentions of dryness of the throat. This is synonymous with sore throat or with dehydration.

We may recall that this region corresponds to the "route of the liquids," chengjian (CV-24), and is essential in the physiology and the treatment of body fluid disorders. Whether or not the origin is infectious, the fact that dryness of the throat is a symptom of maladaptation by the liver is significant to the hypothesis that the liver is involved in the metabolism of the body fluids. We may recall that "If the energy of Shao Yang and Jue Yin is knotted, this is visible in the throat." We may hypothesize about a good many pathological correspondences based on such a statement, since the Wood viscera, liver and gallbladder are closely linked to the thyroid function, the parathyroid function and the energization of the larynx and the pharynx.

Ophthalmological Pathology

Semiological Aspects

The eye is related to the element Wood, as has been said many times and as we have confirmed in our discussion of the ophthalmological pathology of Shao Yang, where we studied the physiological relations between eyesight and the gallbladder, notably in the absorption of vitamin A, and their consequences in pathology. We may recall the aphorism of Qi Bo:

> The energy of the liver is linked to the eyes. When the liver is healthy, the eyesight is normal.

All ophthalmological pathology, however, is not related to a disturbance of the element Wood, or to imbalances in Shao Yang and Jue Yin. Since all the meridians meet at the eyes and since it is here that we may observe the individual's xing, his personal harmony of the five elements in the jing ming, it is normal to find a sectorial distribution of ocular pathology.

It is stated in the *Da Cheng:*

> Within the five circles of the eyes flowers the sexual energy {jing qi} of the five organs and the six bowels. There, the meridians all meet. . . .
> The whites of the eyes depend on the lungs {Metal}. If the white circle becomes scarlet, it is because the fire has risen to the lungs. The flesh depends on the spleen-pancreas; if the circle of flesh is scarlet and swollen, the fire has risen to the spleen-pancreas. The black, the consciousness, the shine, depend on the water of the kidneys.[509] If the black, the water, the consciousness, the shine are veiled, the fire has risen to the liver and the kidneys. The scarlet depends on the heart. It depends also on the liver. If there are red vessels across the eye, the fire is intense.[510]

This passage resembles Qi Bo's remarks in Chapter 80 of the *Ling Shu:*

> The essential energy of the five organs and the six bowels is concentrated in the eyes. The pupil represents the essence of the bones {kidneys}, the iris, that of the muscles {liver}. The sclera represents the overall essential energy {lung}. The little capillaries located on the cornea represent the essence of the blood {heart}.
>
> The pupil and the iris represent the Yin, the sclera and the little capillaries represent the Yang.[511]

On the one hand, we have the kidney and the liver, the Yin organs, and on the other, the lungs and the heart, the Yang organs.

These remarks make it obvious that various organs and meridians are implicated in ophthalmological pathology. Thus, the eye is also helpful for diagnosis and prognosis. The liver, which rules over the eye, has the predominant role. The physiology of the blood is again fundamental. Comparative observation of the complexion and the conjunctiva allows us to make a prognosis:

> When the complexion is at variance with the pulse, if the face is yellow and the eyes are blue,[512] red, white or black, the patient will survive.
>
> However, death will occur in the following cases: red face and white eyes, green face and black eyes, black face and white eyes, red face and green eyes.[513]

Zhang Zhi Cong comments on this passage:

> In this paragraph, the blood of the five organs flows into the liver, which appears in the eyes, and which we may observe because the eyes govern the blood and the complexion, the face governs the energy and the complexion.[514]

If the five shades of the eyes appear in a face that is slightly yellow, this is because the Yin of the five organs still contains the Yang energy of the stomach {see Physiology of Yang Ming}. This is a sign of life.

If, for example, the facial complexion is black or reddish, it is because the perverse energy has overcome the Yang of the stomach; there is nothing but Yin left, and this means death.[515]

The blood is thus indicative of the liver function and we may judge the qualitative diagnostic and prognostic value according to the color of the conjunctiva.

Qi Bo states clearly in the *Ling Shu:*

Red conjunctiva, this means that the heart is affected. If they are white, it means the lungs; if they are green it is the liver, if they are yellow, it is the spleen; if they are black, it is the kidneys, if they are neither red nor yellow but rather orange, it is the chest that is affected.[516]

In short, through the complexion we may observe the state of a patient's energy, through the conjunctiva we may observe the state of the blood, depending on the five organs. If the complexion is slightly yellow but with a shade of the organ that is predominant or affected, this means that the energy has not been affected quantitatively, only qualitatively. The prognosis is positive, independent of the shade of the conjunctiva that show the state of the blood. However, if the complexion loses its healthy quality and the color changes to indicate a pathological state, we must closely observe the eyes. A disturbance of the energy of the heart and of the blood of the lungs is fatal (*i.e.,* red face, white eyes). The same is true of the energy of the liver and the blood of the kidney, the energy of the kidney and the blood of the lung, and the energy of the heart and the blood of the liver.

While there is an interest in the qualitative aspects of the blood in the eyes for diagnosis and prognosis, the quantitative aspect is fundamental in ophthalmological pathology. The *Da Cheng* reminds us that "the liver is coupled with the artery of the eyes."[517] In our discussion of multiple sclerosis, we have briefly seen the importance of the relationship between the blood and the physiology of the eyesight. In Chapter 10 of the *Su Wen,* it is written, "During sleep, the blood goes to the liver, which allows us to see."[518] Chamfrault translates this passage as follows:

When we sleep, the eyes close, the blood enters the liver {which governs the eyes}, and this is why, when we wake up we can see clearly again, because the blood has been renewed.[519]

This is undeniably a fundamental physiological indication of the role of the liver in the sense of vision. The comparisons with retinol and retinal purple have been discussed in the chapter devoted to the physiology of Shao Yang. It would be interesting to study the nyctohemeral chronology of the enzymatic function of hepatic carotenase, or of any other mechanism concerned in this physiology.

Myopia, Presbyopia, Hemeralopia, Optical Neuritis

In any case, a disturbance in the physiological function of the blood attributed to the liver is likely to lead to disorders in the eye and of the eyesight. Qi Bo states, without ambiguity, "If the liver is deficient, there is a reduction in visual acuity."[520] We have already seen the case of optical neuritis in our discussion of multiple sclerosis; the relationship with the liver remains valid whatever the etiology. In this case, there is an insufficiency of blood of the liver. But there is also an insufficiency of blood of the liver in myopia, in amblyopia, in presbyopia and in hemeralopia.[521]

The *Da Cheng* indicates:

> If there is too much blood in the eye, this means that the bladder (Tai Yang) and stomach (Yang Ming) meridians are in excess. If the blood doesn't get to the eye, it is because the liver (Jue Yin) is deficient.[522]

The myopic eye is too long: the image forms in front of the retina. It is understandable that Jue Yin subjects, who have a constitutional tendency towards a deficiency of the liver, are more likely to have less visual acuity and to be myopic. It is so true, that in practice we consider myopia to be quasi-pathognomonic of the Jue Yin temperament, especially when it is congenital. Functional amblyopia (and only the functional affection interests us here) is most often discovered during the school year, as we examine and explore the strabismus that it causes. A drop in visual acuity — in a single eye — of an average of about 4/20°, with at least a 6/20° difference compared to the other eye, more often than not, justifies convergent strabismus.

Because of compensation by the motor and central nervous systems (neutralization), the common combination of myopia, a drop in visual acuity, amblyopia and strabismus is one aspect that enables Chinese medicine to make a connection between the eyesight, the blood and the muscles, all governed by the element Wood and the liver. As for hemeralopia, when it is primitive, it is most often due to tapetoretinal degeneration, an affection of the retina that takes the form of retinitis pigmentosa, whose origin is genetic. We may also mention the heredodegenerations that affect not only the retina, but also the medulla, the brain stem and the cerebellum, such as Friedreich's ataxia or Marie's disease. The comparison deserves to be made between the cerebellar syndrome with dysarthria, the pyramidal and posterior cordal syndromes of these affections, and the anatomo-clinical aspects of multiple sclerosis. Nonetheless, the affection is certainly genetic. For this reason it is interesting to notice the direct genetic relationships among the eye (the retina), the vestibule, the cerebellum and the medulla. In Chinese medicine these structures are closely linked to Jue Yin, as we have seen in our discussion of neurology.

Among the many etiologies of optical neuritis, we may note the neuritis due to ophthalmic zona (see Shao Yang), or due to neuroanemic syndromes, where there is a direct link between the blood, the nerves and the eye. Here, the concept of deficiency of the blood of the liver takes on a very modern look.

As for myopia, or "blurred vision" as it is called in the ancient texts, the *Da Cheng* indicates ququan (LV-8). As we might have expected, "Dizziness and pains in the eyes, blurred vision. . . "[523] This point is certainly to be associated with the protocol of the Shanghai authors, who recommended fengchi (GB-20), hegu (LI-4), jingming (BL-1), chengqi (ST-1) and xiajingming (N-HN-2). According to these authors, "in cases of myopia from natural causes, if undertaken in time, acupuncture treatment gets certain results."[524] Describing hemeralopia, Tong Fun writes:

> If the patient is at once anxious and angry, it means that his liver lacks blood; for this reason it is absolutely contraindicated to bleed him. On the contrary, we must tonify the liver and the stomach at the same time.[525]

The *Da Cheng* indicates the external orbital point, tongziliao (GB-1) the first point on the gallbladder meridian for hemeralopia, which is called, in this work, "green blindness" or "hen blindness."[526] The stomach (zu yang ming) is also involved in presbyopia as is indicated by Zang in speaking of zusanli (ST-36): "This point needled with three moxas improves the elderly's visual acuity."[527]

In treating neuritis and atrophy of the optic nerve, which the Chinese called "violent blindness" and later, "green blindness," the Shanghai authors remind us, in justifying their choice of points, that these syndromes are caused by "a lack of Yin {jing qi} in the liver and the kidneys and to a disturbance of the Yang of the wind."[528] They blame "a deficit of blood and of energy" for the physiopathology of optic neuritis and recommend these points: fengchi (GB-20), qiuhou (M-HN-8), jingming (BL-1), hegu (LI-4), chengqi (ST-1), ganshu (BL-18), shenshu (BL-23), zusanli (ST-36) and guangming (GB-37).[529] They use just about the same points for concomital strabismus: fengchi (GB-20) and hegu (LI-4). If the strabismus is convergent, we are to add qiuhou (M-HN-8) and zhongzhu (TB-3). If it is divergent, we add jingming (BL-1) and needle the point sibai (ST-2) in the direction of and up to, jingming (BL-1). The Shanghai authors add that it is useful to combine this treatment with corrective glasses.

In my opinion, it is of primary importance to balance Jue Yin as well as the blood by needling ganshu (BL-18) and ququan (LV-8) in all cases of ophthalmic pathology. Orthoptic re-education is an indispensable therapeutic element in the cases of strabismus just seen, but it may be facilitated, in cases of amblyopia from neutralization, by the application of a recent acupuncture technique, craniopuncture. There is a reflexotherapy zone opposite the occipital visual area, on both sides of the occipital protruberance, that can reduce visual disorders whose origin is central and facilitate reeducation. Balancing Jue Yin and craniopuncture are certainly useful in correcting heterophoria or pathological tendencies towards the deviation of the visual axes.

Inflammatory and Infectious Pathology

The constitutional or temporary weakness of the viscera linked to the element Wood, be it the gallbladder (Shao Yang) or the liver (Jue Yin) influences the conflict between perverse energy and the body's defense energy in the region of the eye. This conflict may cause inflammatory or allergic pathologies or infectious pathology, whether viral, bacterial or mycotic. In Chinese medicine, of course, this is codified as cold, heat or dryness. The perverse energy may attack the eyelid and cause blepharitis, chalazions or sties. It may attack the conjunctiva and cause conjunctivitis; attack the lacrymal canal and cause dacryocystitis; attack the iris and cause iritis and iridocyclitis (eyelashes); attack the cornea and cause keratitis; attack the sclera and cause episcleritis or scleritis. All these symptomologies may be analyzed according to the eight principles. We may predict, in each case, a specific vulnerability of Jue Yin or of Shao Yang, but once the diagnosis has been made by a specialist, we may begin our analysis according to the five elements.

Apart from a technical diagnosis, an inventory of the symptoms with a diagnosis of any general pathology with which it might be associated, along with a study of the behavior of the patient to determine his temperament, allows us to make an educated guess as to the affected sectors and the meridians we will use to balance the patient. The behavior and symptoms of a patient suffering from herpetic keratitis, or from conjunctivitis or from gouty iridocyclitis, who is of Jue Yin or Shao Yang temperament, are totally different from those of a patient suffering concomitantly from Sjogren's syndrome[530] and a rheumatoid polyarthritis. The latter is typical of Tai Yin or Shao Yin temperaments. In therapy, the choice of points to treat will depend on these differences. In the inflammatory and infectious pathology of Jue Yin, the perverse energy is more often than not the wind. The locations that are the most common are the eyelid, the conjunctiva and the cornea. The form is most often allergic, viral or bacterial, but almost always in a contact of hypersensitivity to the causal agent (allergy).

• Blepharitis and Conjunctivitis

The pathology of blepharitis and conjunctivitis[531] is linked to the penetration of the perverse wind that dominates in the springtime. In most cases, the wind is a warm wind. This defines pollen as a perverse wind. It is rare to find conjunctivitis in isolation. There is an obvious allergy context, more often among Jue Yin patients than Shao Yang patients, and we most often find this pathology associated with rhinitis, asthma, migraine or urticaria. Whether it is allergic or viral, conjunctivitis is caused by perverse wind energy. Now and then it is cold wind, rather than warm wind, which is perhaps the case in idiopathic or follicular conjunctivitis, those forms where there is not always proof of a virus. In any case, acupuncture treatment often gets good results, calms the patients and stops corticodependency.

We proceed by balancing zu jue yin and stimulating the he point, which is also the cold point. We needle taichong (LV-3), ququan (LV-8), ganshu (BL-18) with moxa, hegu (LI-4), jingming (BL-1), tongziliao (GB-1) or taiyang (M-HN-9), as well as shuaigu (GB-8), towards fengchi (GB-20) and fengchi (GB-20) itself. There is a perfect correlation with the trace elements:

> Conjunctivitis and eczema of the eyelids are treated with manganese
> and sulfur. . . the allergic behavior is often obvious.[532]

Inflammations of the cornea may be of viral, allergic, microbic or traumatic origin. In cases of general affection, as in syphilis, the etiological treatment will affect its evolution. It is not always easy to overcome allergic keratitis, or viral keratitis, the most common forms of which are herpetic or zonal. As was the case with syphilis, we are dealing with cold-hot diseases. A cold dryness assaults Wood, because of insufficiency of wind, and is followed by the vengeance of Fire (see Dermatology).

In these conditions, not only zu jue yin is concerned with the insufficiency of the liver, but also shou jue yin, which is a part of the Fire Minister, within which resides the pathological phenomenon and through which we may act upon it, as in cases of eczema and other dermatological affections seen above. It would be logical to think that along with the usual points of zu jue yin (liver) that were indicated for conjunctivitis, certain points of shou jue yin (pericardium) would be indicated. And this is confirmed by the *Da Cheng*. Indications for the luo point neiguan (PC-6), for example, are "Inflammation of the eyes, congestion of blood in the eyes."[533]

Herpes, an illness whose recurrence among women patients is often concurrent with their periods (catamenial herpes), involves the entire pathway of Jue Yin and its envelopes. The lesions that occur in multiple locations (genital, anal, around the eyes and lips) prove this fact. In the eye, the most characteristic lesion is keratitis. Given the participation of the pericardium and lesions all along the Jue Yin meridian, the beishu point of the back specific to the pericardium, jueyinshu (BL-14) is indicated by Soulie de Morant for "herpes of the vulva or of the glans penis."[534] The red and painful eyes common to keratitis, with characteristic tears and photophobia are clear signs of a Fire disorder.

In the dermatological pathology seen above, an imbalance of Fire in its vengeance upon Metal caused a congestion of blood in the skin that took the form of eczema. Here, the congestion of blood is located in the eye — more precisely, in the cornea. The cornea is the part of the eye that corresponds to the lung, Metal, and thus to the skin. In dermatology, the vengeful Fire was the Fire Minister, but also the Imperial Fire. The same is true in ophthalmology. The *Da Cheng* indicates that "the artery of the eyes depends on tongli (HT-5)."[535] This confirms that Shao Yin plays a role in retinal hemorrhages. The mixed symptomology of tongli (HT-5) is "Pain and congestion in the eyes."

One last point is worth mentioning, shangxing (GV-23). This point is indicated in the *Da Cheng* for "troubles of the eyes, cataract, corneal inflammations," and, Soulie de Morant adds, "keratitis."[536] This point seems specifically indicated for ophthalmological disorders, since it is also indicated for "congestion and hardness of the eyeball (glaucoma), pupil pain, headaches, dizziness, myopia."[537] This tends to prove the close anatomical link between the cephalic branch of zu jue yin (liver) and the points of du mai as we had noticed in the physiopathology of angioneurotic edema, as well as in the pathology of the scalp. It is remarkable that this point is indicated for "ascension of energy to the head, to the face, to the throat, congestion of the face, and also coryza and rhinitis."[538] In conclusion, the behavior of patients suffering from keratitis is more often Jue Yin than Shao Yang, with a predominance of Fire, and thus dystonic. The perverse heat energy dominates the wind. We are dealing with a cold-hot affection.[539] This is why the complexion of the face and especially the cheeks is so often reddish.

• Keratitis

Keratitis is so unpleasant, so chronic and without hope of a cure (particularly the herpetic form since it is not possible to use corticotherapy), that it is indeed a miracle that acupuncture is able to bring comfort to the patients and to bring about the healing of the lesions. The points to use are: taichong (LV-3), ququan (LV-8), neiguan (PC-6), daling (PC-7), jingming (BL-1), shangxing (GV-23) and jueyinshu (BL-14), as well as ganshu (BL-18), using moxibustion. The prescription of trace elements is again correlative. Menetrier confirms this by saying:

> Keratitis appears linked to a dystonic personality, often with a hyposthenic antecedent.[540]

This justifies treatment by manganese-cobalt and sulfur, but also manganese-copper, according to the author, when there are patent hyposthenic (Metal-lung) aspects.

• Iritis, Iridocyclitis, Choroiditis

We might think that since the iris is the ocular sector that corresponds to the element Wood, the specific disorder of the liver or of the gallbladder, would be located in the iris. This is not so. The study of the etiologies of iritis and iridocyclitis shows that various meridians are involved. It is useful to point out that the innervation of the iris and of the ciliary muscle is assured by the common ocular motor nerve and that the cervical sympathetic nervous system determines both the dilation of the iris and exophthalmia.[541] According to Soulie de Morant, the points xuanlu (GB-5)[542] and fubai (GB-10) command the common ocular motor nerve, and fengchi (GB-20) commands the cervical sympathetic nervous system.[543] Most of the time the inflammatory affections of the iris concern an inflammation of the ciliary body. Then we speak of iridocyclitis, synonymous with anterior uveitis. Choroiditis is an inflammation of the posterior uvea, but most of the time the whole uvea is affected, including the iris, ciliary body and choroid. That is why we speak of posterior uveitis.

• Anterior Uveitis, Iritis, Iridocyclitis

The causes of anterior uveitis may be infectious or allergic. The hypersensitivity to various antigens, microbes, virus and allergens is a good sign of the specific vulnerability of the element Wood. This corresponds to the allergic diathesis. The affection may be caused by the herpes virus, the zona virus or even that of syphilis. It may be secondary to keratitis. The treatment is identical to the Jue Yin and Shao Yang protocols, just like the microbic (staphylococcus, streptococcus) infections, whose origin may be a gynecological focal infection or a urinary infection, and which is the result of an association with a shan characteristic of Jue Yin. Once more, this is the direct repercussion of a disturbance in zu jue yin which strikes its own cephalic and ocular branch.[544] However, the causal agent of iridocyclitis may also be that of tuberculosis, the mump virus or perhaps a germ localized in the sinus or in the teeth. In these cases, we are faced with a patient whose temperament is Tai Yin or Yang Ming.[545]

In so-called diathetic iridocyclitis, if the origin is gouty, we are faced with a Shao Yang patient,[546] or to a lesser extent one who is Jue Yin. If the origin is

272

diabetic, the temperament is Tai Yin or Yang Ming. If it is stiffening spondylarthritis, the temperament is Tai Yang or Shao Yin. In common cases of acute iritis resulting from hypersensitivity, with ocular pain spreading sometimes to half of the head, photophobia and variable visual disturbances, the meridians that are affected are almost always Shao Yang and Jue Yin.

These etiologies are specific to these temperaments. In such cases, when the eye is red the pupil on the affected side is in miosis and contracts insufficiently in bright light. We may attempt a treatment on the opposite side concentrating on the Shao Yang and Jue Yin meridians in combination with a general treatment identical to that for keratitis. As for anterior uveitis caused by exogenous infection from an eye wound, or secondary to an ocular contusion, the problem is not the same. It is necessary to determine the temperament of the patient and to reinforce the vulnerable meridians. All in all, the treatment of anterior uveitis is variable according to the temperament of the patient and to the causal pathology.

• Choroiditis

The problem posed by posterior uveitis and choroiditis is the same in every respect, since the etiologies are exactly the same, with the exception of posterior uveitis of rheumatic origin, which does not exist. The functional signs, however, are different: there is the classical impression of fog, of flies or of spots before the eyes. Here too, the treatment is etiological. The symptomology points to a perverse energy that is less violent, less Yang than is the case with acute iritis, and seems to be more exactly a cold wind or a humid wind, rather than perverse heat. The treatment is based on this difference, and we recommend the sequential shu-antique points.

Glaucoma

The Shanghai authors note that glaucoma was called "wind of the half of the head," by the ancient Chinese and later "internal obstruction of a green wind." These names evoke a disturbance of the element Wood. Nonetheless, with glaucoma we must make the same reservations and distinctions as with the rest of ocular pathology. In Western medicine, we discriminate between congenital glaucoma,[547] acute primitive glaucoma, chronic primitive glaucoma and secondary glaucoma.

These elements define glaucoma: ocular hypertension, an essential sign that leads to the degradation of the visual field and the alteration of the optic disk. In Chinese medicine, glaucoma raises the question of hypertension of the "organic fluids" in the eye (aqueous humor) and forces us to take a closer look at the mechanism of the organic fluids and at the meridians in question.

• Acute Primitive Glaucoma

This is violent intraocular hypertension, determined by the closing of the iridocorneal angle. The excruciating frontal pain radiating into one-half of the head gave it its Chinese name. Among the triggering circumstances we often find a strong emotion or the prescription of medicine that dilates the pupil, such as atropine. This may, if the iridocorneal angle is acute, bring on an attack of acute glaucoma. In Chapter 10 of the *Ling Shu*, which develops the symptomology of

273

the meridians, we find mention of ocular symptoms related to the physiology of the fluids for the following meridians: shou tai yang (small intestine), zu tai yang (bladder) and shou shao yang (triple burner). These three meridians are in fact those responsible for the general physiology of the body fluids, along with zu shao yang (gallbladder).[548]

In reality, the temperament Tai Yang seems to be just as emotional as Shao Yang — passionate and coleric, respectively. Emotion, of course, is likely to dilate the pupil and to trigger an internal mechanism that will lead to glaucoma in predisposed patients. The pupil, as we have seen, is under the dependency of the element Water (kidney and bladder) and may be influenced by their meridians, zu tai yang and zu shao yin.

The iris, on the other hand, is under the dependency of the element Wood and the meridians Shao Yang and Jue Yin. Two miscellaneous meridians that converge at the eye at the point jingming (BL-1), also rule over the ocular fluids. These are yang qiao mai and yin qiao mai:

> Yin qiao mai is an annex of the primary channel[549] of the kidneys. It corresponds to the energy of the Earth. It goes, consequently, from down to up, and brings the fluids to the eyes.

> Yang qiao mai is an annex of the primary bladder channel. It receives the energy from yin qiao mai at the point jingming (BL-1), and from there returns towards the inferior members. It corresponds to the energy of Heaven. It goes, consequently, from up to down.[550]

These two miscellaneous channels also shunt into the Water meridians, since the yang qiao mai key point is shenmai (BL-62) on the bladder meridian and the yin qiao mai key point is zhaohai (KI-6) on the kidney meridian. An imbalance of the fluids in a meridian seems to relate to a disturbance at its shu point.[551] This was the hypothesis of the modern authors at the Tai Yuan hospital in China. They were able to confirm their hypothesis by measuring the variations in intraocular pressure while they needled the shu points of the twelve meridians in a healthy subject.[552] They were thus able to prove the importance of the shu points of the liver and the triple burner to treat acute glaucoma.

In acute primitive glaucoma among adult patients, the perverse energy does not seem to be the determining factor, but yields to emotional energies and to alimentary or toxic (medicinal) factors. The role of the temperament in this pathology is fundamental. The first place goes not only to the Wood temperaments, but also to one associated with Water, Tai Yang. The onset of the attack, of course, is explained by the abnormal closing of the iridocorneal angle. The symptoms, Yang and violent, evoke the specific vulnerability of the Yang temperaments. They are typically Shao Yang. There is a violent hemicranial pain located on the territory of the triple burner and the gallbladder. This pain might pass for a migraine, but there is also nausea and frequently vomiting and prostration, specific signs of a Wood disorder. Also in this disorder, the eye is red, the cornea cloudy; the anterior chamber diminished; the eyeball is hard. But without a doubt, the most typical aspect visible in the ophthalmic examination is the greenish glint of the crystalline lens.[553] This color is, without question, a sign of the element Wood and explains the Chinese analogy (green-Wood) according to which glaucoma was known as "internal obstruction of a green wind," well before the invention of our modern instruments.

Acupuncture treatment may be considered alongside classical local (pilocarpine) and general (Diamox, glycerin, even mannitol in perfusion) treatments, to bring down the ocular pressure, particularly in rebellious cases, and to prepare the patient for surgery. It is certainly useful when there are contraindications to surgery. As the pathway of the fluids is obstructed within the eye, we must unblock its descent by opening yang qiao mai using shenmai (BL-62), and needling the xi point of zu tai yang (bladder), jinmen (BL-63). Locally, we needle jingming (BL-1), tongziliao (GB-1), shuaigu (GB-8) and taiyang (M-HN-9)[554] to make the energy flow in Shao Yang and to make it penetrate from fengchi (GB-20) into the other miscellaneous shunt channel, yin qiao mai, which "hides the Yang." Xuanlu (GB-5), which we have already mentioned as a useful ophthalmological point, unites the energy of the three Yang and is also to be needled. Its symptomology in the *Da Cheng* is, "Migraine that spreads to the corners of the eyes."[555]

The words of Qi Bo concerning the physiology of the ocular fluids and tears may inspire us to choose the point tianzhu (BL-10):

> When we have trouble, worries and the heart is disturbed, and when
> consequently the five organs and the six bowels are equally disturbed,
> as well as the ancestral channels yin qiao mai and yang qiao mai, we
> must disperse the point tianzhu {BL-10}. If tears do not come to the
> eyes, on the contrary, we must tonify this point.[556]

We will balance the fluids in the meridians involved by needling their shu points. We will needle taichong (LV-3), zhongzhu (TB-3), taixu (SI-3) and sanyinjiao (SP-6) to balance the ascending Yin within the Yin meridians. If the temperament of the patient or the disturbance itself is dominated by Tai Yang, we will needle houxi (SI-3) for "red eyes with a veil before the eyes."[557] To recapitulate, the points useful for treating acute glaucoma are: BL-1, BL-10, BL-62, BL-63, TB-3, GB-1, GB-5, taiyang (M-HN-9), LV-8, KI-3 and SP-6. The modern Shanghai authors advise that we treat the patient once or twice a day during the acute attack.[558] The choice of points may be varied from one session to another.

• Chronic primitive glaucoma among adults

This affection takes on a different form. Here the iridocorneal angle remains open. The hypertonia is caused by modifications of the secretion, circulation or evacuation of the aqueous humor, the reasons for which are unknown. There are also vascular modifications of the head of the optic nerve that sensitize the optic nerve to a minimal hypertonia.[559] Chronic primitive glaucoma among adults is a hereditary disease. In other words, even more than in the acute form, the nature of the terrain is preponderant, may be transmitted from one generation to the next and must be defined.

This terrain is related to a characteristic psychological profile that is well known in classical medicine. It has been defined in many works on pathology and corresponds to the temperament Jue Yin. It has been described as being "vagotonic" with nervousness and "emotional instability" to such an extent that the unanimous recommendation is to cut out stimulants — tea, coffee, tobacco — and to take neurosedatives (barbiturates).[560]

The symptoms are not so violent, not so Yang, as in acute glaucoma. On the contrary, they consist of a visual fog, of halos around sources of light, or morning tears for no apparent reason. There is a progressive drop in visual acuity and an equally progressive shrinking of the visual field. This should be examined every three months. These symptoms do not bring to mind a Yang etiology such as warm wind, nor a disturbance of the Yang meridians, but rather a cold wind and a Yin meridian, Jue Yin. One revealing sign is the presence of headaches instead of hemicranial pain, as seen in the acute form.

The classical description is a subacute attack against a chronic background, triggered by the cold, by emotions or even by the darkness.[561] This confirms the cold wind etiology. The increase in pressure is characterized by the elevation of the resistance to the outflow of the endo-ocular fluids and is caused by the cold represented by water. There is a clear correlation with the endolabyrinthic hyper-pressure of Meniere's disease. The two affections occur, as if by chance, on the same psychological profiles and are sensitive to the same triggering circumstances. We may say that in Chinese medicine chronic primitive glaucoma in adult patients is to the eye what the dizziness associated with Meniere's disease is to the ear. We find the same combination of a favorable genetically transmitted temperament, the perverse energy, the psychic (emotional) energy and even an alimentary energy (stimulants). This is why the treatment differs from that of acute glaucoma.

During the attack, we will perform the same treatment as we did for Meniere's disease: with dadun (LV-1) and zhongchong (PC-9), either on the opposite side or bilaterally. Dadun (LV-1) corresponds to the symptomology, "Chill with headache or nosebleed,"[562] which fits the present case. The only ophthalmological indication for zhongchong (PC-9) given by the *Da Cheng,* however, is "child cannot see at dusk." For general balancing we may act upon the liver and the emotions by needling xingjian (LV-2), taichong (LV-3), tianchi (PC-1), jianshi (PC-5), neiguan (PC-6) and daling (PC-7). These points have all been noted in our discussion of Jue Yin psychiatry. We needle xingjian (LV-2) because it is the heat point that counteracts the perverse cold wind. We needle the shu point of the meridian, taichong (LV-3), because it is opposed the penetration of the perverse energy. The rong and shu points treat organic disease. The *Da Cheng* indicates xingjian for "the patient does not want to look, always closes his eyes."[563] Hua Tuo mentions it for all eye disorders: "taichong {LV-3}: unclear vision."[564] Tianchi (PC-1), the "heavenly window point of the blood of the liver," as we are fond of calling it, corrects vagotonia in the cardiac sphere and is indicated for "dizziness, unclear vision."[565] Jianshi (PC-5): "chill, fear of the wind and the cold, following a chill, sensation of great malaise in the chest which seems knotted."[566]

Apart from these points we may stimulate tongziliao (GB-1), fengchi (GB-10), tianzhu (BL-20), shenmai (BL-62) and jinmen (BL-63) to facilitate the drainage of the eye fluids. The points recommended for chronic primitive glaucoma among adult patients are: PC-9, LV-1, LV-3, PC-1, PC-5, PC-6, PC-7, GV-23,[567] GB-1, GB-20, BL-10, BL-62 and BL-63. Their dystonic behavior makes these patients, depending on their age, prime targets for manganese-cobalt or manganese.

• Secondary Glaucoma

Here, the etiology is all-inclusive and consequently, problematic. The affection may be secondary to a crystalline lens trauma, to an intra-ocular disturbance or to a tumor, which we will not study here. Chronic uveitis may lead to a secondary glaucoma. All the etiologies and the temperaments mentioned in the discussion of iridocyclitis and choroiditis need to be examined. Glaucoma may also be secondary to hypertensive iritis or to diabetes. In this case, the most probable temperaments are Yang Ming and Tai Yin. It is indispensable to needle hegu (LI-4), a point that is generally useful in all ocular affections. An obliteration of the retinal artery, a rare cause of secondary glaucoma, evokes Jue Yin only when the spasmodic element is dominant. This occurs among young subjects (Shao Yang or Jue Yin), during an attack of paroxystic high blood pressure in cases involving a severe neurovegetative disorder. Clinically, this means the sudden loss of an eye.

Acupuncture treatment focuses on the cardiovascular and neurovegetative imbalances.[568] Locally, we needle jingming (BL-1), tongziliao (GB-1) and, regionally, fengchi (GB-20), tianzhu (BL-10) and the heavenly window point, tianyou (TB-16). There is an obvious correlation with the trace elements, Diathesis I and manganese; the two therapies may be combined with classical emergency treatments. As we have just seen, ophthalmological pathology is often influenced by the element Wood; by the two viscera, liver and gallbladder; and also by the two meridians, Shao Yang and Jue Yin. Nonetheless, ocular disorders are not limited to these two temperaments as we learn by carefully studying the ancient Chinese texts, and especially the *Nei Jing Ling Shu.*

Hematological Pathology

Here we will consider the physiological aspects of coagulation attributed to the liver, as well as its role in hemorrhage.

Traumatology and Hemorrhage

"The liver produces the blood," we learned in the *Su Wen,* and "the spleen regulates the blood." Production and regulation of the the blood are kept in balance by a Wood-Earth equilibrium. Wood triumphs over the Earth, but the Earth turns against Wood. In Chapter 67 of the same work we read about the close relationship that exists between the kidney, the adrenal gland and the liver through the interaction of the five elements. As far as the blood is concerned:

> The north engenders the kidney. The kidney feeds the bones and the marrows, which transmit life to the liver.[569]

One parallel of this relationship, but certainly not the only parallel, is represented by the renin-angiotensin system.

Note that Earth maintains a relationship of opposition and equilibrium with Water as well. The Earth triumphs over Water (the spleen over the kidney) and Water may turn against the Earth. The hematological equilibrium is thus dependent on the Wood-Earth-Water triangle and the mutual influences of activation and inhibition of the kidneys, the liver and the spleen. Apart from the role of perverse wind, three aggressions are likely to disturb this equation of the blood.

Wood, Earth and Water Etiologies

The Wood etiology concerns external trauma, which causes bruises; the Earth etiology concerns the aggression of perverse humidity against the spleen; and the Water etiology concerns perverse cold, which affects the kidney, and indirectly the energy and the circulation of the fluids. Depending on the intensity of the disorder, there will be repercussions that we may observe by examining the complexion (pallor, waxen color) and the pulse, if only in its Western aspect (rapid or little and fleeing).

> Huang Di asked, "Chronic illnesses of the five organs influence the complexion and the pulses. How may we distinguish them from the acute illnesses?"
>
> Qi Bo answered, "Your question is pertinent. Chronic states are differentiated from acute states through the examination of complexions and pulses.
>
> A little pulse and normal complexion mean recent illness. A normal pulse and abnormal complexion mean chronic illness.[570] Normal pulse and five normal complexions mean recent illness. Abnormal pulse and five abnormal complexions mean very old illness."[571]

To explain his comments, Qi Bo gives the following example:

> The pulses of the liver and the kidneys are tense and deep {simultaneously}, and the complexion is green and red. This is the result of a "demolition" of the energy {juy thuong}, although the blood is still intact.[572] If the blood is diminished, it is because the destruction is accompanied by an aggression of perverse humidity or by the energy of water.[573]

The energy of water is rendered by Husson as "qi of water" and corresponds to exudates, edemas or ascites.

Nguyen Van Nghi quotes from the commentaries of Zhang Jing Yao concerning this passage:

> Contusions, with or without ecchymosis, impede the circulation of blood and energy, causing swelling, as is the case in disorders caused by perverse water energy and disorders resulting from perverse humidity, edema or ascites[574]

We may conclude that the liver, which produces the blood, is the first organ affected in external trauma (ecchymosis, hematoma). But the kidney, mother of the liver, which engenders the marrow and gives life to the liver, will be affected next by the "demolition" of the energy. The analysis of pulse and complexion given by Qi Bo in the same chapter is comprehensible:

A strong, hard and long pulse of the liver, if the face is not greenish, signals an accumulation of blood beneath the ribs[575] subsequent to a fall or a contusion. The patient is dyspneic.

If the pulse becomes soft and sluggish, and if the complexion is fresh, the patient will be very thirsty. Drinking copious amounts of liquid will cause the illness known as *gia am* {an edema}.[576]

This is an exudate caused by a substantial deficiency of blood cells or to hyperproteinemia. In the *Ling Shu,* Qi Bo goes compares a liver disorder of emotional origin to a traumatic disorder:

If we take a great fall, the black blood of the hematoma stays within the body, or if we get too angry, the energy rises and may no longer descend, and accumulates in the sides of the body. These two causes may wound the liver.[577]

In the minds of the Chinese, emotional energy is powerful and capable of doing great damage.[578]

Acupuncture treatment consists in powerfully tonifying the liver and the blood with moxas on ganshu (BL-18), "when the liver lacks blood,"[579] geshu (BL-17), the hui point of the blood related to the spleen, gaohuang (BL-38)[580] and shenshu (BL-23). We will, of course, stimulate ququan (LV-8) regularly (and for a long time) with moxa, as this point strengthens the deficiency of the liver and of the blood. It is also to be stimulated when there is a deficit of coagulation factors, either constitutional or acquired, caused by a "wound of the liver." This is according to Soulie de Morant who describes the symptomology of ququan (LV-8):

Insufficient coagulation, bleeding at the slightest scratch, with a delay and for a long time, the patient is very easily bruised.[581]

The *Da Cheng* indicates ququan for "digestive hemorrhage."[582]

We may note in passing, as we did in the case of extrauterine pregnancy in our discussion of gynecology, that the signs of insufficiency of the liver and of the blood at a functional state include pallor, asthenia, lipothymia, anxiety, sticky perspiration and syncope.

When there is a localized congestion of blood, we apply a technique described by Qi Bo in the *Su Wen:*

If there is blood congestion, it is necessary to bleed the points of the secondary vessels to prevent the black blood from penetrating the vessels.[583]

On the other hand, a deficiency of blood should be treated by discerning the deficient meridians and inserting a needle into them; withdrawal of needle should be suspended for a prolonged period of time so that the acupuncturist can observe the reticular meridians as they become enlarged at which moment the needle should be drawn out quickly without excreting the blood {without bloodletting}.[584]

The close relationship between Jue Yin, the blood, the energy, the liver and the muscles with the lunar cycle makes it necessary to take into account the celestial phenomena:

> At the new moon, the blood and the energy begin to purify themselves, the defensive energy (wei) begins to flow. At the full moon, the blood and energy are in abundance, the muscles become firm.[585]

> As the moon wanes, the muscles relax, the meridians and the secondary channels empty, the defensive energy is dispersed, the container no longer adapts to the contained. This is why the regulation of the blood and the energy must be based on the celestial phenomena. . . never disperse at the new moon, never tonify at the full moon, never needle as the moon wanes.[586]

> At the new moon, dispersion might weaken the internal organs. During the full moon, tonification is likely to lead to an increase in the volume of the blood and the energy, causing stasis of the blood in the secondary channels, forming what we call *trung thuc,* a superimposition of excesses {chong chi}.[587]

In conclusion, Jue Yin through the liver plays an important role in the physiology of the blood and in hemorrhage syndromes. The regulation by acupuncture of the aftereffects of hemorrhages or the treatment of hematomas, ecchymosis or any other hemorrhage of lesser abundance, obeys very precise laws. It calls for a careful observation of the celestial phenomena, especially the lunar cycle. We should recall the curious position of the point gaohuang (BL-38), "envelope of the portion included between the heart and the diaphragm," located on the horizontal of jueyinshu (BL-14), the shu point of the pericardium (shou jue yin). It plays an important part in vasomotricity. The properties of gaohuang in relation to hemorrhage and to anemia have been known at least since the *Da Cheng* was written and have been mentioned by Soulie de Morant, Nguyen Van Nghi and others. We will say more about this point in the discussion of hematology in the chapter devoted to the pathology of Tai Yin.

Chronobiology of Jue Yin

Diurnal Rhythm

Shou jue yin's hour is xu: from 5 p.m. to 7 p.m. Its animal is the dog. Zu jue yin's hour is chou: from 1 a.m. to 3 a.m. Its animal is the ox.

Annual Rhythm

> From Jue Yin come orchitis and gynecological tumors. Jue Yin carries the number five {in the twelve terrestrial branches}. The third month is that of Yin within Yang, the xie is in the interior, whence come lower abdominal pains and swellings.

280

Impossibility of flexing and straightening painful limbs: the third month gives impetus to the flourishing of the creatures that bend like branches under the weight of new vegetation. Genital and lymphatic pain: Yin is still abundant and the dilated vessels are no longer permeable. This is called tui long shan {orchitis, lymphatic swelling, spasmatic pain}. In serious cases, there is dryness in the throat, the consequence of the struggle between Yin and Yang.[588]

Terrestrial Duodecimal Rhythm

The second and sixth years correspond to Jue Yin.[589]

Monthly Rhythm

Shou jue yin corresponds to the third month of autumn; zu jue yin to the third month of winter.[590]

Rhythm of Jue Yin in the Inferior and Superior Limbs

The ninth month corresponds to the meridian zu jue yin (liver) in the right leg.

The tenth month corresponds to the meridian zu jue yin (liver) in the left leg, this is the end of Yin.[591]

Shou jue yin, which is not associated with a material organ, does not take part in the ten day rhythm.

Synthesis of the Temperament Jue Yin

Jue Yin subjects correspond to the nervous personality profile as defined by Gaston Berger and to the dystonic diathesis defined by Menetrier. Their behavior is characterized by a nervous and emotional instability as well as dystonic syndromes such as dizziness, headaches, spasms, trembling, jumpiness and fits of tears. These people are often dilettantes, aesthetes, who talk a lot and often try to focus attention on themselves to the point of being hysterical or mythomaniacal. This instability is manifested physically as a tendency toward cardiac erethism and high blood pressure. As far as digestive pathology is concerned, visceral spasms, gastralgia, right-sided colonopathy, flatulence, constipation and diarrhea are predisposed.

An allergic terrain is also characteristic of Jue Yin subjects. Asthma, rhinitis, conjunctivitis, keratitis, eczema, lichens, angioneurotic edema, all sorts of allergens (sun, insects, shellfish, medications), as well as fronto-orbital headaches, which may or may not be catamenial, are the likely results of aggressions. The vulnerability of their veins predisposes them to varicose veins and hemorrhoids. Among women who do not tolerate oral contraceptives, affections such as dysmenorrhea, fibromas, memory problems, asthenia, fright, insomnia, anxiety and even epilepsy may occur. We have shown how all these syndromes are driven by the same energy mechanism, a deficiency of Yin or jing of the liver with a corollary deficiency of blood. The blood descends and accumulates in the lower part of the body, causing a surge of energy, or Yang of the liver, in the upper part of the body. Among Jue Yin subjects, the penetration of cold or of cold wind is likely to cause a whole range of specific syndromes: headaches, back pains, leukorrhea, impotence, frigidity, pollakiuria and cystitis. Meniere's disease and chronic glaucoma among adult patients are two other results of perverse cold water penetration of Jue Yin, one located in the labyrinth, the other in the eye; two territories that are energized by the liver as are the genitals and the lower urinary tract.

We may say that the pathology of Jue Yin is dominated by the physiology of the blood and the liver, and that this temperament is disposed to deficiency. This is why, when there is an aggression of the liver (viral hepatitis, contraceptives, medicine or toxic substances) or aggression against the blood (hematomas, trauma, post-partum, extra-uterine pregnancy), the deficient tendency is amplified, the morbidity is reinforced and aggravated. This may lead to grave illnesses such as multiple sclerosis, delirium tremens or Korsakoff's syndrome. Psoriasis of the scalp, Duhring's disease and dishydrosis are other syndromes that affect patients of the Jue Yin temperament. These, too, result from the same global imbalance of blood within the meridian.

This whole range of syndromes is in perfect correlation with the definition of Diatheses I and III in their Yin modality, thereby justifying the association of the two therapeutic paradigms and the prescription of manganese and manganese-cobalt, as well as sulfur, iodine and cobalt trace elements in treating patients of this temperament.

Notes

¹ *Su Wen* (8), Chapter 8, p. 46.

² *Su Wen* (28), p. 95.

³ *Su Wen* (8), Chapter 21, p. 95.

⁴ *Ling Shu* (8), Chapter 4, p. 326.

⁵ Husson (28), p. 85, translates this as celestial obscurity. Xuan, "before the light of day," is translated by Schatz (104) as anterior heaven.

⁶ Husson (28), p. 85, translates, "in man, it is the Tao that leads to wisdom."

⁷ *Su Wen* (8), Chapter 5, p. 33.

⁸ *Su Wen* (28), Chapter 9, p. 99.

⁹ *Ling Shu* (8), Chapter 65, p. 515.

¹⁰ For the relationship between the liver, the blood and the channels, see Physiology of the gallbladder, Shao Yang.

¹¹ *Su Wen* (28), Chapter 5, p. 85.

¹² Tremollieres (110).

¹³ Kappas (30), p. 378.

¹⁴ Husson (28), p. 367, translates this as "the most noble."

¹⁵ *Su Wen* (8), Chapter 79, p. 298.

¹⁶ *Ling Shu* (8), Chapter 16, p. 391.

¹⁷ Yin means body energy, as opposed to perverse energy (Yang), which does not contradict the comments by Nguyen Van Nghi.

¹⁸ *Su Wen* (28), Chapter 79, p. 369.

¹⁹ Hanania (25).

²⁰ Rideller and Colognac (96), pp. 41-50.

²¹ Dessertene *et.al.* (15).

²² Rideller and Colognac (96).

²³ See discussion further on in this chapter on spasmophilia.

²⁴ *Su Wen* (28), Chapter 5, p. 85.

²⁵ Internal imbalance of energy, Jue Yin. (See Introduction.)

26 *Su Wen* (28), Chapter 19, p. 127.

27 Husson (28), pp. 139-140, translates this as "the emotions."

28 *Su Wen* (66), Chapter 21, pp. 351-355.

29 *Ibid.*

30 Husson translates, "In the ruining of the essence due to terror." Terror here corresponds to fear, to stress.

31 Nguyen Van Nghi (66).

32 That is, Tai Yang, Shao Yang, Yang Ming, etc. Here the taking of the pulse is not only located at the left gate for the liver and the right inch for the pericardium, it is a global measure of deficiency and excess on the left compared to the right, which allows us to determine the disorder of Tai Yang or of Jue Yin. It is understandable that the information gathered is only of value if we compare the two systems.

33 Husson translates as "vain sweat."

34 *Su Wen* (66), Chapter 21, p. 150.

35 Chamfrault (7), pp. 578-579.

36 *Ling Shu* (7), Chapter 5, p. 335.

37 Soulie de Morant (107), p. 446.

38 *Ibid.*

39 *Da Cheng* (7), p. 576.

40 *Ibid.*, p. 638.

41 In light of the dystonic context and the origin of the behavior of these subjects with spasmophilia, it would be useful to look for the origin of the repolarization difficulty in the ion mechanisms of calcium in the myocardial cell. The jing of the liver represents the endocrine aspect of the organ linked to the thyroid and parathyroid. See Endocrinology.

42 Chamfrault (7), p. 497.

43 See Spasmophilia, below.

44 Menetrier (44), p. 75. According to certain authors, says Menetrier, phosphorus may have a positive action in certain cases of asystolia. The phosphorus ion is prescribed in cases of spasmophilia and is a part of the phospho-calcic metabolism.

45 Soulie de Morant (107), p. 486.

46 Nguyen Van Nghi and Picou (67), Chapter 19, p. 287.

[47] *Ibid.* See also, Shanghai (105).

[48] Jagger and Braunwald, referenced in Harrison (26), p. 1297.

[49] See Shao Yang and below, Neurology.

[50] Menetrier (44), p. 46.

[51] *Ibid.*, p. 75.

[52] *Ling Shu* (8), Chapter 10, p. 366.

[53] Soulie de Morant (107), p. 884. See also the role of ququan (LV-8) in all other hepatic insufficiencies.

[54] See Arteritis, Yang Ming.

[55] *Su Wen* (28), Chapter 45, p. 204.

[56] *Ibid.* See also, *Ling Shu* (8), Chapter 21, pp. 407-408.

[57] *Da Cheng* (7), p. 479.

[58] Be careful, this sign seems to correspond to the neuropathies in the lower limb, too. (See Tai Yin.)

[59] Soulie de Morant (107), p. 884.

[60] *Ibid.*

[61] *Da Cheng* (7), p. 348.

[62] Soulie de Morant (107), p. 436. The author states that the venal tissue ought not to have lost its elasticity.

[63] *Da Cheng* (7), pp. 566-580.

[64] Menetrier (44), p. 76.

[65] These describe cases that may correlate with acrocyanosis and Raynaud's Syndrome, where the vasomotor disorders depend on shou jue yin (pericardium).

[66] All are circumstances in which Jue Yin and the element Wood are involved, especially thyrotoxicosis, studied in Shao Yang.

[67] Fitzpatrick and Haynes, referenced in Harrison (26), p. 281.

[68] Kay (31).

[69] Caen (4).

[70] *Ling Shu* (8), Chapter 21, p. 422.

[71] The pulse stretched like a violin string means that it no longer has the softness of the stomach energy that normally makes it more flexible, more like a bow-string. In other words, the essential energy is exhausted and can be seen in the pulse. This is a sign of gravity and possibly of death. See Physiology of Yang Ming.

[72] *Da Cheng* (7), p. 579.

[73] *Ibid.*, p. 587.

[74] Quoted by Nguyen Van Nghi (66), p. 72.

[75] See Epistaxis in Tai Yin, Jue Yin chapters, ORL in Yang Ming chapter.

[76] Best and Dale, quoted by Malmejac (42), p. 227.

[77] "When the wind insinuates a vicious emanation, if the essence fails, the perversion gains the liver" *Su Wen* (28), p. 79. It is the essence jing qi that is failing, as we say.

[78] *Da Cheng* (7), pp. 423-424.

[79] *Ibid.*

[80] Picard (75), p. 96.

[81] Fabre (18).

[82] Translated as "anterior heaven" by Schatz, the expression is used in the translation of the *Yi Jing* by Wilhelm and Perrot, 1973, and also used by Lu Tsu in *The Secret of the Golden Flower.*

[83] *Su Wen* (28), Chapter 67, pp. 265-266.

[84] This may correspond to the genetic program of a subject, as we suggested in discussing physiology.

[85] We must remember that the hun (qi of the liver) is the advisor of the shen (qi of the heart in which the spirit dwells), and that this hun is the "spiritual soul" that dwells in the liver and that gives its name to zhangmen (LV-13), "door of the shelter."

[86] This may evoke respiratory symptoms as well as cardiac symptoms.

[87] *Ling Shu* (8), Chapter 67, p. 473.

[88] Requena (92), p. 148.

[89] Shanghai (105).

[90] The gastralgia of Tai Yin and Yang Ming origin are studied in the corresponding chapters.

[91] *Su Wen* (66), Chapter 22, p. 373.

[92] Menetrier (44), p. 78.

[93] This protocol deserves rigorous experimentation in hospital circumstances.

[94] Sensitization eczemas belong to Diathesis I and are treated with manganese and sulfur. They often accompany the allergy series: asthma, rhinitis, migraines, Quincke's edema. In Chinese medicine the correlation with Wood is obvious.

[95] Caroli and Hecht (5), p. 86.

[96] *Ling Shu* (8), Chapter 4, p. 326.

[97] *Su Wen* (28), Chapter 45, p. 206.

[98] Vietnamese term in Nguyen Van Nghi's translation that corresponds to the Chinese term sun xie: diarrhea. Quoted in Husson (28), p. 119.

[99] *Su Wen* (66), Chapter 17, p. 241.

[100] *Ibid.*

[101] Husson translates, ''When the wind insinuates a vicious emanation (yin qi) and the essence fails, the perversion gains the liver.'' This shows once more the constitutional predisposition at the origin of the aggressivity of a perverse energy.

[102] *Su Wen* (8), Chapter 3, p. 25.

[103] Nguyen Van Nghi (59), p. 108.

[104] Husson (28), p. 79.

[105] See semiology of the *Da Cheng* in Chamfrault (7) pp. 427, 576-587.

[106] *Ibid.*

[107] *Ibid.*

[108] *Ibid.*, pp. 580-583.

[109] This is true when the symptomology indicates an excess, for example, where a deficient organ is invaded by perverse energy yielding excess and consequent impingement.

[110] ''The attack of the wind in the spring brings on a perversion that causes abdominal upset (dong xie) or diarrhea (sun xie).'' *Su Wen* (28), Chapter 3, p. 79.

[111] Menetrier (44), p. 46.

[112] Shanghai (105).

[113] The terms ''infectious'' and ''serum'' hepatitis are now obsolete concepts.

[114] Koff and Isselbacher, referenced in Harrison (26), p. 1603.

[115] Shanghai (105).

[116] Remember that Jue Yin in the cosmos symbolizes the wind.

[117] Nguyen Van Nghi (66).

[118] Koff and Isselbacher, referenced in Harrison (26), pp. 1603-1610.

[119] *Ibid.*

[120] *Ibid.*

[121] There is a clear connection between the spleen (zu tai yin) and the lung (shou tai yin) by way of Tai Yin, which is visible in the increase of appetite when patients stop smoking, as well as the accompanying gain of weight.

[122] Koff and Isselbacher, referenced in Harrison, 1975, pp. 1603-1610.

[123] *Ling Shu* (8) Chapter 74, p. 536.

[124] *Su Wen* (8), Chapter 17, p. 71.

[125] The bilateral pulses of the foot (LU-7 left and right) explore the Yin in the body.

[126] *Su Wen* (8), Chapter 18, p. 77.

[127] The specific epidemic aspect of the affection is discussed in the text *Dan Xi Xin Fa,* quoted by Shanghai (105). The factors responsible for epidemics are included among virus, microbes, parasites. See *Trung Y Hoc* of Hanoi, quoted by Nguyen Van Nghi; see also the concept of curious perverse energy.

[128] The channels are relatively Yin (jing) compared to the gallbladder (curious bowel). See physiological considerations in Shao Yang concerning alkaline phosphates.

[129] Quoted by Requena and Rat (95), pp. 219-229.

[130] *Su Wen* (66), Chapter 19, p. 305.

[131] Let us mention the onset of glomerulopathy or of rheumatoid arthritis in the course of active chronic hepatitis.

[132] *Su Wen* (66), p. 304.

[133] *Su Wen* (8), p. 85. Husson speaks of nerves and of vessels.

[134] Koff and Isselbacher, referenced in Harrison (26), p. 1068. Among other rare complications, we may note acute hemorrhagic pancreatitis, atypical pneumonias and also polyneuritis (disorder typical of Tai Yin). See Neurology, Tai Yin.

[135] Shanghai (105), p. 150.

[136] Green jaundice (Wood) is different from yellow jaundice (spleen).

[137] See below, in the treatment section following, the local points of this region for the treatment of fulminant hepatitis.

[138] This impression signals the escape of energy caused by the deficiency of the organ and announces the coma. This is different from the primitive upsurge of Yang energy (neurology of Yang Ming).

[139] *Su Wen* (8), Chapter 22, p. 214.

[140] See Infectious Pathology of Tai Yin.

[141] *Su Wen* (8), Chapter 22, p. 215.

[142] We have rapidly seen the results of this, as has our colleague, P. Rat, in his experimentation.

[143] Requena (95), pp. 219-229.

[144] Quoted by Chamfrault (7), p. 599.

[145] This point is one distance beneath yanglingquan (GB-34) and it is specific for acute infections of the bile ducts (Shanghai).

[146] Chamfrault (7), p. 580.

[147] See Urticaria in Shao Yang.

We have sponsored experimentation on the treatment of the common form in hospital practice, which was the subject of a thesis (Rat, P., "Essai de traitement par acupuncture dans certaines affections hepatiques"). These pour le Doctorat en Medecine. Marseille, France, 1977.

[148] The action on the central nervous system of renzhong (GV-26) has been proven as far as the cerebral PaO_2 is concerned.

[149] These points have been described in our work, Requena *et.al.* (92).

[150] Quoted by Soulie de Morant (107), p. 647 and Shanghai (105).

[151] Requena (94), pp. 295-297.

[152] Menetrier (44), p. 93.

[153] *Ling Shu* (8), Chapter 35, p. 447. Swelling and distension are more precisely translated as exudates and edemas.

[154] *Ling Shu* (8) Chapter 4, pp. 325-326.

[155] Alpers and Isselbacher, quoted in Harrison (26), p. 1589.

[156] This is the flapping tremor.

[157] *Su Wen* (28), Chapter 32, p. 167.

[158] Perspiration is the criterion for amelioration. The backwash of qi described is also called escape of Yang upwards, and results in coma caused by the exhaustion of Yin that no longer balances the Yang, whose natural tendency is to rise. (These Yin etiologies of comas are treated in the discussion of cerebrovascular accidents and comas in Yang Ming.) Headaches and dizziness are symptoms of the liver related to the internal channel that arrives at baihui (GV-20) at the summit of the skull.

[159] Leung Kwok Po (38), pp. 27-32.

[160] *Ling Shu* (8), Chapter 10, p. 376.

[161] *Ibid.*

[162] Leung Kwok Po (38), p. 29.

[163] This chapter is the one we quote from at the end of each temperament, in the discussion on cosmic rhythms and meridians. Each paragraph describes a pathological series in function with the meridian (Shao Yang, Jue Yin, etc.) and the month.

[164] *Su Wen* (28), Chapter 49, p. 216.

[165] Husson quotes Yang Shang Shan in saying that the fox cannot urinate at night. In fact, each time Chinese medicine speaks of foxes, we are dealing with symptoms that come and go. Here it is probably pollakiuria.

[166] *Su Wen* (28), Chapter 64, p. 254.

[167] This is the same fox shan wind.

[168] See migraines, in Shao Yang.

[169] *Su Wen* (28), Chapter 33, p. 170.

[170] *Ibid.*, Chapter 43, p. 200.

[171] *Ibid.*, Chapter 36, p. 181. We believe that the translation ''malaria'' is an improper extrapolation of ''intermittent fever'' as given by some authors.

[172] *Su Wen* (8), Chapter 45, p. 170. There may also be retention of fecal matter, constipation. This chapter has already been quoted from, in Gastroenterology.

[173] *Ibid.*

[174] *Ibid.* See also, Tai Yang, Intestinal Occlusion.

The opposite of this profile is urinary incontinence, as is said in the text on the pulsology of the liver, ''If the pulse is slightly sliding, there is urinary incontinence.'' *Ling Shu* (8), p. 326.

[175] *Ibid.*, Chapter 63, p. 510.

[176] Quoted by Chamfrault (7), p. 584.

[177] See Physiology of Yang Ming.

[178] Nguyen Van Nghi (67), p. 333. There is no pyuria here, which is why the Eastern semiologists say ''clear urine.'' Nonetheless, we must recognize that in cystitis, the urine is often quite pale.

[179] This means the pulse of the liver.

[180] *Su Wen* (28), Chapter 10, p. 102.

[181] Menetrier (44), p. 46.

[182] *Ibid.*, p. 82.

[183] See pathology of this meridian in the corresponding chapter.

[184] Zhang Zhi Cong, quoted in Nguyen Van Nghi (59), p. 97.

[185] Dewan and Rock, *American Journal of Obstetrics and Gynecology.*

[186] Compare with the work of Jonas, E., ''Predetermining the Sex of a Child,'' in Ostrander and Schroeder, 1966.

[187] *Su Wen* (8), Chapter 79, pp. 298-299.

[188] Nguyen Van Nghi (59), pp.342-343.

[189] Zhongji (CV-3) is considered to be one of three linking points of the three tendino-muscular channels (Yin) of the lower limb (spleen, liver, kidney).

[190] Nguyen Van Nghi (59), pp. 342-343.

[191] As for the solar plexus, it seems perfectly represented by the three mu points of the triple burner, shangwan (CV-13) upper burner, zhongwan (CV-12) middle burner, and xiawan (CV-10) lower burner. The two other mu points of the triple burner, shimen (CV-5) and yinjiao (CV-7), might correspond to the hypogastric plexus, and would overlap with qihai (CV-6) and guanyuan (CV-4), hypogastric and sacral respectively. Yinjiao (CV-7) is a passage point of dai mai, and guanyuan (CV-4) and qihai (CV-6) are the mu points of the two fundamental points of the kidney energy qi. Haishu (BL-24) is the beishu point of the sea of energy and guanyuanshu (BL-26) is the beishu point of the "origin of the gate." For these reasons, we understand that the pericardium and the triple burner were taken for the neurovegetative system and for its ortho and parasympathetic polarity, which is far from representing its only function.

[192] Soulie de Morant (107), p. 480.

[193] See Shao Yang.

[194] *Ling Shu* (8), Chapter 2, p. 315.

[195] We do not go into dysmenorrhea due to organic stenosis.

[196] See also Tai Yin, Yang Ming, Tai Yang.

[197] Shanghai (105).

[198] This mechanism has been widely treated. See Pernice (73), pp. 163-171; also, Nguyen-Recours (57), pp. 117-127.

[199] *Su Wen* (28), Chapter 64, p. 254. That is, spasms and migraines (ophthalmic), or fronto-orbital headaches (see Neurology in Shao Yang).

[200] Leung Kwok Po (38), p. 28.

[201] Michel-Wolfromm (51).

[202] Qihai (CV-6) and sanyinjiao (SP-6) are two of the four points indicated by Dr. Zhang as basic treatment for all shan.

[203] Chamfrault (7), p. 345.

[204] *Ibid.*

[205] *Da Cheng* (7), p. 434.

[206] This point is used by the Shanghai authors in association with qihai (CV-6), xuehai (SP-10), sanyinjiao (SP-6) and taichong (LV-3) in the treatment of endometriosis, whose clinical manifestation may be dysmenorrhea. We believe endometriosis and fibroma to be common to shan qi.

[207] The pericardium is part of the Fire Minister in the system of five elements and Shao Yang is the Fire Minister in the six energies. This is why pericardium and triple burner are the Yin and Yang function of the Fire Minister.

[208] Shanghai (105). See Pernice (73), p. 167.

[209] *Da Cheng* (7), pp. 389-581.

[210] *Ibid.*

[211] *Ling Shu* (8), Chapter 10, p. 375.

[212] For neiguan (PC-6), see Obstetrical Pathology below.

[213] *Da Cheng* (7), p. 500, 579, 583, 584.

[214] Leung Kwok Po (38), p. 28.

[215] *Da Cheng* (7), p. 577.

[216] *Da Cheng* (107), p. 569.

Another sign, a strange one, is described for zulinqi (GB-41): "Numbing of the lower limb after orgasm." In this case, we must needle on the opposite side. This sign foretells of the neuritis of the lower limb discussed in the chapter devoted to Tai Yin, where dai mai and zong jin (big muscle) are active in its constitution.

[217] Alpers and Isselbacher note that the disturbances of the catabolism of the estrogens are at the origin of spider angioma and of gynecomastia. The estrogens can act directly on the liver, inhibiting its secretory functions. Estradiol and its derivatives, particularly those used as oral contraceptives, interfere with the excretion of BSP and sometimes boost the alkaline phosphate level. Harrison (26), p. 1592.

[218] In this case, we may think that it is eclampsis.

[219] *Da Cheng* (7), p. 555.

[220] Pregnancy is not mentioned.

[221] *Da Cheng* (7) p. 556.

[222] Shanghai (105).

[223] The physiological vulnerability of these meridians explains the frequency of constipation among women patients. Yemen (TB-2), the rong point (Water), means "door of the fluids."

[224] *Su Wen* (28), Chapter 39, p. 188.

[225] *Su Wen* (66), Chapter 19, p. 130.

[226] *Su Wen* (28), p. 130.

[227] This text has been mentioned, in the discussion of viral hepatitis, as a model of the penetration of perverse wind and of its evolution in the body which creates pre-jaundice symptoms, those of jaundice itself and of the complications. The

wind was associated with heat. The same mechanism applies for cold wind, but then the symptoms are different.

[228] Leung Kwok Po (38), p. 28.

[229] Zong jin is the muscle that "governs the cohesion of the bones and the articulations." It is the energy of dai mai that holds it. It seems to correspond to the psoas muscles (iliac), to the pelvic belt, to the hernial orifices and to the abdominal wall.

[230] *Su Wen* (28), Chapter 44, p. 203.

[231] See etymology of frigidity in Gynecology, Shao Yin.

[232] Pernice (73), p. 167.

[233] *Da Cheng* (7), p. 577.

[234] *Ibid.*, p. 588. This mentions "all post-partum affections; precious point in difficult deliveries."

[235] This partly covers the Shao Yin dysmenorrheas (see Shao Yin).

[236] See zulinqi (GB-41) and Pneumonia and Tuberculosis, Shao Yang.

[237] See sun xie, seasonal diarrhea, *Su Wen* (28), p. 79 & 119.

[238] See Acne, Tai Yin.

[239] See Epistaxis in Jue Yin, Yang Ming.

[240] Chamfrault (9), p. 238.

[241] Nguyen-Recours (57), p. 131-132.

[242] Menetrier (46), p. 92.

[243] As Menetrier comments about dystonic (manganese-cobalt) patients, and as we commonly see in practice regarding female Jue Yin and Shao Yang patients, these are the patients who most often present premenopause malaises. These are the temperaments for whom the menopause transition is the most difficult.

[244] *Da Cheng* (7), p. 582.

[245] Wood represents the muscles, muscular contraction.

[246] Chamfrault (7), p. 582.

[247] For details, Leung Kwok Po (38), p. 28-29.

[248] Eczema is a stagnation of the energy of the blood in the skin. (See Dermatology, below.)

[249] *Ling Shu* (8), Chapter 10, p. 376.

[250] Leung Kwok Po (38), p. 20.

[251] Wood indicates muscles.

252 Leung Kwok Po (38), p. 20.

253 Soulie de Morant (107), p. 891.

254 *Ibid.*

255 *Ibid.*

256 *Da Cheng* (7), p. 897.

257 *Ibid.*

258 This point is indicated by the Shanghai authors in treating impotence.

259 Qichong (ST-30) is the middle point of the zong jin (chief muscle), which we have mentioned above. It is indicated in the *Da Cheng* (107), p. 891, for "excess of licentiousness," by dispersion.

260 Leung Kwok Po (38), p. 29.

261 Quoted by Soulie de Morant (107), p. 890.

262 Picard (75), p. 145. Here it refers to impotence among the elderly.

263 *Su Wen* (59), Chapter 7, p. 318. Feng jue translates literally as "disease determined by the wind." In his translation, Husson makes the following note: "The breath is suddenly blocked as if by a burst of wind." (28), p. 92.

264 Husson (28), p. 92.

265 Zhang Jing Yao, quoted by Nguyen Van Nghi (66), p. 319.

266 Husson notes, "The failure of Wood gives rise to the dryness of cold. The qi of birth (spring); when not on time, the vegetation will be late."

267 *Su Wen* (8), Chapter 69, p. 268. Husson also speaks of cold-hot affections, ulcers, dermatitis, abscesses and pimples, especially when the Fire comes to avenge Wood (see below, Dermatology and Infectious Pathology).

268 Chondrocalcinosis coincides with diabetes and hypoparathyroid, related to a metabolic failure of Tai Yin (see Diabetes in Tai Yin).

269 *Su Wen* (28), Chapter 10, p. 102.

270 *Su Wen* (8), Chapter 45, p. 206.

271 *Su Wen* (28), Chapter 43, p. 200-201

272 This has already been mentioned in the introduction to Genital Pathology.

273 The physiology of the huang points has been explained by J.M. Kespi, in relation to the pelvic and heart envelopes. J.M. Kespi, "Conference au premier weekend post-universitaire," AFA Paris, 1978.

274 Juliao (GB-29) is indicated here just as we gave it for dysmenorrhea (dark liver) and fibroma (gynecologic shan).

275 *Su Wen* (28), Chapter 55, p. 223.

276 *Ibid.,* Chapter 49, p. 216.

277 The bowstring is the classical aspect of the radial pulse of the liver.

278 *Su Wen* (28), Chapter 41, pp. 193-195.

279 *Ibid.*

280 *Da Cheng* (7), p. 581.

281 D'Omezon (17).

282 Roustan (99), p. 14.

283 *Su Wen* (8), Chapter 5, p. 33.

284 *Ling Shu* (8), Chapter 4, pp. 324-326. The term contractures varies according to the passages: contractures, spasms, jumps, convulsions. The analysis we make of their physiopathology is not limited to spasmophilia but concerns also the muscular disorders of epilepsy, diseases that may involve the liver, as well as those of different neurological diseases such as polio, multiple sclerosis, amyotrophy and metabolic myopathy. To limit muscular pathology to a single affection would be to misinterpret Chinese medicine.

285 *Ling Shu* (8), Chapter 4, pp. 324-326.

286 The closing chapters of the *Ling Shu* give the general laws of the cosmic variations that influence all diseases. See *Ling Shu* (28), Chapter 71, p. 409. In a modern view of the world, we might imagine that these variations would concern the factors of pollution of the environment, just as the Chinese grouped all the factors of imbalance under the term ''perverse energy.''

287 *Ling Shu* (8) Chapter 63, p. 509.

288 *Ibid.*, Chapter 8, p. 347.

289 D'Omezon (17), p. 61.

290 *Ibid.*

291 Perlemuter and Cenac (70).

292 *Ibid.*

293 D'Omezon (17).

294 Among the etiologies of hypoparathyroidism, we will mention the surgical causes, the DiGeorges syndrome, the autoimmunity etiologies and those said to be idiopathic, such as the aftereffects of Basedow treated with Iodine 131. The hemochromatosis etiology will certainly not surprise an acupuncturist. We may also mention, among the etiologies of hypocalcemia, the malabsorption syndromes, notably in cirrhosis, as well as the anticonvulsive drugs (barbiturates and especially phenylhydantoin) that lead us to greater caution in treating Jue Yin epileptic syndromes.

295 *Ling Shu* (8), Chapter 5, p. 335.

296 *Ibid.*, Chapter 10, p. 366.

297 *Su Wen* (66), Chapter 21, p. 360.

298 To be compared to phosphocalcic disorders (conduction).

299 *Ling Shu* (8), Chapter 10, p. 374.

300 *Su Wen* (8), Chapter 65, p. 243.

301 Husson (28), p. 259.

302 D'Omezon (17), p. 61.

303 *Da Cheng* (7), p. 503.

304 Mou Tse Tsao, cited in Chamfrault (9), p. 140.

305 Nguyen Van Nghi translated, "If we are so often anxious."

306 *Su Wen* (28), Chapter 148, p. 148.

307 See Gynecology.

308 This is partly Shao Yang territory.

309 *Su Wen* (8) Chapter 4, p. 26.

310 *Su Wen* (28), Chapter 32, p. 167.

311 *Ibid.*, Chapter 22, p. 143.

312 Precordialgia and hypochondriacal pain.

313 *Su Wen* (66) Chapter 10, p. 89.

314 Zhang Zhi Cong, quoted by Nguyen Van Nghi (66), p. 92.

315 It is not rare, however, to find an association of the two affections (liver and spleen) and in the interrogation we find signs such as compulsive eating, cravings, etc. These signs necessitate the treatment of both meridians and the prescription of zinc-nickel-cobalt for these patients who have often shown an ambivalent temperament at an early age (Jue Yin/Tai Yin). In the same way, if we account for the presence of cold, the associated affection (liver-kidney) is found among patients who show the ambivalent temperament Jue-Yin/Shao Yin — copper-gold-silver (see Gynecology; also Multiple Sclerosis).

316 Nguyen Van Nghi (66), p. 401, adds, "which are the signs of excess."

317 Weak, according to Nguyen Van Nghi.

318 *Su Wen* (28) Chapter 22, p. 143.

319 This term, tian wang, is sometimes translated as irritability, anger, forgetfulness, amnesia, as does Nguyen Van Nghi, who gives the commentary by Wang Bing: "The word 'wang' {forgotten, wandering} was probably introduced into the text by error. The right word was nu, anger." This comment is not necessarily convincing.

320 *Su Wen* (28), Chapter 19, p. 127.

321 See Gastroenterology, control of the liver over the spleen. As this text states further on, ''The qi of maturity (Earth) is unable to do its job, the qi of birth (Wood) is despotic.''

322 This involves the relations between the planet and the excess or the deficiency of the invited element (Wood).

323 *Su Wen* (28), Chapter 69, pp. 278-280.

324 See dysmenorrhea, leukorrhea and headaches caused by cold damp.

325 Mars = Fire = summer.

326 Venus = Metal = autumn. *Su Wen* (28) Chapter 69, pp. 278-280.

327 Perlemuter and Cenac (70).

328 This syndrome is developed in Tai Yang.

329 Excluding multiple sclerosis (see below) and metastasis of visceral cancer (see Apoplexy, Yang Ming).

330 Perlemuter and Cenac (70).

331 For a traditional Chinese semiologist, the sensation of inebriety associated with peripheral dizziness with vestibular hypoexcitability (associated or not with alcohol), is only the chronic aspect of such a sensation felt as if under the influence of alcohol, and betrays the liver as being the imbalanced organ.

332 This is the equivalent of the term tian wang (''forgotten''), to be compared with memory problems.

333 Victor and Adams, quoted in Harrison (26), p. 326.

334 *Ling Shu* (8), Chapter 4, p. 326.

335 The territory of the ear and auditive acuity depend partly on the kidney (see Table I and pathology in Shao Yin), but not exclusively. Vomiting (of vestibular origin, as it is here) excludes the kidney from the picture, indicating that the pathology is related to the liver.

336 An excess of cold, implying Water, enables us to comprehend the mechanism of hyperpression of the fluids in the ear.

337 *Ling Shu* (7), Chapter 24, p. 423.

338 *Da Cheng* (7), p. 506.

Meniere's disease and cold wind or cold humid headaches are similar, and belong to the same etiology, approaching gan bi.

339 Victor and Adams, referenced in Harrison (26), p. 1820.

340 Sal (103), p. 136.

[341] *Yi Xue Ru Men,* quoted by Soulie de Morant (107), p. 710.

[342] There is another possibility of the epileptic syndrome due to "escape of energy" in the case of deficiency of liver (as of any other organ) from profound causes, metabolic or degenerative (see Organic Coma, Yang Ming).

[343] Poskanzer and Adams, referenced in Harrison (26), pp. 1903-1906.

[344] Husson translates, "The vision suddenly fogged with instability of vision, blindness, deafness. . ." (28), p. 102.

[345] *Su Wen* (66), Chapter 10, p. 85.

[346] Lhermitte (39). These are all signs of Jue Yin nature.

[347] Poskanzer and Adams, in Harrison (26), p. 1904.

These would be due to the demyelinization of the subcortical fibers.

[348] As far as urinary symptomology is concerned, the semiological analogy is obvious, and goes beyond the etiological differences in this text, be they infectious or neurological.

[349] The equivalent of meridians, for Husson.

[350] A deficit of blood in the liver may also lead to a drop in visual acuity, in particular to myopia, frequent among Jue Yin subjects (see Ophthalmology, below).

[351] Husson notes, "painful congestion attributed to an accumulation of perverse breath."

[352] Husson notes, "lack of fluidity, comparable to a mixture of snow and water."

[353] Meaning the main acupuncture points: ting, rong, shu, jing, he.

[354] *Su Wen* (28), Chapter 10, p. 101.

[355] Poskanzer and Adams, in Harrison (26).

[356] *Ibid.*

[357] See Shao Yin; the correlations with copper-gold-silver are obvious.

[358] *Ibid.,* p. 1904.

[359] See Hematology at the end of the chapter.

[360] Poskanzer and Adams, in Harrison (26), p. 1904.

[361] This explains the value of the prescription of cerebral phospholipids for demyelinizing diseases like this one, as H. Baruk suggested at the Bichat conference in 1972.

[362] Poskanzer and Adams, in Harrison (26), p. 1903.

[363] *Ibid.*

[364] D.C. Poskanzer. "Epidemiological Evidence for a Viral Etiology for Multiple Sclerosis." pp. 52-63. "Slow, Latent and Temperate Virus Infections." U.S.

Department of Health, Education and Welfare. NINDB. Monograph No. 2, 1965.

[365] Poskanzer and Adams, in Harrison (26), p. 1903.

[366] See Neurology of Tai Yin. See also, Requena (87).

[367] *Ling Shu* (8), Chapter 80, p. 556.

[368] As well as the pelvic deficiency pathologies such as impotence, pollakiuria and incontinence (see Gynecology, Rheumatology and Urology, above).

[369] We find the same symptomology as with "congealed blood in the vessels" mentioned above.

[370] *Su Wen* (28), Chapter 43, p. 202.

[371] See Shao Yin.

[372] *Ling Shu* (8), Chapter 80, p. 556.

[373] Poskanzer and Adams, Harrison (26), p. 1906.

[374] Lhermitte (39), p. 1176.

[375] Perlemuter and Cenac (70).

[376] See remark on this subject in the physiology of Yang Ming.

[377] Heat disperses the wind; see Vascular Accidents, Yang Ming.

[378] *Da Cheng* (7), p. 578.

[379] *Ibid.*

[380] *Ibid.*

[381] Soulie de Morant (107), pp. 447-448.

[382] *Ibid.*

[383] *Su Wen* (28), Chapter 43, p. 204.

[384] As needling this point disperses the blood of the meridian (see Psychiatry, below).

[385] Soulie de Morant (107), p. 451.

[386] Chamfrault (7), pp. 474-583.

[387] *Ibid.*

[388] Soulie de Morant (107), p. 556.

[389] *Su Wen* (28), Chapter 24, p. 148.

[390] Nguyen Van Nghi (66), p. 450.

[391] There is an increase in blood and energy in Jue Yin as the moon waxes, a decrease as it wanes.

[392] *Universal Calendar,* in Nguyen Van Nghi (62), pp. 133-139.

[393] Nguyen Van Nghi. "Mouvements et energies; utilisation des troncs et des branches en medecine." Le mensuel du medecin acupuncteur, no. 38, February 1977, pp. 287-301. The whole technique is taken from the *Nei Jing Su Wen* and the *Nei Jing Ling Shu.*

[394] *Universal Calendar* (62).

[395] 3 a.m. to 5 a.m., China time, corresponds to 4 a.m. to 6 a.m. in the winter, and 5 a.m. to 6 a.m. daylight savings time, in France. (See note in our discussion of cyclic rhythms in the chapter devoted to Shao Yang.)

[396] See Tai Yang.

[397] *Su Wen* (28), Chapter 22, p. 142.

[398] All these laws of chronobiology, whose importance is demonstrated more and more often (even concerning pharmacological effects of medicines), are even more refined when applied to the energy system of acupuncture. The ancient Chinese, we must believe, were able to master these refinements to perfection.

[399] For these two ions, see memory deficit discussion.

[400] Menetrier (46), p. 90.

[401] See Endocrinology, Cardiology, Gynecology, Gastroenterology of Jue Yin, Psychiatry of Shao Yin.

[402] See the introduction in Psychology of the Six Temperaments, for the concept of constitution in Chinese medicine.

[403] *Su Wen* (8), Chapter 62, p. 222.

[404] Also translated as "principle of conscience." The hun is the vegetative soul or visceral qi of the liver.

[405] *Ling Shu* (8), Chapter 8, p. 348.

[406] See Psychiatry of Tai Yang and of Yang Ming.

[407] Perlemuter and Cenac (70), "Alcoolisme aigu."

[408] See Psychiatry of Shao Yang.

[409] Perlemuter and Cenac (70), "Delirium tremens."

[410] See below, dream activity and hun.

[411] Perlemuter and Cenac (70).

[412] *Ibid.*

[413] *Su Wen* (8), Chapter 17, p. 70. Husson translates this as "overabundance of both," and "dreams that people kill each other." (28), p. 117.

[414] See Neurology of Shao Yin.

[415] Perlemuter and Cenac (70).

[416] Chamfrault translates this succinctly as "madness."

[417] *Ling Shu* (8), Chapter 22, p. 411.

[418] Nguyen Van Nghi (58), pp. 11-21.

[419] *Ling Shu* (8), Chapter 22, p. 412.

[420] Nguyen Van Nghi (58), p. 16.

[421] See Psychiatry of Tai Yang.

[422] *Su Wen* (8), Chapter 62, p. 224.

[423] See deficiency of liver and intense asthenia, in the discussion of gynecology.

[424] This would also be the case in Korsakoff's syndrome, where the anatomopathological study shows that the mamillary tubercle and the postgemina are affected.

[425] In the physiology of the blood, of the psyche and of the arteries, the element Fire, to which these three sectors correspond (especially the heart, with its pericardial envelope), is incontestably active, notably in memory disorders. This is confirmed by the indications of the tongli (HT-5), shaohai (HT-3), etc. (see Shao Yin). These statements do not contradict, but complement, each other.

[426] Quoted by Soulie de Morant (107), p. 633.

[427] See Ophthalmology, below.

[428] See the expressions mentioned at the beginning of the chapter, "to have heart in the guts" and "to have the livers."

[429] *Su Wen* (8), Chapter 5, p. 33.

[430] The precise correspondences between Chinese medicine and the Taoist philosophy imply a memory other than the genetic memory, one that is related to yuan qi, a memory programmed before conception. Husson translates, "In heaven, the East is the mysterious obscurity, xuan, before the light of day (anterior heaven)."

[431] *Da Cheng* (7), p. 446.

[432] To compare with Barlow's disease, seen above in Cardiology.

[433] Shanghai (105).

[434] Soulie de Morant (107), p. 633.

[435] Chamfrault (7), p. 598.

[436] Terms according to which Rubin translates yanggang (BL-43) precisely (101), p. 150.

[437] See Physiology of the Gallbladder in Shao Yang.

[438] *Da Cheng* (7), p. 447.

439 *Ibid.*

440 Menetrier (46), p. 108.

441 Only the Yin form is described here, which survives among Jue Yin subjects belonging to the Fire Minister. Yang form is discussed in Tai Yang.

442 Perlemuter and Cenac (70), "La nevrose hysterique."

443 See Tai Yang.

444 Soulie de Morant (107), p. 750. Feng tian signals cerebrovascular accident and other yang excess etiologies.

445 *Su Wen* (8), Chapter 62, p. 221. See analysis of psyche and shen in Shao Yin.

446 *Ling Shu* (8), Chapter 10, p. 366.

447 *Ibid.*, Chapter 24, p. 420.

448 Soulie de Morant (107), p. 750

449 The semiology of the *Da Cheng* for ximen (HT-4) is, "Convulsions, fear, sadness, groaning, sudden atony of the tongue, suddenly mute." (7), p. 388.

450 Chamfrault (7), pp. 388-503.

451 Soulie de Morant (107), p. 483.

452 Translation by Rubin (101). The character for "space" is to be understood as an interval. Its second name, erbai, is translated by Shanghai (105) as "space or interval of the 100."

453 Soulie de Morant, Chamfrault, Shanghai.

454 We may compare this to the hypersensitive and receptive behavior of the pithias at Delphi, who lent their name to hysterical people whom we call pithiatic.

455 Soulie de Morant (107) and Chamfrault (7).

456 Chamfrault (7), p. 388.

457 Renzhong (GV-26), gui (ghost) point; lieque (LU-7), luo point of shou tai yin; and yangxi (LI-5), jing point of shou yang ming, have precise psychiatric indications discussed in Tai Yang and Tai Yin.

458 *Encyclopedia Universalis* (113), p. 768.

459 Hysteria in Greek: hustera means uterus.

460 Roustan (99), p. 19.

461 *Ibid.*

462 See Physiology of Yang Ming and Tai Yin.

463 See Rheumatology, Dermatology, Hematology in Tai Yin.

[464] *Ling Shu* (8), Chapter 52, p. 488.

[465] *Su Wen* (28), Chapter 42, p. 197.

[466] Norman, referenced in Harrison (26), p. 387.

[467] *Su Wen* (8), Chapter 62, p. 224.

[468] *Ibid.*

[469] Soulie de Morant (107), pp. 937-938.

[470] *Ibid.*

[471] *Ibid.*

[472] *Ibid.*, p. 451.

[473] Quoted by Chamfrault (7), p. 927.

[474] *Ibid.*, p. 503.

[475] See below, pathology of the scalp.

[476] Menetrier (46), p. 83.

[477] *Ibid.*

[478] Chamfrault (7), p. 504.

[479] Menetrier (46), p. 85.

[480] There is, however, a Shao Yin aspect that we frequently find, and that we must not underestimate.

[481] See Ophthalmology below and Infectious Pathology in Shao Yang.

[482] *Su Wen* (28), Chapter 2, p. 74.

[483] This is associated with GV-23, SP-4 and LI-11.

[484] Quoted by Chamfrault (7), p. 609.

[485] Chamfrault (7), p. 611; Soulie de Morant (107), p. 645.

[486] *Su Wen* (28), Chapter 17, p. 119.

[487] *Ibid.*, Chapter 69, p. 280. If the wind is insufficient, the dryness-cold triumphs (Metal triumphs over Wood, which is deficient) then the son comes to the rescue: heat triumphs over the dryness-cold (Fire controls Metal).

[488] *Ibid.*, Chapter 42, p. 197.

[489] *Ibid.*, Chapter 17, p. 119. Other passages in the *Su Wen* do evoke these two etiologies, translated as such by Husson.

[490] *Ibid.*, Chapter 42, pp. 197-198.

[491] *Ibid.*

[492] *Su Wen* (8), Chapter 58, p. 204.

[493] *Su Wen* (28), p. 229.

[494] The larynx again (''throat'' in the Jue Yin imbalance, see hyperthyroidism in Shao Yang).

[495] Shepard, referenced in Harrison (26), pp. 908-911. See also, Perlemuter and Cenac (70), ''La lepre.''

[496] Geshu (BL-17), hui of the blood, is indicated for ''cold abscess'' in the *Da Cheng*.

[497] Chamfrault (7), pp. 387-499 and 503-504.

[498] *Ibid.*

[499] *Ibid.*

[500] *Ibid.*, p. 503.

[501] Asthenia, headaches and especially articular pain are signs of Jue Yin disorder.

[502] *Ling Shu* (8), Chapter 10, p. 370-372.

[503] Compare this to Qi Bo's remark, ''When the celestial presidency returns to Jue Yin, the predominance of the guest buzzing in the ears, dizziness, a fall; the predominance of the master gives pain in the chest, difficulty speaking because of the tongue.'' *Su Wen* (28), Chapter 74, p. 347.

[504] These pains are probably accessible to acupuncture because one of the treatments consists in local anesthesia at the painful spot.

[505] Small intestine (Tai Yang) and heart (Shao Yin) make up the Imperial Fire and are closely linked to cardiovascular pathology (see Tai Yang and Shao Yin).

[506] *Su Wen* (28), Chapter 49, p. 216.

[507] That the tongue is affected here indicates its link with the peribuccal cephalic branch. This is why it was logical to find lichen planus localized in the tongue, with its motor difficulties, in syphilis. The tongue is not, then, the exclusive territory of Shao Yin (heart) and Tai Yin (spleen).

[508] *Su Wen* (28), Chapter 16, p. 114.

[509] The xing corresponds to the individual mixture of jing of the viscera and is visible in the sparkle of the eye, in the pupil, which is black. The pupil and its sparkle correspond to the kidney, the storage house of jing qi, which is produced throughout the body. This allows us to identify the sing with the jing, which is visible in the jing ming, as we said in the introduction.

[510] *Da Cheng* (107), p. 762.

[511] *Ling Shu* (8), Chapter 80, p. 556.

[512] The exact color of Wood is blue-green. This is why we sometimes find one, sometimes the other, or both, to define the element.

[513] *Su Wen* (28), Chapter 10, p. 103.

[514] Nguyen Van Nghi (69), p. 97.

[515] *Ibid.*

[516] *Ling Shu* (66), Chapter 74, p. 97.

[517] Soulie de Morant (107), p. 762.

[518] *Su Wen* (28), Chapter 10, p. 101.

[519] *Su Wen* (8), p. 51.

[520] *Ibid.*, Chapter 22, p. 100.

[521] See Ophthalmology of Shao Yang.

[522] *Da Cheng* (107), p. 762.

[523] Chamfrault (7), p. 583.

[524] Shanghai (105).

[525] Chamfrault (7), p. 536.

[526] The hen, or the chicken, is the animal of the element Wood. Tong Fun says, "the mode of treatment of renowned physicians," quoted by Chamfrault (7), p. 804.

[527] Chamfrault (7), p. 353. See Presbyopia in Tai Yin.

[528] Shanghai (105).

[529] *Ibid.*

[530] Although this syndrome is not strictly speaking infectious, it is a collagenosis (connectivitis).

[531] Requena (91).

[532] Menetrier (46), p. 103.

[533] Chamfrault (7), pp. 503-510.

[534] Soulie de Morant (107), p. 580.

[535] *Ibid.*, p. 645.

[536] *Ibid.*

[537] *Ibid.*

[538] *Ibid.*

[539] Except for suppurative parenchymatous keratitis, a rare form that is nonetheless very serious, and one that usually leads to a septic necrosis of the cornea and to the loss of the eye. In this case the energy is perverse heat or Fire. As an adjuvant treatment, we may try needling the shu and he points of Jue Yin and of Shao Yin.

[540] Menetrier (46), p. 103.

[541] See hyperthyroidism.

[542] See Ophthalmology in Yang Ming.

[543] Soulie de Morant (107), p. 762.

[544] However, the temperament may also be Shao Yin and Tai Yang and is worth meticulous analysis.

[545] See ORL in Yang Ming.

[546] See Shao Yang.

[547] It goes without saying that we are not interested in expanding on congenital glaucoma with megalocornea, whose origin is often genetic and whose sanction is surgical.

[548] See Physiology of Body Fluids in Shao Yang and Tai Yang.

[549] Here the dialectic Yin—Yang opposes the energies jing and rong, as we have seen concerning the physiology of the curious bowels linked to the Earth in Shao Yang.

[550] *Ling Shu* (8) Chapter 28, p. 433. See also, *Ling Shu,* trans. Nguyen Van Nghi, ''Le mensuel du medecin acupuncteur,'' No. 52, juin 1978, p. 52.

[551] The shu point, ''transport to offer.''

[552] Experiment mentioned by Nguyen Van Nghi *et.al.* (65), p. 687.

[553] Hamburger *et.al.* (24).

[554] BL-62, BL-63, GB-1, GB-8, M-HN-9 are included in the Shanghai treatment with qiuhou (M-HN-8). Shanghai (105).

[555] Chamfrault (7), p. 539.

[556] *Ling Shu* (8), Chapter 28, p. 433.

[557] *Da Cheng,* (7), p. 399.

[558] Shanghai (105), ''Le glaucome.''

[559] Perlemuter and Cenac (70), ''Glaucome primitif chronique de l'adulte.''

[560] *Ibid.*

[561] Hamburger *et.al.* (24), p. 1025.

[562] Soulie de Morant (107), p. 445.

[563] Chamfrault (7), p. 497, 500-501, 577-578.

[564] *Ibid.*

[565] *Ibid.*

566 *Ibid.*

567 For shangxing (GV-23), refer to treatment of keratitis, above.

568 See Cardiovascular Pathology in Jue Yin.

569 *Su Wen* (28), Chapter 67, p. 267.

570 Husson (28), p. 120, translates chronic as ancient.

571 *Su Wen* (66), Chapter 17, p. 244.

572 Husson translates these terms as ''wound without hemorrhage'' (ecchymosis) (28), p. 120. We think we may also say hematoma.

573 *Su Wen* (66), Chapter 17, pp. 244-245.

574 *Ibid.*

575 This might be expressed in modern terms as hemoperitoneum, or it might represent portal hypertension as a result of a presinusoidal blockage whose origin is traumatic.

576 *Su Wen* (66), Chapter 17, p. 236.

577 *Ling Shu* (8), Chapter 4, p. 321.

578 This is what makes Nguyen Van Nghi say, ''The demolition of the energy is caused not only by psychic causes but also by external elements (contusions).''

579 Chamfrault (7), p. 428.

580 See Tai Yin.

581 Soulie de Morant (107), p. 451.

582 Chamfrault (7), p. 583.

583 *Su Wen* (8), Chapter 62, p. 222.

584 *Ibid.*

585 Remember the opposite mechanism, behind multiple sclerosis.

586 This is what is called *de chi* (choose the moment). Husson (28), p. 152.

587 *Su Wen* (66), Chapter 26, pp. 473-474.

588 *Su Wen* (28), Chapter 49, p. 216.

589 *Su Wen* (8), Chapter 66, p. 250.

590 *Su Wen* (28), Chapter 7, p. 91. p. 91.

591 *Ling Shu* (8), Chapter 41, p. 459.

Yang Ming

Physiology of Yang Ming

Gastric Functions

• Gastric Secretions

We commonly define the two phases of gastric secretion as the cephalic phase and the gastric phase. The cephalic phase involves the direct vagal stimulation of the fundic cells, eliciting the secretion of gastric fluids rich in pepsin. There is also an indirect production of antral gastrin and the production of gastrin and histamine. Indirect constituents facilitate these secretions, as do the cholinergic reflexes linked to the distension of the fundus and the presence of alkaline solutes.

All these factors are dependent on the cholinergic nerves. The neurohumoral relationships are the key to the mechanics of gastric secretion. The physiological data from modern research allow us to establish the following relationships:

> 1) There are oxyntic cells that secrete HCl and are particularly concentrated in the mucosa of the fundus.

> 2) There are gastrin secreting cells particularly concentrated in the antrum.

The secretion of HCl from the oxyntic cells depends exclusively on the liberation of histamine by the mastocytes in the fundic mucosa. These mastocytes liberate histamine upon reception of two sorts of messages and therefore possess two types of receptors for these different messages: a cholinergic receptor and a gastrin receptor. In normal circumstances when the secretion of HCl by the fundus is sufficient, the secretion of gastrin in the antral cells is inhibited.

There are, therefore, two stages of the secretion of HCl by the oxyntic cells, with two sorts of messages (Figure 10). The first stage concerns the mastocyte. The cholinergic message may be inhibited by anticholinergic substances, such as atropine, or by vagotomy. The gastric message may also be inhibited by substances antagonistic to gastrin such as proglumide.

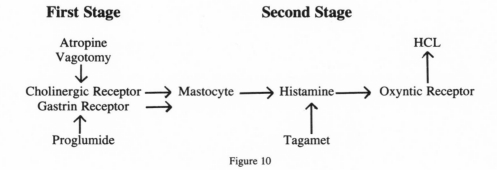

Figure 10

The second stage involves the action of the histamine on the appropriate receptors of the oxyntic cell, which may be inhibited by antihistamines, such as Tagamet.[1]

We might add that the antral cells in the stomach are not alone in secreting gastrin. There are also gastrin secreting cells in the endocrine pancreas. This is why, in Zollinger-Ellison's syndrome, a tumor in the endocrine pancreas causes multiple ulcers in the stomach. Gastrin does many things:

— Stimulates acidic and peptic secretion in the stomach;

— Stimulates gastric and intestinal motility;

— Increases the tonus of the esophageal sphincter;

— Increases the hepatic bile production, as well as the pancreatic volume and enzyme concentration;[2]

— Increases the production of the intrinsic factor that facilitates the absorption of vitamin B12.

The small intestine is active in the inhibition of gastric secretion (via entero-gastrone), as we may observe in resections of the small intestine that lead to gastric hypersecretion. Under normal conditions the gastric mucosa is remarkably resistant to aggression. Autodigestion is avoided by the production of mucus by the epithelial cells. Mucus has the notable property of absorbing pepsin. Cortisone and aspirin cause qualitative changes in the mucus that facilitate its breakdown by the pepsin. They also diminish the flow of mucus. The small intestine protects itself against the acidity of the gastric chyme by the production (in the duodenal Brunner's glands) of an alkaloid mucoid secretion that acts as a buffer.

In Chinese medicine, the role of the stomach and the pancreas (spleen-pancreas) in the assimilation of the energy of the nutrients and the flavors is fundamental:

The spleen-pancreas and the stomach are the granaries, the depositories of food.[3]

Husson translates this passage as:

The spleen and the stomach are the officials in charge of food storage and from whom the five flavors are derived.[4]

Nguyen Van Nghi translates this as follows:

The spleen and stomach are providers and constitute the source of the five flavors.[5]

The difference between the Chinese view and Western notions of digestion is that in acupuncture there are specific networks. The spleen (zu tai yin) and the stomach (zu yang ming) meridians form a network with the secondary channels, the internal channels and the great luo channels, all of which are active in the direct distribution of the assimilated energy (rong qi and wei qi) into the anastomotic circuit of the primary channels (jing luo). While the alimentary bolus continues on its way down the anatomical pathway, it goes through other energy extractions. This happens in various organs that either circulate the energy

310

through their own meridians or pass it to other organs and meridians with which they maintain anastomoses (see Shao Yang, Shao Yin).

• Gastric Motility

Studies of gastric electrical activity have shown there is a veritable "pacemaker" in the cardia that produces peristaltic waves. These are propagated as far as the antrum, which contracts upon their arrival. In Chinese medicine, the production of nutritious alimentary energy, as well as its circulation, depends on the great luo channel of the stomach, xu li. The cardia is located very near the dwelling of zong qi, the ancestral energy. According to the *Su Wen,* the beating of xu li drives this circulation and overlaps the arterial circulation.[6] We may note that the etymology of cardia and cardiac is the same, coming from the Greek, *cardiakos,* and from the Latin, *cardia,* meaning heart. There are then two automatisms: an automatic cardiac reflex and gastric peristalsis. Each functions in much the same way and is located in the thoracoabdominal region between the cardiac plexus, above, and the cardia, below. That these two automatisms are controlled by xu li and by the energy zong qi greatly contributes to the explanation of the Yang Ming subjects' cardiovascular pathology. The projection point of this privileged zone is, of course, the he point of the energy, the dwelling of zong qi, shanzhong (CV-17).

• Physiology of the Colon

The terminal portion of the digestive tube, the colon, is about 1.20 meters long and secretes very little mucus. Its main activity is the active transfer of sodium, which induces the osmotic reabsorption of water and the dehydration of the matter contained within the colon.[7] It may also absorb certain salts and certain nutritive substances (about 10) that have not been absorbed in the preceding stages of digestion.[8] Bacterial fermentation helps to break down the glucides. About one half of the cellulose can be absorbed. Because of the action of the bacteria, there is also putrefaction as the proteins are attacked, with the production of ammonia. The reduction of the bile into urobilinogen and stercobilin allows its passage and reintegration into the enterohepatic cycle. Certain vitamins produced by the bacteria are absorbed and can play a non-negligible role in cases of vitamin deficiency.[9]

In Chinese medicine, the role of the colon is defined in the *Su Wen:*

The colon transforms.[10]

Nguyen Van Nghi translates this more precisely:

The large intestine has a transit function, but also participates in the transformations.[11]

The relationships established in acupuncture between the large intestine and its coupled organ (the lung) within the element Metal attributes to this viscera and to its meridian an original physiological role in the circulation of the blood and energy. This is in accord with the Yang Ming bowel, the stomach, which we will now examine.

Physiological Relationships Between Yang Ming and Wei Qi

• Connection with the Capillary Microcirculation

Immunological studies have shown the existence of a circulating gastrin with a high molecular weight. Its functional and physiological purpose, however, remains unexplained. In the Chinese texts, we may read:

> The defensive energy (wei qi) comes from the inferior burner.[12]

The inferior burner is located in the region of the pylorus, at the point xiawan (CV-10).[13] As we have seen in the introduction, wei qi is the fierce defensive energy:

> The energy comes from the stomach and from there passes to the lungs to feed the five organs and the six bowels. Pure energy is called rong qi, impure energy is called wei qi. Rong qi flows within the meridians and wei qi flows outside of the meridians.[14]

Thus, there is a circulation of wei qi outside of the meridians and great vessels of the arterial trunks. Its defensive role is incontestable:

> The errant energy that does not follow the meridians is known as the defensive energy, wei qi.

Other passages of this text indicate that wei qi circulates within the flesh and in the tiny capillaries.

This is the terrain on which, according to the ancient Chinese, the conflict between the perverse energy (xie) and the defensive energy (wei qi) takes place:

> When a patient is affected by perverse energy, it is always the defensive energy wei qi that is first to be affected, and the perverse energy almost always lodges in the tiny capillaries. If you disperse them and bleed them, you will always do well.[15]

From the standpoint of immunology, we now understand very well the meaning of this therapeutic technique, although we might wonder what inspired the ancient Chinese to do such a thing. We know that in cases of aggressions, vasodilation is for the most part the result of a concentration of mastocytes and the liberation of histamine and various kinins. These are the origin of the activity of the leucocytes and the macrophages. The piercing of the capillary endothelium by way of the brutal bleeding needle (trocar) naturally intensifies the defense reaction.

There is also an important clinical observation. We notice in examining Yang Ming and certain Tai Yin-Earth patients that their capillary circulation is often altered. This is manifested by a marbled network over the whole surface of the body, most often in the face and in the legs, where the skin takes on a pinkish, pearled aspect. We might wonder what physiological connection might exist among Yang Ming subjects between this capillary vulnerability and their vascular morbidity. Yang Ming is determined by a physiological tendency toward excess of the stomach — the circulating gastrin — certain effects of which are related to the liberation of histamine by the mastocytes and may explain this connection.

This is a hypothesis that might serve to orient fundamental research where the action of acupuncture could prove very useful.

• Connections with the Encephalon

Recent neurobiochemical research has astonishingly revealed the presence of gastrin in cerebral tissue, establishing still other connections between gastrin and wei qi. We quote Qi Bo:

> The energy of the stomach, after passing through the lungs, assails the head. It is a violent, fierce, warlike energy. It passes to the eyes, to wind up in the brain (like a spring), passes back to the face, following the meridian zu yang ming from the lower jawbone, and passes to the point renying {ST-9}.[16]

Notice the clear link between wei qi, cerebral circulation, regulation of the arterial pressure and the cerebral flow rate.[17]

• Connections with the Main Blood Vessels

Yang Ming's most fundamental connection is certainly with the primary blood vessels, the trunks and big arterial axes:

> The earth is moistened by the water from heaven; the five organs and the six bowels are moistened in the same way by the organic fluids. The heaven is Yang, the earth is Yin. The upper part of the body is Yang, the lower part Yin. There is Yin and supreme Yin: Tai Yin; Yang and supreme Yang: Tai Yang. There is also Yin within Yang and Yang within Yin.

> To apply these concepts to man, we must remember that zu yang ming {the stomach} is the sea of the five organs and the six bowels. The arteries that are in its pathway are big and are full of blood. Its heat is strong; its energy always full. If we needle this meridian to disperse it, we must insert the needle deeply and leave it in place for a long time.[18]

We may thus understand the comment in the *Su Wen:*

> We must needle Yang Ming whenever we want to disperse the energy and the blood.[19]

In Chinese medicine, the stomach assimilates the nutrients and transforms them into energy and blood with the aid of the colon. Yang Ming makes the energy and blood flow. Here, wei qi comes into the picture, this time entering the meridians, or the arteries, which are in some ways indistinguishable.

On one hand, the texts say that wei qi flows specifically through the transverse luo (secondary channels), which are likened to the capillaries.[20] On the other hand, they indicate that the pulse is largely due to the energy of the stomach, more exactly, to wei qi:

> In a healthy subject, the "breath" is continually nourished by the stomach. The emanation of the stomach {wei qi} is a constituent

> element {two thirds} of the ''breath'' of the subject. One who has no wei qi is in disorder (ni), which is fatal.
>
> In the springtime {the pulse that has} wei qi is slightly like a rope in the healthy subject. If it is more like a rope than {soft, due to the presence of} wei qi, this means that his liver is ill. If it is vibrant with no softness, it is fatal. . . [21]

The other third represents the specific energy of the organs, radially palpable in their respective place at the wrist and measured qualitatively with the flesh of the finger. The anatomical and physiological connections between the blood vessels and Yang Ming are substantial and deserve attention. It was said that two thirds of wei qi corresponds to the basic arterial tone. Once more, we may wonder about the role of the circulating gastrin and of all the molecules involved in arteriolar motoricity.

In practice, the relationships between Yang Ming and the physiology of the blood are an important part of diagnosis. They include observation of the capillaries, the radial pulses, the specific peripheral pulses and the pulse of Yang Ming:

> The energy and blood that circulate within the arteries and the meridians are brought, by the energy created by the stomach, to the meridian shou tai yin{lung} in the radial groove. [22]
>
> But the energy and the blood of the five organs that circulate within the body, outside of the arteries and meridians, is also brought by the energy created by the stomach, not to the radial groove, but in the tiny capillaries of the meridian shou yang ming {large intestine} under the arm, in the space that we have called the one-meter pond. [23] There is always a correlation between the quality of the pulse {of the meridian shou tai yin} and the quality of the skin at the one-meter pond (fish belly). [24] Thus when the arteries of the radial pulse are tense, the skin of the one-meter pond is equally tense. If the beating of the pulse is slow and soft, the skin is lax and soft. This may be true to such an extent that, for an expert acupuncturist, it is enough to examine the skin of the one-meter pond without even taking the pulse. [25]

This paragraph of the *Ling Shu* sheds light on the physiology and the circulation of Yang Ming as well as on its diagnostic consequences.

In some European works on acupuncture, too much emphasis has been placed on taking pulses. This is the most delicate and subjective factor of the Chinese diagnosis. The observation of complexion and of the quality of the skin is a much more objective diagnosis and was valued just as highly by the ancient Chinese authors.

In the chapter on ''Pulses and Illnesses,'' Huang Di asked:

> ''I would like to be able to establish a diagnosis by examining only the one-meter pond, without taking the pulse or looking at the complexion of the patient. Is that possible?''
>
> Qi Bo replied, ''Yes, it is partly possible, however you must all the same examine the pulse of the 'foot' at the wrists and see if it is slow

314

or rapid, small or ample, sliding or raspy; we always find a correspondence between the qualities found in the pulse and the state of the skin at the one-meter pond.

If the pulse is frequent and tense, the skin will seem tense. If the pulse is slow, the skin will seem relaxed. If the pulse is ample, the skin will seem swollen. If it is little, it will be lax. If it is sliding, the skin will be equally sliding. If it is raspy, the finger will feel as if it passes over sandpaper.

If the skin of the one-meter pond is slippery and moist, or slightly greasy, the patient is affected by feng. If it is rough or raspy, he is affected by feng-wei.[26]

The subtleties of the qualities of the skin are naturally difficult to distinguish, but a good acupuncturist who is used to observing this region is supposedly no longer in need of taking the patient's pulse, and doesn't even have to observe his complexion. The best formula, however, is to practice the three examinations: the pulse, the complexion and the physical symptoms. The pulse, complexion and symptoms are parts of an inseparable whole. They are associated as is the echo to the voice, the root to the leaf. We cannot imagine the one without the other.''[27]

The circulation of the blood and the body's energy comes from the stomach. It rises through the meridians and the arteries, taking the pathway of Tai Yin (lung), and goes through the flesh and the tiny capillaries by the pathway of Yang Ming, then spreads throughout the body. The state of the energy and of the blood depends on the force, the vigor and the power of assimilation of the stomach. This is reflected in the one-meter pond, which shows us the state of the capillary circulation. It is visible in the radial pulse, which reflects the state of the circulation of the blood and the energy within the meridians and the arteries.

The radial pulse is directly proportional to the vigor of the stomach. Qi Bo says this in another way:

The energy that we feel in a healthy man's pulse corresponds to the energy of the stomach. If this stomach energy is lacking, it is a sign of gravity, which may lead to death.[28]

The characteristics of each organ's pulse that have been discussed in the chapters devoted to the pathology of Tai Yin, Shao Yin and Jue Yin (and that involve the lung, the spleen and the heart, the kidney and the liver, respectively), depend, in part, on the stomach. This is why, when we take each organ's pulse, we feel the modulation of the organ pulse against a background of the energy of the stomach. Let us give an example:

When the pulse of the lungs appears and its waves, its pulsations, are calmer, the pulse is light; but if we perceive the energy of the stomach, the pulse is normal. If it seems to be too light, like the down of a hen, if it no longer feels elastic, if it does not go up and down, if it no longer undulates, this means that the lungs are affected.

315

If it seems extremely light, like something floating in the air and that the wind will take away, it means death; it is the end of the lungs.[29]

This means there is no more stomach energy, thus no more ancestral energy, and death is imminent. As Qi Bo said, "A pulse that contains no stomach energy is called Yin-organ. The strictly Yin pulse indicates complete exhaustion of the stomach energy, which means death."[30] This state of major deficiency seems to correspond, considering all that has been said, to circulatory arrest. The total exhaustion of zong qi corresponds to the end of the beating of xu li, or cardiac arrest, which had been for ages the sign of death prior to the advent of modern reanimation techniques.

The Yang Ming pulse is described as follows:

> When Yang Ming is visible in the pulse, it is superficial, ample and short. In this case, the energy of the stomach is good.[31]

The *Su Wen* goes on to describe an excess of the Yang Ming pulse:

> If the pulse of Yang Ming is the dominant pulse, this is a sign of an excess of Yang energy. We must disperse the Yang and tonify the Yin by needling the shu points in the lower limbs.[32]

Therefore, an excess of Yang Ming energy is pathological. We may infer that this corresponds, at least partly, to high blood pressure. There is another way of taking pulses. This method considers that the right radial pulse[33] reflects all the Yin meridians (Tai Yin, Shao Yin, Jue Yin) and that the Yang meridians are felt on the artery that passes over the stomach meridian, the carotid, at the point renying (ST-9). To this effect we may quote Qi Bo:

> The three Yang are to be found in the head; the three Yin in the hand. In spite of this distinction, they are one.[34]

The commentary by Zhang Jing Yao maintains:

> Renying {ST-9} is located on the external carotid, one and a half distances from the Adam's apple. It is also called the three Yang of the head.[35]

There is no possible confusion. He continues:

> According to the *Nei Jing Su Wen,* the five flavors are kept in the stomach to maintain the energy of the five organs. The energies appear at the mouth of energy {qi hao, right radial pulse}. Here we may determine the states of excess or of deficiency of the three Yin meridians.[36]

These considerations partially illuminate Chinese pathology and dispel our doubts about the complexity of diagnosis based on the pulse.

Elsewhere, we may read that ren ying (the radial pulse in the left wrist) explores the Yang energy in general, the energy of the three Yang.[37] Therefore, it must be of semiological value comparable to renying (ST-9), necessitating the taking of peripheral or specific pulses. For the stomach, however, there are two peripheral pulses: renying (ST-9) and chongyang (ST-42).[38] Chongyang (ST-42) means the ''assault of Yang.'' Apart from the lung meridian, which receives the energy of the stomach and passes it on to the other meridians, as its origin lies in the conception vessel points (CV-12, CV-10, CV-13), what are the other pathways of the stomach energy? Let us follow the stomach meridian, shou yang ming. At the internal canthus of the eye, where the anastomosis of the large intestine meridian (zu yang ming) and the stomach meridian are located, the external descending pathway of the stomach meridian begins to descend to the clavicle, quepen (ST-12). Here it splits and follows two pathways, one internal and one external. The external channel passes over the thorax to the mamilla, then follows the external edge of the rectus abdominis muscle as far as qichong (ST-30). As the *Ling Shu* says:

> A secondary channel descends in a straight line from the clavicle straight to the mamilla, passes next to the navel and stops at the point qichong {ST-30}.[39]

The internal channel descends from quepen directly to the stomach and to the spleen.

> Another secondary channel begins at the stomach, inside the abdomen, goes to qichong {ST-30} and from there descends to the anterolateral side of the thigh, etc.[40]

The Shanghai authors say:

> The external pathway descends as far as qichong and from there penetrates into the false pelvis.[41]

Following the twelve meridian energy cycle, the energy gathered by the lung meridian passes to the large intestine meridian, then to the stomach meridian. From there it follows an external pathway that heads inward, first at quepen (ST-12) (clavicle), and a second time at qichong (ST-30). This explains the phrase, ''The Yang Ming meridian opens inwards.'' The stomach energy may go directly from the viscera through its own internal pathway to the point qichong (ST-30) and down the leg through the external pathway. This point, which intersects chong mai, means ''assault of the energy.'' There are thus two different points on the stomach meridian that bear the name ''assault.'' This expresses the idea of energy rising in chongyang and qichong.

Apart from the centrifugal flow of energy from the head to the feet, there is apparently a centripetal flow of energy from the feet to the head. This centripetal flow will be more or less active according to the relative excess of stomach energy. This is confirmed by modern authors:

> We must not consider the energy circulation theory to be absolute. The Yin energy (rong qi) may flow in different directions within a given meridian.[42]

This conforms to the ancient texts, particularly as concerns the stomach:

> The essential role of acupuncture consists in balancing the circulation of the energy. As we have seen, the energy comes partly from the stomach, where it is transformed into wei and rong energies. The

essential energy (yuan qi) comes from chong mai and rises, as does the energy from the stomach, to the upper part of the body.[43]

We read also, "The stomach is the sea of nourishment; the point of diffusion of its energy is the point qichong {ST-30} above, and zusanli {ST-36} below."[44]

This physiological phenomenon is very likely to intensify to the point of creating a pathological circulatory inversion, as is confirmed in the *Ling Shu:*

When we are faced with disturbed energy that rises back up again, we must needle the points located in the hollow of the chest[45] and those located over the artery in the lower part of the stomach meridian.[46]

This may be, as Chamfrault states, qichong (ST-30), located over the femoral artery. It may also be, as we believe, zusanli (ST-36), over the anterior tibial artery, or chongyang (ST-42), the "assault of Yang," the point located over the dorsalis pedis artery. It is by stressing the possibility of an upward circulation of stomach energy that we are able to explain cardiovascular pathology resulting from an imbalance of Yang Ming.

This pathology may occur only when there is an overflow of energy. This is more likely to affect Yang Ming subjects than others, particularly the sanguine subjects (Yang Ming-stomach). Based on the traditional texts, Chamfrault wrote:

The pulse of the dorsalis pedis artery at the point chongyang shows the state of the Yin. That of the Yang is examined on the carotid artery at the point renying {ST-9}.[47]

We have come full circle. This shows that if there is an excess of Yin in the body's energy, the energy descends. At the same time, the pulse in the foot is ample and the carotid pulse normal or weak. If there is an excess of Yang, the energy rises. The carotid pulse is full and the foot pulse weak. Thus, the foot pulse at chongyang has the same semiological value as the right radial pulse (qi hao). The carotid pulse, at renying (ST-9), has the same value as the left radial pulse (renying). The use of the two systems of reference has another advantage that enables us to diagnose a relative excess or deficiency of Yang Ming on either side (unilateral) in order to assess the vascular risk of cerebral thrombosis (hemiplegia) or of peripheral thrombosis (uni- or bilateral arteriopathy).

The semiological value of taking the carotid, femoral and pedis pulses in Chinese medicine is parallel to the diagnostic interests of Western medicine, but immediately implies specific therapeutic action using acupuncture. The choice of points to needle, and particularly the choice of which side of the body to treat ("opposite side" technique), stems directly from this analysis.

Our discussion of the physiology of Yang Ming would be incomplete were we to leave out the point wuli (LI-13):

All the energies and all the bloods {circulating within and outside of the meridians} of the five organs and the six bowels meet around the meridians shou tai yin {lung} and shou yang ming {large intestine}, concentrating at the point wuli {LI-13}, the most important of all the points of the meridians.[48]

This point, three distances above quchi (LI-11, inside the elbow), is located at the angle formed by the humero-stylo-radial vastus internus and brachialis internus muscles. Just beneath lies the deep brachial artery. The Chinese physiological explanation may be inferred from Qi Bo's commentary:

> The beating of the pulse of the foot and of the radial pulse correspond to the energy of the lungs. Wuli {LI-13}, located three distances over the inside of the elbow, and the five organ beishu[49] points are the most important points.

> If there is the slightest disturbance in the energy, we will be able to feel it in the two pulses {radial and foot}. The lungs govern the energies that circulate within the meridians and the large intestine governs the energy and the blood circulating outside the meridians. The point wuli must not be needled more than five times, as the energy we feel in the two feet of the radial pulses comes from this point.[50]

Based on this passage, we may suppose, among other hypotheses, the possible existence of a vasomotor reflex with an effect on the autonomous nervous system, something like the vagal reflex belonging to this privileged zone of the humeral artery.

The importance of the lung (Tai Yin) and of the large intestine (Yang Ming) in the physiology of the circulation of blood and energy must be mentioned. Qi Bo expressed this in the following terms:

> The lungs follow the lead of the large intestine, as it is a transit bowel.[51]

> In the body of man, it is within the meridians and the arteries that energy and blood flow.

> With acupuncture, we may tonify them or disperse them; we may bring energy, or we may strengthen it after its passage. But there is one very important notion that we must not forget, which is that we must not needle the point wuli {LI-13} more than five times, for it is the point in which is concentrated the most energy. If we needle more than five times, we won't kill the patient immediately, but we will harm his vitality.[52]

The large intestine, a bowel of transformation and of transit, is in accord with the lungs on the one hand,[53] and the stomach on the other. With these it makes the unit pair meridian Yang Ming in order to put energy and blood into circulation. Thus, the large intestine is a link between two opposites: Tai Yin, opening outward, and Yang Ming, closing inward. However:

> All the energies, the blood, the Yang and the Yin of the organs and bowels pass through the lung and stomach meridians to rise to the upper part of the body or to descend to the lower part, to go outwards from the body or to go inwards into the body, exactly like the energy of the heavens that flows everywhere. Of all the meridians, these two are the most important.[54]

319

Perhaps we understand why Yang Ming subjects, whose temperament is favorable towards the circulation of blood and energy, are as Xia Se describes them:

> They are easy to treat. If they show signs of excess, we disperse them. If they show signs of deficiency, we tonify them. With them, we must needle the jing points.

A universal treatment for energy imbalance, no matter what the temperament of the patient, but particularly for Yang Ming patients, is needling the famous associated points, hegu (LI-4) and zusanli (ST-36). Hegu (LI-4) is the yuan point of the large intestine meridian and balances the circulation of blood and energy in the meridians and arteries in connection with lieque (LU-7), luo point of the lung. It balances the energies outside of the meridians and arteries because of the specific physiology of the meridian it commands. Zusanli (ST-36) is the he point of the stomach meridian, special action point for the meridian and the viscus itself. As Qi Bo says:

> The he point of the stomach meridian is the point zusanli {ST-36}. All the he points govern the energy circulating within the meridians.[55]

Zusanli, then, regularizes the stomach in its role of production and circulation of energy, as well as its meridian, zu yang ming.

If our discussion of the physiology of Yang Ming seems overly long or complicated, it is because we feel this is necessary to understand the pathologies we will examine. First, it is important to keep in mind that the very close ties between the stomach and wei qi, on the one hand, and between wei qi and the organic fluids, on the other, enables us to explain the frequency of wei qi disturbances and organic fluid disturbances when Yang Ming is imbalanced. These imbalances are more or less related to the kidney. A common denominator in Western physiology may be the carbon anhydrase enzyme, which is present and active in both of these viscera.

Cardiovascular Pathology

Among Yang Ming subjects, it is certainly those who are sanguine, often plethoric, who are most often at risk of cardiovascular difficulty. We find in practice, however, that other Yang Ming subjects, the phlegmatic ones, are almost every bit as exposed. Physiologically, those who are exposed to this pathology do not have balanced Yin and Yang, but rather a tendency towards a stomach excess. When young, they are distinguishable because their skin is rather pale and marbled by capillaries.[56] They eat well and are optimistic. As they get older, these tendencies are accentuated. Their cheeks become red as does their general complexion.

Coronary Disease

Our discussion of the physiology of Yang Ming will enable us to understand the mechanism of the accident described in the *Su Wen:*

> When the upper and lower burners fail to function, the hot energy
> (Yang) from the stomach heats up the chest.[57]

In other words, an excess of production (blood and energy) from the stomach,
coupled with an insufficient circulation among the organs (lung, kidney, liver)
leads to accumulation. This accumulation causes heating. This heat of internal
origin[58] is responsible for coronary disease.

The repercussions of this accumulation will be seen in the annex thoracic
channel, xu li, as well as in the stomach meridian. The energy will flow through
the internal gastro-inguinal pathway to qichong (ST-30).[59] At this point, the
"assault of energy" (the excess of Yang), will spurn the lower limb and rise again
through the abdomen, through the thorax to the head, by way of the stomach meridian, zu yang ming. This ascension of Yang energy is responsible for the sensation felt by the patient at the moment of a heart attack. Within the trunk, the
excess stomach heat passes directly to the thorax by way of xu li. The physiology
of this channel is defined in Chapter 18 of the *Su Wen:*

> The great luo {secondary channel} of the stomach meridian is called
> xu li, the open path.[60] From the stomach it passes to the diaphragm to
> join the lungs, exiting beneath the left breast at the point rugen
> {ST-18}. Its beating may be communicated to the clothing[61] and this
> is how we may examine the ancestral energy (zong qi).
>
> If the beating is very strong, rapid and with strong breathing {as in
> dyspnea} and starts and stops, this is a sign of a disorder of shan-
> zhong {CV-17}.
>
> If the beating has the aspect of a knotted pulse {slow, which stops}
> whose energetic current spreads within the intercostal space, it is a
> sign of an accumulation of energy.[62]

In his study of the great luo of the stomach, Nguyen Van Nghi gives the following symptomology:

> Pain in the epigastrium and in shanzhong {CV-17} with respiratory
> trouble, precordial pains.

Thus, any excess of stomach energy with a circulatory incapacity may cause a
coronary accident and also, I believe, certain rhythm disturbances. In Chinese
physiology, ischemia is portrayed by the terms, "arrest of the circulation of the
blood" and "stagnation and heating up of the blood," as is the case in abdominal
emergencies, a mesenteric infarction, for example.

For therapy, we must follow the advice of the *Ling Shu:*

> If the energy rises back up again, we must needle the points located in
> the hollow of the chest and those located on the artery in the lower
> part of the stomach meridian.[63]

This passage, quoted in our discussion on the physiology of Yang Ming, now
takes on its full meaning. There is now no doubt which points are located on the
arteries. It must be qichong (ST-30) and zusanli (ST-36), the "sea of

321

nourishment'' points, which are capable of orienting the circulation. Qichong (ST-30) is also called qijie, ''street of energy.'' It is indicated in the *Da Cheng* for:

> Energy that rises back upwards in the body, energy that assails the heart, preventing normal breathing.[64]

Zusanli (ST-36) is indicated by the same source for:

> Sensation of energy that rises back upwards, excess in the heart and in the belly, brutal pain in the heart; arteriosclerosis, high blood pressure.[65]

Thus, the two energy diffusion points may be used to regulate the direction of energy flow, but only if we needle deeply, to disperse the excess.[66]

In the *Su Wen* we find another point located on an artery: tianshu (ST-25). This point means ''celestial hinge.'' It is also called gumen, ''the door of the nutrients.'' The hinge can be celestial only if it links the lower part of the body with the upper part. The contrary would give the point the name, ''terrestrial hinge.'' The ''door of the nutrients,'' then, is a heavenly window, through which the energy of the stomach may rise. When there is an excess of stomach energy, the door is forced open. It is no surprise that this point is indicated as follows:

> Excess in the chest, energy that assails the heart and the chest.[67]

This point must also be deeply needled to shut the door against an untimely rise of energy.

The point located in the hollow of the chest must be burong (ST-19). Located just beneath rugen (ST-18), the terminal point of xu li, this point means ''uncontaining, cannot contain, cannot tolerate.'' These terms certainly express an excess in the thorax that is looking for a way out and which will choose the path through burong (ST-19) if needled. Its symptomology as described in the *Da Cheng* is:

> Pain in the heart, with, at the same time, pain in the shoulders and back.[68]

This is the first point to needle among those located in the hollow of the chest, though not necessarily the only one[69] for cases of cardiac pain with dyspnea. For bronchopulmonary dyspnea, chengman (ST-20) seems to be indicated.

Another method of regularizing an excess of stomach energy related to ischemic attack is indicated in the Chapter 24 of the *Ling Shu*. This treatise deals with ''energy disturbances, energy that stops flowing, energy that becomes stagnant and upstream energy.'' The method consists of drawing the energy downwards by needling the distal points:

> In cases of pain in the heart with swelling of the belly and of the chest, it is not the heart that is affected, it is the stomach. We must needle yinbai {SP-1} and dadu {SP-2}.[70]

By needling yinbai (SP-1), we draw energy into the small communication channel of chongyang (ST-42),[71] ''assault of Yang,'' and into the spleen meridian. With

322

dadu (SP-2), the rong point, we accelerate the movement to get the energy flowing in the Yin channel. The main points to remember are: ST-30, ST-36, ST-25, ST-19, SP-1 and SP-2. These points are useful in ischemic pathology, as well as in cardiac conduction disorders that result from an excess of stomach energy. This therapy has the advantage of being usable in a preventive manner.

As for the correlations with the trace elements, in this pathology we will not prescribe zinc-nickel-cobalt, the classic Earth trace element. In this instance, where there is an excess of energy and blood that has accumulated and been heated up, and where the complexion (sign of the heart) is red, there is an obvious connection with manganese-cobalt. This paradoxical situation shows that we must open our eyes and use our heads, and not blindly follow the formal correspondences. The same exception is mentioned in the *Ling Shu:*

> If the subject is of the Fire type, we must regulate the blood and energy in the large intestine meridian (shou yang ming).[72]

This confirms the solid connection between the element Fire (manganese-cobalt) and the Yang Ming temperament. The description of Fire subjects applies as well to Shao Yin subjects as Yang Ming-stomach subjects. That is, those who are sanguine, which is, we must admit, a good name for them.

High Blood Pressure

The arterial hypertension that occurs among Yang Ming subjects follows the same pattern as that of the coronary diseases: excess of Yang in the stomach. This is an internal mechanism and, as in coronary disease, it may be amplified or triggered by perverse heat or cold energy.[73] The rise in blood pressure is proportional to the accumulation of stomach energy. It overpowers the circulatory capacity of the lung and creates a blockage of energy in the thorax. When we read that the energy no longer rises to the upper part of the body, this concerns the internal and external pathways of the lung meridian and not the excessive energy in the stomach meridian, which tends to circumvent the obstacle by leaving the body at qichong (ST-30). This is why we read, as an introduction to the paragraph in the *Ling Shu* that deals with the heavenly window points:

> All the Yang energies come from the Yin {Yin engenders Yang} and always rise from the bottom to the top. If the flow of these energies is disturbed, they cannot rise beyond the abdomen, and we must know how to discern the affected meridian. We tonify the Yin meridian, as Yin engenders Yang, and we disperse the Yang meridian to draw the energy once again towards the upper part of the body.[74]

This is a good definition of the protocol mentioned in the discussion of coronary disease. It is the same pattern we will adopt in the present case, dispersing zusanli (ST-36) and tonifying yinbai (SP-1) and dadu (SP-2). If we read further, we find:

> The arterial point of the meridian is renying {ST-9}.[75]

> We needle the point renying {ST-9} in case of great pain in the head, when there is a sensation of excess in the chest, with trouble breathing. All these symptoms indicate that the energy is unable to rise to the upper part of the body.[76]

In this picture of great thoracic oppression we understand the headache as associated with the rise in blood pressure. We better understand the semiology of Yang Ming in its chronology:

> The meridian Yang Ming corresponds to the fifth month: this is the period of maximum activity of Yang energy, but this energy begins to enclose a bit of Yin energy (this is the Yin in the Yang). At this moment there may be swelling in the lower limbs, pains in the chest, edema and pains in the head, because the Yin energy enters into conflict with the Yang energy.[77]

The fifth month (starting from the beginning of the Chinese year, at the end of January or the beginning of February) coincides with summer. It would be interesting to compare the *Ling Shu* observation with epidemiological studies of cardiovascular accidents.

It is certainly not by chance that zusanli (ST-36), needled in dispersion, is a key point in treating high blood pressure, or that one of the specific action points that lowers blood pressure (*ap huyet* in Vietnamese), is located on this meridian, between (ST-36) and shangjuxu (ST-37).[78] It lies between the two he points and exerts a special action on the stomach and the large intestine, the two bowels of Yang Ming.

As far as edemas are concerned, we know that the stomach produces the organic fluids: "The stomach is the granary of the organic fluids."[79]

> The kidneys are the valve of the stomach. If the valve functions poorly, the water accumulates and overflows towards the epidermis, the ankles swell and show signs of edema.

Since we are dealing with an excess of Yang, the Yin battles against the excess and functions poorly. This coincides with the pathology of Shao Yin (see Urinary Pathology of Shao Yin). To confirm this pattern of physiopathology, we quote Qi Bo's advice concerning edema in the *Ling Shu*:

> For all cases of edema, we must disperse zusanli {ST-36} as rapidly as possible.[80]

The physiopathology of edema is complex and is also studied in the various chapters dealing with the pathology of the other temperaments. Here it involves a disturbance of the circulation of rong qi and wei qi. Huang Di asks the following question:

> If the defensive energy wei stops flowing and stagnates in the belly, the patient has a sensation of swelling in the stomach and his breathing is labored. How can we cure him?

Qi Bo replies:

> If the wei energy accumulates in the chest, we must needle the points renying {ST-9} and tiantu {CV-22}.

This simultaneous disturbance of rong and wei energies, with excess and blockage, is related to the arterial disorders that we are now going to examine. The

324

important points for treating high blood pressure among Yang Ming subjects are: ST-36, SP-1, SP-2, ST-9 and ST-37, and the special point, *ap huyet*. The correlation with manganese-cobalt does not vary.

Arterial Occlusion of the Lower Limbs

This pathology is also discussed in the chapters devoted to Tai Yang and Shao Yang. In the chapter of the *Su Wen* dealing with meridians and arteries, Qi Bo has this to say about Yang Ming:

> If the pulse of Yang Ming is dominant, this is a sign of an excess of Yang energy. We must disperse the Yang and tonify the Yin by needling the shu points of the lower limbs.[81]

This clearly refers to the plethora of Yang energy of the stomach, and its tendency to stagnate in the thorax when excess, or to rise outside the body to the head, dominating the Yin, which is both incapable of drawing the Yang downwards to the lower part of the body and of making it rise through the Yin meridians to the head as it should. Thus arterial diseases represent, like the coronary diseases, high blood pressure and even cerebral congestions, as we will study below as one different modality of the same pattern. These affections may be isolated or combined, depending on each patient's specific weaknesses.

In the lower limbs energy circulation involves more than Yang Ming, although this is the predominant meridian, as we may read in the text:

> Yang Ming, the stomach, is the sea, the ocean of the five organs and the six bowels; it feeds the muscles and waters the whole organism. The miscellaneous channel, chong mai, is the ocean of the arteries and the meridians; its energy infiltrates into the ki or the kou {small and large valleys between the muscles}. These two meridians, Yang Ming and chong mai, meet at the genitals. In this region the meridians Shao Yin {kidney}, Tai Yin {spleen}, ren mai and du mai also meet, to rise to the abdomen and to meet again at qichong {ST-30}. It is the meridian of the stomach that is the most important.[82]

At the same time as it attributes a predominant role to the stomach meridian, this text accords great importance to the physiological role of chong mai in the circulation of the energy. Elsewhere, this is confirmed many times and must be mentioned here.

> Huang Di asked, ''Does the meridian chong mai not go to the lower part of the body?''
>
> Qi Bo answered, ''No, it does not go to the lower part of the body. The miscellaneous channel, chong mai, is the sea of the five organs and the six bowels.[83] This means that the five organs and the six bowels receive their energy from chong mai. This channel rises to the upper part of the body, and along the way it waters the various organs. Down below, chong mai enters the capillaries of Shao Yin, in the region of qichong {ST-30}. It passes down the inside of the thigh and of the calf at the malleolus, where it enters the Shao Yin meridian.[84]

It waters the three Yin meridians, passes back to the ankle, then down to the big toe. At the ankle it enters the little capillaries that are there to warm the flesh. This is why, when the little capillaries are knotted, we cannot feel the beating of the pulse there, and the patient certainly feels that his feet are frozen.''[85]

It is interesting to note that this pulse corresponds to the posterior tibial pulse, whereas the pedis pulse corresponds to chongyang (ST-42). The relative deficit of one or the other will enable us to determine whether the chong mai or Yang Ming meridian is most involved in the circulatory deficit of the lower limb in a given patient. Qi Bo has more to say:

As for the circulation of the energy, we know only that rong qi flows within the meridians and that the defensive energy wei flows outside of them. The essential energy (jing) of chong mai circulates at once with rong and with wei. The material energies are represented by the blood, the immaterial energies by the energy.

The miscellaneous channel chong mai springs from the genitals. It rises towards the upper part of the body,[86] circulates outside of the body and disperses on the chest. It circulates within the meridians as well, and passes into the arteries, which we feel beating beside the navel. Through these arteries, chong mai enters the energy ramifications in the abdominal region as well as the ramifications of the stomach meridian.[87] The energy of chong mai enters the kidney meridian to descend along the inside of the lower limb, to penetrate into the energy ramifications in the calf.[88]

It is clear now that arterial affections of the lower limbs result from an excess of Yang energy, either Tai Yang, Shao Yang[89] or more frequently, Yang Ming. This energy regulates the distribution of rong qi and wei qi throughout the body from their area of production, the stomach.

These affections are also the result of an imbalance of the miscellaneous channel, chong mai, which distributes jing qi[90] up and down the body. It is the vector of the motor energy, yuan qi. Chong mai is in anastomosis with zu shao yin, which brings the energy back upwards through the lower limb. This is all summarized by Qi Bo himself:

When the lower limbs are cold, we must start by warming up the body — by rubbing the palms of the hands, the insides of the elbows, the armpits, the feet, behind the knees, the neck and the back with rock salt, which we have roasted beforehand and wrapped in a cloth. Then we examine the body in detail, and if we find spots where the energy seems stopped up, we disperse, as the essential role of the acupuncturist is to regularize the flow of energy. This energy comes, as we have seen, from the stomach, where it is transformed into defensive wei energy and into the nutritious rong energy, and from the original energy of the meridian chong mai, which rises also, like the stomach energy, to the upper part of the body, then descends to the lower limb to link up with the meridian zu shao yin.

326

> If we have the feeling of frozen feet, it is because the ancestral energy
> is unable to link with the meridian zu shao yin. In this case, we must
> treat with moxa and by rubbing with hot salt.[91]

Once again, we find the combination of stomach and kidney meridians important
in resolving an imbalance of rong, wei and jing energies, just as we saw this association evoked to solve the problem of organic fluids that cause edema, since the
kidneys are the "barrier of the stomach."

It is not surprising that the therapeutic indications of the *Ling Shu* read as follows:

> If there is imbalance of all the Yin energies, with cold limbs, we must
> needle the points of the meridians zu yang ming and zu shao yin, and
> leave the needles in until they become warm.[92]

It is said in the *Su Wen:*

> When the Yang energy is deficient in the lower part of the body, the
> limbs are cold.[93]

To summarize, the treatment of occlusive arterial diseases of the lower limbs consists of deeply needling qichong (ST-30) and zusanli (ST-36), or in applying moxa
to zusanli (ST-36), as is indicated in the *Ling Shu:*

> When the legs are cold from the feet to the knees, or just below the
> knees, we must apply moxas to zusanli {ST-36}.[94]

Needle the shu points of the lower limbs, particularly taixi (KI-3), which is also
the shu-yuan point, to draw the Yang energy towards the lower part of the body
and to help the Yin circulate. To follow the idea of dispersing the Yang and tonifying the Yin, we may needle the luo points of the Yang meridians, especially
feiyang (BL-58) and fenglong (ST-40). This treatment is in keeping with the concept of excess of Tai Yang in arterial disease as is discussed in the corresponding
chapter (see Arterial Disease, Tai Yang). Subsequently, we needle the yuan
points of the coupled biao-li Yin meridians, *i.e.* zu shao yin (kidney) and zu tai yin
(spleen). As we have already spoken of taixi, next we needle the yuan point,
taibai (SP-3). Thus, we create the attraction of the Yang in the Yin through the
transversal luo channels, from the Yang meridians (bladder and stomach) to the
Yin meridians (kidney and spleen). Needling gongsun (SP-4) will open chong
mai. Xuanzhong (GB-39), the luo point of the three yang of the lower limbs, is
also useful to disperse the excess of these meridians toward the upper part of the
body and aid the descent of the qi. We understand, thanks to the passage quoted
above, the reasons for leaving the needle in place for a long time.

In daily practice, the results of acupuncture treatment of occlusive arterial
disorders is very satisfying. Without changing the oscillometric readings considerably, we enable the patient to move about more freely and we diminish or eradi-
cate the subjective symptoms of pain and paresthesia. The limbs warm up and the
patient no longer feels cold. The useful points to retain are the following: ST-36,
SP-4, KI-3, BL-58, ST-40, SP-3 and GB-39.[95] As with coronary disease and
arterial hypertension, this pathology of excess of Yang is correlated with
manganese-cobalt and also cobalt alone.

Respiratory Pathology

Asthma

There is no point going over the biao-li relationships between the large intestine (Yang Ming) and the lung (Tai Yin). The origins of asthma may stem from one or the other. It is not unusual when questioning a Yang Ming-Metal patient (more often colitic than the asthmatic) to find a case history of respiratory sensitivity, with frequent episodes of rhino-pharyngitis, particularly during his early childhood. This does not mean that the Yang Ming-Earth patients do not have similar past histories; they could very well have been Metal in their early childhood. As we will see in the discussion of otorhinolaryngologic (ORL) pathology, rhinitis, rhinopharyngitis, angina and otitis may all result from a primitive affection of the large intestine. It is often difficult during childhood, and even sometimes among adults, to distinguish Yang Ming-Metal patients from Tai Yin-Metal patients. For example, the onset of asthma in a Yang Ming patient may come about from the penetration of perverse energy into the luo channel of the large intestine:

> If the perverse energy lodges in the secondary channel of the large intestine (shou yang ming), there is excess of energy, dyspnea, the sides are swollen, and there is heat in the chest. In this case, we needle the points shangyang {LI-1} and shaoshang {LU-11}. In half an hour, the condition will be healed.[96] Needle on the opposite side if there is no result.[97]

As far as trace element therapy goes, the correlation with manganese-copper is in keeping with the correspondence with Metal.

Acute Pulmonary Edema and Chronic Cor Pulmonale

This pathology fits here because of the susceptibility of the Yang Ming subjects to cardiovascular problems caused by excess, and to the close ties that exist between Yang Ming and the lungs. Qi Bo is very clear about this:

> The suffering of Yang Ming is manifested in the heart and in the spleen. If the illness is transmitted from the large intestine to the lungs, it becomes an incurable suffocation.[98]

Nguyen Van Nghi[99] and Chamfrault[100] clearly note in their translations that when the illness becomes chronic, corresponding to the passage of the illness from the large intestine to the lungs, it is transformed into "destruction by the wind." This is also called fong tieu, "fast and short respiration," which reflects the violence of the symptoms.

At worst, this gives an attack of acute pulmonary edema, as described in this passage from the *Su Wen:*

> If the carotid pulse is agitated[101] the patient presents a cough with rapid dyspnea; the internal canthus of the eye is a bit bulging;[102] there is a disturbance of the balance of the organic fluids.[103]

Husson translates this as "overflow of breath, qi of water."[104]

In short, we may say that an excess of energy in Yang Ming, located in the chest, ends up turning into "destruction of wind." This tells us that the energy mobilizes suddenly and is surging upwards, causing an acute pulmonary edema. It may also cause hematemesis, if the energy is concentrated in the stomach (abdomen, see below). It may also cause hemoptysis. Elsewhere, in the chapter "The Normal and Abnormal," Qi Bo confirms this pathology and teaches Huang Di the difference between asthmatic dyspnea and cardiac dyspnea:

> Those who cannot stay calmly in bed and whose breathing is strong and wheezing have a disturbance of the energy of the Yang Ming meridian (large intestine, stomach). The energy of the three Yang meridians normally goes to the lower part of the body, but among these patients it rises back upwards. This is why we hear their breathing.[105]

> Yang Ming is the stomach, which is the mother of the six bowels; if the energy of the stomach rises back to the upper part of the body, one may no longer stay calmly in bed. Those who may stay in bed when they are out of breath have a disturbance of the energy of the lung meridian; it does not circulate normally, and stagnates in the secondary channels. Now the disturbance of the circulation on the secondary channels is not serious, which is why the patients can rest normally.

> Those who cannot stay in bed calmly because of dyspnea have a disturbance of the fluids.[106] The kidneys govern the water. When there is a stasis of fluids, it is because the energy of the kidneys is disturbed.[107]

This remarkable passage shows us once more what fine semiologists the ancient Chinese were. Many centuries ago they were aware of the gravity of dyspnea decubitus. The passage also shows that energetic physiopathologies are numerous and subtle. Here, we have come a long way from the standard therapeutic response of needling one point or another, depending on its virtues.

The destructive upward surging of stomach energy,[108] known as the "destroyer wind," induces a disturbance of the circulation of wei qi, which stagnates and invades the meridians and disturbs the qi of water, that is, the normal circulation of the body fluids. We may complete this picture by quoting from the *Ling Shu* chapter entitled "Five Sorts of Disorders":

> When there are troubles, that means that the pure rong energy of the meridians, instead of flowing in the Yang, passes into the Yin, while the impure energy wei, instead of flowing in the Yin, passes into the Yang. . . it flows in the wrong direction. If this happens in the lungs, the patient has trouble breathing, he shouts, he jumps about.[109]

This is obviously a picture of respiratory distress such as we find in cases of acute pulmonary edema. The symptomology is enriched by Qi Bo's description in the chapter "Energy Troubles Due to Blockage (Jue)"[110] in the *Su Wen:*

> When there is imbalance in the lung meridian (shou tai yin),[111] with coughing and dyspnea (fullness in the chest) and a tendency to vomit foam, we must needle the points of the lung meridian.[112]

The observation is precise, and leaves no room for doubt. If we take into account the description of dyspnea decubitus and the role of the kidney in the physiology of organic fluids, we will not be surprised by the therapeutic advice given by the ancient physician in the chapter, "Five Sorts of Disorders," from the same source:

> In such a disorder of the lungs, we must needle the rong points of the lungs and the shu points of the kidneys.[113]

These are the points yuji (LU-10), the rong point that makes the energy circulate, and taixi (KI-3), the shu point that tonifies the kidney and causes the kidney energy, which is blocked down below, to rise to the upper part of the body and help the Yang go back down.

Again, the role of qichong (ST-30) is not to be neglected. This point recalls the semiology, "Energy that assails the heart, hindering respiration."[114] Clearly the bleeding of qichong (ST-30), on the femoral artery, is far more energetically judicious than bleeding inside the elbow, in the region of chize (LU-5), the dispersion point of the lung, when the energy in that meridian is almost exhausted. In treating cases of respiratory emergency of cardiac origin we will retain the points LU-10, KI-3 and the stomach dispersion points discussed in the preceding paragraphs, in particular qichong (ST-30).

Pulmonary Infarction and Hemoptysis

Among all the possible etiologies of hemoptysis, the form that corresponds to the Yang Ming etiology will, of course, be of cardiac origin, with an excess of Yang Ming heat and "destruction by the wind." We can include in this category the hemoptysis that occurs during a myocardial infarction, or that associated with an insufficiency of the left ventricle leading to chronic hemoptysic pulmonary edema. We must not underestimate the pulmonary infarction in the thoracic cardiovascular context. Here too, we are face to face with Yang Ming excess heat and an upsurge of the destructive wind.

In Chapter 45 of the *Su Wen,* we find descriptions of most classical medical emergencies, spoken of in Chinese as jue, or energy blockages. One of these immediately sparks our admiration:

> In disturbances of the energy of Yang Ming,[115] with coughing accompanied by dyspnea, fever, anxiety and vomiting blood, we must needle the points of the stomach meridian.[116]

From 15 to 20 centuries before Laennec, the Chinese were able to associate these symptoms that perfectly describe the pulmonary infarction. Maybe we should pay attention to how they treated this affection. We are told to needle the points on the stomach meridian. Which ones? Apart from qichong (ST-30), which is, of course, to be chosen, we will also retain renying (ST-9), which in this clinical context addresses the agitated carotid pulse. If we look again at the chapter on

"The Disorders of Wei Energy" in the *Ling Shu,* we find the Yellow Emperor's question:

> If the defensive energy wei does not circulate and stagnates in the belly, the patient feels that his stomach is swollen, his breathing is labored. How can we cure him?

Qi Bo answers:

> If the defensive energy wei accumulates within the chest, we must needle the points located over the chest; if it accumulates within the belly, we must needle the points located under the belly. If both the chest and the belly are swollen at the same time, we must needle the points located on the sides of the chest and on the belly.
>
> If the energy is accumulated in the chest, we must needle the points renying {ST-9} and tiantu {CV-22}.[117]
>
> If it is accumulated in the belly and the chest, we must needle the point zhangmen {LV-13}.[118]

Thus, it will be a good idea to combine renying (ST-9) with tiantu (CV-22), a very well known point that has a reputation for efficacy in pulmonary dyspnea.[119]

Another point that has a good reputation in treating thoracic and pulmonary emergencies of Yang Ming origin is chengman (ST-20). While the point burong (ST-19) is of value for excess stomach energy in the thoracic region, and means "uncontaining, cannot contain," it relates to cardiac symptomology. Chengman (ST-20), meaning "full containing," on the other hand, is indicated for pulmonary symptomology.[120] The *Da Cheng* announces:

> Dyspnea, spits blood as well as much phlegm and pus.[121] When he breathes, the shoulders rise to accompany the respiration.[122]

Among the other emergency points of thoracic energy along the stomach meridian, we must mention kufang (ST-14), whose symptomology in the *Da Cheng* is as follows:

> Fullness in the chest, in the sides, in the flanks. Coughing with dyspnea. Spits blood, pus and phlegm.[123]

The emergency points in cases of hemoptysis and pulmonary infarction are: ST-30, ST-9, CV-22, ST-20 and ST-14. We may add the point kongzui (LU-6), a point on the lung meridian that is needled in emergencies affecting the lung.

Digestive Pathology

Hiatus Hernia, Nausea, Dyspepsia, Abdominal Distension, Vomiting and Hiccups

> For the stomach, the symptoms of energy imbalances include the sensation of energy that rises back up to the upper part of the body, nausea.[124]

331

We must keep in mind, apart from nausea,[125] a particular sensation of energy that rises to the upper part of the body. It may have very different pathological meanings, as we have seen in the *Ling Shu* and in the *Su Wen* — digestive, cardiac, pulmonary, as well as neurological, as we will see further on. We have discussed the cardiac and respiratory correspondences. In gastroenterology, this rising sensation may include dyspepsia, vomiting or gastroesophageal reflux. It may correspond to a hiatus hernia. What we must remember is that this specific form of dyspepsia and hiatus hernia always corresponds to excess heat of the stomach. This common mechanism explains why we sometimes find coronary or cerebral arteriosclerosis and hiatus hernia together.

To study the specific digestive pathology of Yang Ming, we must understand that the pathology of Yang Ming is the excess-deficiency pair, or, if you prefer, the hot-cold alternative. Qi Bo gives a very good example of the semiological distinction in the *Ling Shu:*

> When there is Yang heat in the stomach, the patient is always hungry and the skin over the navel is warm. When the Yang is in the large intestine, the skin over the navel is cold. When there is Yin in the stomach, the belly is swollen {abdominal distension}. When the Yin is in the large intestine, the patient has borborygmus or diarrhea, and when there is Yin in the stomach and Yang in the large intestine, the patient has a swollen belly and diarrhea at the same time.[126] When there is Yang in the stomach and Yin in the large intestine, the patient is always hungry and the lower abdomen is swollen and painful.[127]

A patient who has an excess of stomach energy, particularly the sanguine subject, will suffer from dyspepsia with abdominal distension and occasional vomiting.[128] There may be an association with a vascular condition that is caused by the same mechanism.

> When the abdomen is swollen, with fullness in the chest and the sides or the flanks, the patient is dizzy in his head, both his legs are cold. The illness dwells in the stomach or the spleen.[129]

The disorders caused by this excess may be blamed on an excess of rong qi or of the fierce wei qi, as we might have expected. We have already quoted Huang Di's question:

> If the defensive energy wei does not circulate and stagnates in the belly, the patient has the sensation of swelling in the stomach, his breathing is labored. How can we cure him?

And Qi Bo's answer:

> If wei is accumulated in the belly, we must needle the points qichong {ST-30} and zusanli {ST-36}.[130]

In practice we find that this stagnation, this imbalance of wei qi, opens the patient to the penetration of perverse energy. The morbid tendency to accumulate wei qi in the stomach, added to the penetration of perverse energy, is likely to trigger a case of hiccups. Qi Bo explains,

332

The stomach engenders the energy, which rises to the lungs. If the cold Yin energy happens to mix with this newly created energy and tends to head towards the stomach, the stomach is troubled and this induces the hiccups. In this case we must tone up shou tai yin {lung} and disperse zu shao yin {kidney}, as this cold energy, Yin, comes from the kidneys.[131]

We once more find evidence of an intimate link between the stomach, wei qi and the diaphragm. This confirms at once the physiopathology of hiatus hernia and its preponderance among Yang Ming subjects when the stomach is in excess. The connection between xu li and the sensation of energy that rises to the upper part of the body is fundamental. Concisely, stagnation of wei qi from an excessive stomach in combination with perverse cold brings on the hiccups, whereas stagnation of wei qi and perverse heat lead to hiatus hernia.

A deficiency of stomach energy may also be at the origin of dyspepsia. The accompanying symptomology will enable discrimination between excess or deficiency.

The Yang Ming meridian in excess is a sign of excess of energy and lack of blood. If there is an excess of blood and a lack of energy,[132] the patient will often be afraid or will have trouble digesting.[133]

Here, as was the case in Jue Yin, we find the energy-blood balance with an excess of one linked to a deficiency of the other. Yet, there is something else here that is of capital importance. For the Jue Yin subject, the pathology related to psychiatric inhibition and to physiological deficits corresponds to a deficiency of blood and an excess of energy. This is exactly the opposite of what we find among Yang Ming subjects. Might this have something to do with the global movement of blood that is *ascending* in the former and *descending* in the latter?

If we compare the two respective personality profiles, we have the exuberant behavior of the excess of stomach opposed to the fearful, introspective and almost misanthropic behavior of a Yang Ming subject with a deficiency of stomach energy and an excess of blood (see Psychiatry, below). We find all this in the tenth chapter of the *Ling Shu,* in the discussion of the symptomology of the stomach meridian:

Swollen belly, borborygmus. . . when there is an excess, there is heat in the front part of the body. The patient is always hungry and his urine is dark in color.[134] When there is a deficiency, the front of the body is cold and the patient feels his belly swollen.[135]

The radial pulse, of relative importance if we have a good grasp of Chinese semiology, confirms the diagnosis:

If the stomach pulse becomes soft and diffuse, the patient has digestive problems.

If the pulse of the stomach is full, the patient is swollen. If it is deficient, he has diarrhea.[136]

333

Apart from the stomach excess-deficiency alternative, dyspepsia may be caused by an excess in Shao Yang (gallbladder) or in Tai Yang (small intestine). When we are in doubt, a differential diagnosis may be obtained by therapeutic trial.

> If a patient has trouble digesting, we must apply moxas to the points of the stomach meridian. If the treatment is not successful, we must then examine the Yang in excess, and needle several times the beishu points that correspond and give medicinal herbal teas.[137]

Anorexia

Anorexia is a symptom that is full of subtlety. Chinese medicine makes a distinction between loss of appetite and the impossibility of absorbing nourishment, despite marked hunger, because of illness felt in the epigastrium.

> The stomach is the sea of nourishment, the point of diffusion of its energy is qichong {ST-30} above, and zusanli {ST-36} below.

> When the sea of nourishment is full, in excess, the belly is swollen. If it is deficient, the patient is hungry, but may not eat.[138]

The energetic mechanism of this symptom involves the stomach and the spleen, the two viscera related to the element Earth. Huang Di asks for more precision:

> Why do we sometimes feel hunger, when we don't have a good appetite?

Qi Bo answers:

> It is because the energy is concentrated in the spleen, and only warm energy is left in the stomach, which digests food very rapidly. This is why we may feel hungry, but the lack of energy causes a loss of appetite.[139]

In summary, an excess of stomach energy corresponds to the plethoric profile of the sanguine subject: a red face, abdominal distension, occasional trouble eating, even with good appetite, hiccups and possibly a hiatal hernia with associated cardiovascular symptoms. Deficiency of stomach energy corresponds to a moody, phlegmatic profile: frequent bad health, pessimistic, fearful, introspective and alone, a tendency to be sensitive to the cold, cold felt in the abdomen, dyspepsia and often diarrhea.

Gastritis

Most of the time, we are dealing with a typical ulcer. This is not an absolute rule, but we may say that a deficiency, or a deficiency of cold in the stomach, which is the fourth etiology of epigastric pain described elsewhere,[140] causes an ulcer located in the stomach. We may also find atypical gastritis without finding an ulcer through x-ray or endoscopic examination. Excess of energy in the stomach meridian corresponds to the third etiology of the *Trung Y Hoc:* "Excess heat of the liver and stomach." It is more violent, but of shorter duration and the location is more often duodenal. Here, we are in accord with the discussions of ulcers and gastritis from an excess of the liver and gallbladder as presented in the chapters devoted to Shao Yang and Jue Yin. Excess heat in the liver and stomach is manifested by ulcer pain, retrosternal burning that prevents eating, nausea, dry throat and a bitter taste in the mouth.[141] For treatment, we disperse taichong (LV-3) and zusanli (ST-36).

Here, we are most interested in the case of deficiency of cold, as this is the gastritis that is most specific to Yang Ming subjects. It occurs usually among Yang Ming-Metal (phlegmatic) subjects, but it may also affect certain sanguine subjects during times of depression or failure. The psychological profile presented above may be constitutional or temporary, depending on the individual case. It corresponds to the "deficiency of stomach" — fear, misanthropy, easily cold, etc.

These patients may be constitutionally "deficient Yang Ming" and present a specific digestive morbidity:

> "Which are the patients who are likely to suffer from digestive illnesses?" asked Huang Di of his physician Shao Shi.
>
> Shao Shi replied, "Those whose skin is very thin and without lustre,[142] whose flesh is slack, whose stomach and large intestine don't function well, fall ill as soon as they are affected by perverse energy."[143]

The physician Shao Shi's comment is very interesting here, because it tends to support the concept of terrain in Chinese medicine. The text continues:

> We fall ill because of a weakness in this organ or that one, and the perverse energy attacks the organs and the bowels differently, depending on the seasons. If the organs are poorly constituted, the perverse energy may attack them directly.[144]

In this text, this dialogue between the Emperor and his physician follows commentaries on vulnerabilities to bi, which are polysectorial affections, as we have said again and again (see Jue Yin).

Thin, lustreless skin and slack flesh are the signs of a deficiency of Yang Ming (large intestine and stomach) and constitute a terrain that is vulnerable to attack by cold, or cold wind perverse energy. This causes gastritis at first, then more generalized affections (bi) as time goes on.[145] These subjects are often long-lined, thin and dry. Their pulses are as soft as their flesh, and the *Su Wen* indicates:

> Stomach pulse soft and inconsistent, this is alimentary bi.[146]

The *Trung Y Hoc* informs us:

> In case of cold deficiency of the stomach, there may be vomiting of clear fluids or of food, sensitivity to cold, skin, hands and feet frozen, asthenia, pollakiuria, diarrhea with pasty stools.[147]

Cold deficiency, we see, means more than a simple digestive incident that causes gastritis or ulcers, as would occur among Shao Yang subjects (because of their excess of liver and gallbladder). It is, on the contrary, a deep imbalance of the visceral energy facilitated by a terrain of specific vulnerability of the digestive system. The cold penetrates there more easily, finds the deficiency and settles in. This identifies the affection as bi, whose evolution we have every reason to fear will be polyvisceral, for example, chronic polyarthritis.

If the result is only an ulcer, this will not only be a recurring ulcer, but it will also become chronic, possibly even terebrant. These patients are somber, dark complexioned, fearful and depressed. They are introspective misanthropists whom other therapies do not manage to cure. Acupuncture treatment must be intensive and make systematic use of moxa in daily sessions. If this is not possible, treatment must be given at least every other day. We must needle the beishu and mu points of the stomach, weishu (BL-21) and zhongwan (CV-12). Weishu (BL-21) is used for:

> Vomiting, the patient regurgitates everything he eats, eats copiously, but stays thin; Yin (cold) in the stomach; spasms or distension of the stomach, poor digestion, anorexia, loss of weight, cancer of the stomach. . .[148]

Zhongwan (CV-12), the concentration point of Tai Yin, the mu point of the stomach as well as the he point of the bowels, is indicated in the *Da Cheng* for:

> Nausea, vomiting, abdominal pain, gastric distension, stomach spasms, gastric hemorrhage, cancer of the stomach, poor digestion and anorexia.[149]

It is useful to combine the points weicang (BL-45), the "storehouse of the stomach," which is on the same horizontal as weishu (BL-21), and tianshu (ST-25), the mu point of the colon. Weicang (BL-45) is indicated for:

> Sensitivity to the cold, fear of cold, neither fluids nor solids go down {dysphagia or stenosis?}, fullness and distension of the abdomen because of Yin, ascites.[150]

Tianshu (ST-25) is indicated for:

> All the chronic affections of the stomach and intestine; sensation of pain with impression of cold around the navel, etc.[151]

We may combine the beishu and mu points of the spleen, pishu (BL-20) and zhangmen (LV-13), also zusanli (ST-36; moxa) and even shenshu (BL-23) and taixi (KI-3), the shu and mu points of the kidney.

We will retain LV-3 and ST-36 to treat gastritis of excess heat in the liver and stomach, and BL-21, CV-12, BL-45, ST-25, BL-20, ST-36, SP-6, BL-23 and KI-3 with moxibustion for gastritis whose origin is cold deficiency of the stomach and which relates to serious etiologies of chronic or organic nature.

Menetrier makes a distinction between functional stomach disorders and epigastric disorders. The former are included in the allergic diathesis and are comparable to the gastric symptoms of Shao Yang and Jue Yin. Epigastric disorders, with "spasms, blockages, post-prandial abdominal distension, aerogastria," correspond to the dystonic diathesis. The prescription of manganese-cobalt combined with zinc-nickel-cobalt (Earth trace element) is justified. Here again, the excess pathology of the sanguine subject coincides with manganese-cobalt. However, in what could correspond to the deficiency pathology, and to the behavioral profile of Yang Ming-Metal, Menetrier mentions the appearance of ulcerous syndromes, preceded by:

> Vague digestive disturbances; the dominant dystonic behavior is coupled with more ancient manifestations of the hyposthenic profile {such as respiratory fragility or colic fragility}, with the progressive development of anxiety and emotivity.[152]

In this case, alternation between manganese-copper and manganese-cobalt is indicated. Nonetheless, the action of zinc-nickel-cobalt should not be neglected. I find that in dyspeptic disturbances, and in any digestive problem where the Earth (spleen and stomach) is involved, zinc-nickel-cobalt is always useful.

Colitis and Constipation

Among the five most frequent etiologies of these functional disorders, we are interested here in two: excess and deficiency of the large intestine meridian.[153] In the first etiology, the symptomology is very turbulent, with violent pain predominating in the left colon, abdominal distension and borborygmus. Constipation is the rule. There may be mucus in the stools in the form of stercoroma, which are most often dry and very dehydrated. Radiologically, megadolichocolon is frequent. In the second etiology, deficiency of the large intestine meridian, the colon is atonal, sometimes dilated. This occurs often among the elderly, or after the prolonged evolution of the former etiology. There is very little pain, if any. The problem is often due simply to the inhibition of bowel movements. In this case, the stools are normal.

The justification of the treatments indicated is found in the classical texts, as are certain secondary semiological indications.

> When the large intestine is affected, there is pain in the intestines and borborygmus. In the winter, the patient tends to catch colds, which trigger diarrhea and periumbilical pains, making it impossible to stay upright for a long time. As the large intestine and the stomach make a whole {Yang Ming}, we must, in these cases, needle shangjuxu {ST-37}.[154]

It is remarkable to note in this passage that the Chinese recognized the existence of the "irritable colon." Our modern pathologists attribute a particular susceptibility of the large intestine to the cold heat that is specific to functional colons. Shangjuxu (ST-37) is the he point with special effect on the colon. An internal channel connects this point with the colon and through this channel flows the energy of shou yang ming. We may point out here that perverse energy considerably influences this pathology, if only as a triggering factor, as in the role of cold or of heat. Metal (lung and large intestine) corresponds to the autumn. We may expect a recrudescence of this pathology at that time. The paragraph we quoted from above is taken from the chapter devoted to meridian imbalances caused by perverse energy. Elsewhere, in the chapter on the "Energy of the Four Seasons," Huang Di asks:

Perverse energy is variable during the four seasons. This energy may cause all diseases. Will you tell me the points we must needle according to the seasons?

Qi Bo replies:

In the autumn, we needle the jing and shu points; if the perverse energy is located in the bowels (zang)[155] we must needle the he points.[156] In all the affections of the large intestine, we must also needle zusanli {ST-36}; we disperse if the energy is in excess and we tonify if the energy is deficient.

When a patient presents borborygmus and has the sensation that his energy assails the upper part of the body, with trouble breathing and standing up for a long time, it means that the perverse energy has penetrated the large intestine. In this case, we must needle the point qihai {CV-6}, then the points shangjuxu {ST-37}, the he point of the large intestine, and zusanli {ST-36}.[157]

Dyspnea here is related to a disturbance of the pulmonary sphere, as the perverse energy has passed from the large intestine to the lung, its coupled organ. Once again the association of respiratory sensitivity and colic, found among many hyposthenic patients, is confirmed.

Our hypothesis that the dyspnea is of pulmonary origin[158] is supported by Qi Bo's indication of qihai (CV-6). At times this point is indicated alone, but it is also indicated in the *Da Cheng,* in synergistic association with xuanji (CV-21), for dyspnea with pulmonary troubles. The indication of xuanji (CV-21) confirms our therapeutic recommendation:

In dyspnea with pulmonary troubles, needle xuanji {CV-21} and qihai {CV-6}.

Bian Que also indicates:

In dyspnea that prevents sleep, tonify and disperse qihai {CV-6} and xuanji {CV-21}.[160]

Where abdominal pain is concerned, there is a general rule found in the *Ling Shu:*

When the belly is painful, needle and massage the points located next to the navel, on the stomach meridian.[161] The patient will immediately be relieved, but if not, needle and then massage qichong {ST-30}, and then he will certainly be relieved.[162]

There are two points on the stomach meridian that act on all abdominal pain, one of whose polarity is shou yang ming, tianshu (ST-25), and the other whose polarity is zu yang ming, qichong (ST-30). This is an eloquent statement of the role of Yang Ming in gastroenterology.

Yang Ming colitis is the form that tends to become chronic, to settle in for good, predominantly on the left side. Its complications include diverticulosis, diverticulitis, fistulas and fissures. There is a correlation with the findings of diathetic practitioners and the prescription of manganese-copper. Constipation, they note, is often found with nausea, headaches and poor appetite. American authors have shown that these accompanying symptoms are not due to intoxication resulting from the proliferation of colic microorganisms, but are the functional consequence of the distension of the colon and rectum. These symptoms have been artificially induced in normal subjects simply by placing a small balloon in the colon and in the rectum.[163] The observation of poor appetite and nausea establishes a link between shou yang ming (large intestine), zu yang ming (stomach) and the cephalic territory (upper pathway of the two meridians). Whatever the neurovegetative mechanism, in particular, headache, their sedation is achieved by regulating the Yang Ming distal points as we will see in the discussion of neurology.

Diarrhea

Yang Ming imbalance can also give rise to diarrhea. The *Su Wen* says:

> The symptom of energy imbalance in the large intestine is diarrhea.[164]

When diarrhea is caused by an imbalance of the large intestine meridian, perverse cold energy is most often involved in one of three ways. It may accidentally penetrate the large intestine, as is the case with seasonal diarrhea from cold, or the absorption of cold food, such as ice cream. It may penetrate periodically into a sensitive colon, as is the case for irritable colon. Or, it may chronically settle within the viscera, causing chronic diarrhea. This is the case with colitis or more severe organic disorders. Chronic cold is equivalent to the cold deficiency found in gastritis or in chronic terebrant ulcers. Here we are dealing with the same misanthropic, fearful, dark-complexed patients, which indicates that the pathology is that of bi of the colon. This proves, once again, that perverse energy only settles in where there is a predisposing terrain, a deficiency of the bowel, which is responsible for the name, cold deficiency.

These three physiopathologies correspond to the semiological origin of diarrhea we saw at the beginning of the chapter.

> In cases of Yin in the large intestine, the patient presents borborygmus or diarrhea.[165]

However, even in the absence of perverse energy, there is a specific physiopathology that may be responsible for diarrhea. This is the case of internal energy circulation disturbance. Qi Bo explains:

> When there is imbalance, that means the pure energy of the meridians, rong qi, passes into the Yin, instead of circulating in the Yang. The impure wei energy, instead of circulating in the Yin, passes into the Yang and flows in the wrong direction. If this happens in the large intestine and in the stomach, we find chronic diarrhea.

> We must needle the points of the bladder and stomach. If there is no result, we will needle zusanli {ST-36}.[166]

The stomach points Qi Bo speaks of are certainly dachangshu (BL-25) and tianshu (ST-25), the shu and mu points of the large intestine.

In this case, we must neither tonify nor disperse, we must only guide the energy, as there is neither excess nor deficiency; we must insert and slowly withdraw the needle.[167]

In functional colonopathies, irritable colons, colitis and diverticulitis we will use ST-37, ST-36, CV-6, ST-25 and ST-30, as well as the beishu point of the colon, BL-25.

Organic Pathology of the Colon

Hemorrhagic coloproctitis and Crohn's disease are discussed in the chapters devoted to Shao Yin and Tai Yang. Incontinence of fecal matter was considered to be a grave semiological indication related to coma in the ancient Chinese texts. Qi Bo relates this syndrome to an assault on the Earth and on its two viscera:

When the granaries {spleen and stomach} are disinhabited {by the visceral spirits, shen}, the anus is incontinent.[168]

The patients who conserve their shen live, those who cannot, die.

If the head is thrown back and the eyes drown, this means that the shen will fail.[168]

These remarks help us to better understand the role of the shen in cerebral activity, and the specific role of each of the twelve meridians that pass through the brain.

As far as trace elements are concerned in functional and organic colic pathology, manganese-copper is indicated if the diathesis is hyposthenic. This is the case of Yang Ming subjects, among whom a certain reverence for law and order, exacerbated, tends towards obsessional meticulousness. Menetrier, too, signals the exclusive (or at least dominant) localization of functional symptoms on the left side as being pathognomonic of hyposthenia (Metal).

Ascites, Disorders of the Organic Fluids

Here we must remember the importance of the stomach in the production of the organic fluids, on the one hand, and its role in the constitution of the energy wei, which links the stomach to the inferior burner, on the other.[169] This is summarized in the phrase, "The kidneys are the door of the stomach." The physiopathology of ascites or of certain other abdominal emergencies depends on this role, as is explicit in Qi Bo's remarks:

Rong energy circulates within the meridians, wei energy outside of the meridians. If wei qi penetrates into the meridians, the skin becomes swollen. If wei qi is disturbed in the chest or in the abdomen, there will be swelling in the belly and fullness in the chest.[170] If wei qi obstructs the ways of the fluids,[171] there will be immediate swelling in the stomach and intestines. In any case and as quickly as possible, we must disperse the point zusanli {ST-36}, whether there is an excess or a deficiency, as wei qi comes from the stomach.[172]

The therapeutic recommendations found at the end of the chapter are in keeping with the physiology of the stomach:

It is enough to needle zusanli {ST-36}. In recent cases, we may obtain healing in a single session of treatment; in chronic cases, no more than three will be necessary, if we do touch the energy. If we do not obtain results, which is very rare, we must needle the energy points, those located above and below the navel: shangwan {CV-13}, zhongwan {CV-12}, xiawan {CV-10}, guanyuan {CV-4}. If we manage to draw the energy, the patient will certainly be cured.[173]

We must understand that these disturbances in the circulation of wei qi may be associated with the penetration of perverse energy, as we saw with hiccups. If such is the case, exudates are not contradictory to a pathology of vascular ischemia. This might be the case in pericarditis or pleurisy among cardiac Shao Yin or Yang Ming patients. Both the stomach and the kidneys are active in these complex mechanisms. We may also find a neurological emergency where mental disorder is combined with acute abdominal or cardiac symptoms.

When an accumulation of perverse energy brings on madness, the feet are suddenly very cold, the chest and the intestines very painful, the pulse is rasping. If the symptoms are Yang, we needle zu shao yin {kidney}; if they are Yin, we needle zu yang ming {stomach}, which is to say we disperse. We disperse the Yang and we tonify the Yin.[174]

This indicates dispersion of zusanli (ST-36) and taixi (KI-3) or tonification of fuliu (KI-7).

This modification of the patient's mental state, which may go so far as loss of consciousness, can parallel the aberration associated with myocardial infarction, acute pulmonary edema, stroke, or a severe metabolic disorder linked with an abdominal pathology with advanced ascites. There is another way to handle fullness of the abdomen caused by the obstruction of the fluids indicated in the *Su Wen*:

If the belly suddenly becomes swollen, this is because the stomach is in excess. We must needle its mu point, zhizheng {SI-7}, five times and the beishu point of the kidneys, shenshu {BL-23}, using a round pointed needle.[175]

This is evidence of the close rapport between stomach and kidneys in the metabolism of the fluids and enlightens us as to why zhizheng (SI-7) is a mu point of the stomach.[176] As the path of the fluids is obstructed, the stomach and the intestines are in excess. The small intestine is "like a lake that regulates the flow of the river." It has a fundamental role in the transportation and distribution of the fluids (see Tai Yang). If we needle its luo point, we remove the obstruction and also the obstruction of the stomach. Thus, we relieve the plethora. Again, the indications for zhizheng (SI-7) are precise and well defined.

Hematemesis

The most common etiology of hematemesis is perverse heat localized in the stomach. We see this in the excess heat of the liver and stomach etiology of stomach ulcers. The excess heat leads to stagnation and an excess of blood with the tendency to rise. This is nothing other than the exacerbation of the "sensation of energy that rises back up to the upper part of the body." Here, the sensation corresponds to something very concrete: the backwash of blood (xue) associated with hemorrhage. This calls for bleeding. The physician Tong Fun, logically enough, indicated this tactic for qichong (ST-30):

> When there is vomiting of blood, which is in general incurable, we only have to bleed qichong with a triangular needle.[177] The healing is immediate.[178]

Urinary Pathology

Anuria

We have already shown the extent to which the stomach is active in the constitution of the organic fluids. This is why its meridian is concerned in the treatment of problems of severe diuresis.

> With anuria, when the lower abdomen is painful or swollen, it is because the bladder is affected. In this case, we must examine the little capillaries located along the pathway of the bladder and liver meridians, around the malleolus and the calves. If they are congested, we must needle and bleed them. If the swelling spreads all the way to the stomach, we must needle zusanli {ST-36}.[179]

The liver meridian is of interest because of its pathway through the pelvic region, and because of its link with the lower urinary tract, as we have seen in Jue Yin (see also Tai Yang).

Genital and Gynecological Pathology

Amenorrhea, Impotence

This deficiency pathology is sometimes found among Yang Ming patients. A single physiopathological mechanism that affects the meridian Yang Ming causes amenorrhea among women and impotence among men. Modern authors call it the "descent of energy."[180] It is not impossible that this disorder corresponds to a more advanced and organic condition.

> The suffering of secondary Yang {Yang Ming} is manifested in the heart[181] and in the spleen; we find impotence and amenorrhea.

> If the illness is transmitted {from the stomach to the spleen} it becomes chachexia.[182]

The term cachexia is generally translated as "degenerative illness" by Chamfrault, according to whom it either corresponds to diabetes, tuberculosis or to cancer, depending on the context. But the *Su Wen* continues:

> If the illness is transmitted {from the large intestine to the lung} it
> becomes incurable suffocation.[183]

Here we find the thoracic and cardiovascular etiologies of Yang Ming (see cardiac lung). In other words, impotence and amenorrhea may represent a functional stage of Yang Ming imbalance, whose organic stage corresponds either to a degenerative disease with cachexia or to serious cardiac pathology. Apart from the points indicated elsewhere (see Dysmenorrhea of Tai Yin), we will retain quchi (LI-11), which corresponds to the semiology "absence of menses" in the *Da Cheng*.[184]

Rheumatological Pathology

Yang Ming subjects are very sensitive to hygrometric variations, as they are partly Earth and partly Metal, humidity and dryness. Shao Yang and Jue Yin rheumatism patients are, above all, sensitive to the wind and acute inflammatory pathology (arthritis, arthralgia). Tai Yang and Shao Yin patients are especially sensitive to variations in the temperature, mostly fearing the cold, but sometimes the heat (rheumatic fever). Yang Ming and Tai Yin patients are prime victims of hygrometric variations and fear the humidity, which aggravates their discomfort.

Subacute and Chronic Polyarthritis

Evolving chronic polyarthritis is a disorder that associates imbalances of Shao Yin and Tai Yin (see Rheumatology in Shao Yin), but that may also involve Shao Yin and Yang Ming. It is the relationship of Earth and Metal with collagen, which allows for the multiplicity of temperaments in this affection. Let us recall the words of Qi Bo:

> When humidity has affected the articulations for a long time, we must
> heat the needles and needle zusanli {ST-36}.[185]

In the same way, ankylosing spondylitis may occur among Yang Ming patients. In this case, the behavior and morbidity of the subject is very different from the same affection among Tai Yang subjects. For example, the classic spondylitis that strikes a patient who is already suffering from hemorrhagic coloproctitis is certainly Yang Ming in temperament.

One classic physiopathology of dorsalgia involves Yang Ming patients:

> Lumbago of the stomach meridian hinders the torsion of the trunk. If
> the patient tries to look backwards, the heart is tight. We needle
> zusanli three times. Do not bleed in the autumn.[186]

We must remember one last piece of advice: Autumn is the Metal season. The correlation with manganese-copper is developed in the corresponding discussion in Tai Yin.

Scapulo-Humeral Periarthritis

This affection, too, is specific to the Metal constitution.[187] Just as for the lung, the semiology of the primary channel of the large intestine is mentioned in the tenth chapter of the *Ling Shu:*

> Pain in the forepart of the shoulder, in the upper part of the arm, around the thumb and index finger.[188]

Further on, we find:

> In the problems that begin in the arm, we must needle the points of the large intestine and the lung meridians; as soon as we manage to make the patient perspire, he will be relieved.[189]

All acupuncturists have personal knowledge of this phenomenon of perspiration under the arms during treatment, particularly problems of this nature. Our choice of points is hegu (LI-4), quchi (LI-11) and jianyu (LI-15) homolaterally, perhaps combined with shangyang (LI-1) contralaterally. Jianyu (LI-15) must be needled using the hot needle method. The manganese-copper indication is obvious for these patients, who often present a combined pathology of chronic respiratory disorders (asthma, emphysema) or colon disorders (left-sided colitis), and often other associations (sinusitis, rhinitis, tooth decay).

Lumbago

Lumbago is common among Yang Ming patients. It involves the stomach meridian, as we have seen in the case of spondylitis. Pain caused by L4-L5 disk problems often occurs among these subjects and corresponds to a constitutional weakness of the large intestine. This is felt at the beishu point, dachangshu (BL-25), which is located on the horizontal of the L4-L5 intervertebrate space. In practice we often see patients suffering from chronic lumbago whose pain involves L4-L5 and who also suffer from periodic colitis. The onset is either simultaneous, one triggering the other, or they follow an alternating pattern, *i.e.,* when there is lumbago the colitic symptoms are absent and vice versa. It is not always the case, but most of the time sciatic problems found among Yang Ming patients involve L5, with radiation to the big toe where the stomach meridian-spleen meridian anastomosis is found. By way of comparison, S1 sciatica — location of the beishu point xiaochangshu (BL-27) of the small intestine — radiates to the heel and the fifth toe, which corresponds to the end of the bladder meridian (see Rheumatology of Tai Yang). Sciatica that involve considerable functional alteration or organic modification of the corresponding viscera are very difficult to treat since the pain is deep, dull and permanent.

Gonalgia

Gonalgia of articular or bony origin is linked to the stomach meridian. Its pathway travels through the external ligaments of the articulation and the patella. "Painful and swollen knee"[190] is mentioned as part of the semiology of the stomach meridian in the tenth chapter of the *Ling Shu*. In the twenty-sixth chapter we learn:

> When there is pain inside the knee, needle dubai {ST-35} with a needle whose point is very fine and whose body is very thick.[191]

The tendinomuscular channel of the stomach enters the two inferior angles of the patella[192] at the point xiyan, which means "eye of the knee," and at the most external point, dubai (ST-35).[193] These two points are indicated for arthrosis and arthritis of the knee. We must needle deeply, to a depth of 1 or 2 cm. Zusanli (ST-36) is indicated by the *Da Cheng* for "rheumatism in the knee, weak and painful knee."[194] This may explain why knee problems are common among Yang Ming subjects.

Endocrinological Pathology

Hypothyroidism

It goes without saying that dysthyroidism is responsive to acupuncture treatment. I have treated patients with biologically confirmed cases of hypothyroidism and have had success achieving biological normalization. Hypothyroidism coincides with a concurrent deficiency of Yang Ming and Tai Yin. This deficiency causes the inhibition of the phlegmatic subject's activity, rendering him apathetic. He becomes inactive and inhibited, behaving like the amorphous and apathetic Tai Yin, the temperament that is most predisposed to this pathology. I do not pretend to be able to treat the more advanced form of this affection (myxedema), but it is worth describing, if only to demonstrate the relationships between Tai Yin and Yang Ming.

The most frequent form of this disease consists of the progressive atrophy of the thyroid. Although the etiology is as yet unknown, it is probably the result of a viral affection. In acupuncture, we may interpret this as an attack of perverse cold, judging by the resulting symptoms. Perhaps the perverse cold initially invades Tai Yin, then spreads to Yang Ming, or, most likely, vice versa. In the semiology of the *Ling Shu,* we may read of the large intestine meridian:

> If there is cold, the patient becomes sensitive to the cold, and feels cold all along the pathway of the meridian.[195]

And for the stomach meridian:

> When there is a deficiency, there is a sensation of cold in the front half of the body.[196]

This fits well with these patients' sensitivity to cold, their hypothermia and the coldness of the integument. Their bovine obesity, moonlike faces, thick necks, massive thoraces and waxen skin correspond to a cutaneous mucosa infiltration, *i.e.,* a thickening and infiltration of the flesh, which is Tai Yin territory. This is just a morbid exaggeration of the usual amorphous (Tai Yin-spleen) morphology. The tongue is thick and broad (tongue = spleen). There is a loss of body hair, as in cases of lung imbalance (see Dermatology, Tai Yin), the hair is sparse, the fingernails brittle. A very characteristic feature is tooth decay.

In spite of all the "perverse cold" aspects of the symptomology, we find tooth decay and ruddy cheeks (the dwelling of Yang Ming), confirming the

345

possibility of suppuration in general, due to compression of perverse cold that is thus transformed to heat. This is particularly the case in the domains of ORL and stomatology, which are vulnerable among Yang Ming subjects (see sinusitis, rhinitis, angina, tooth decay and otitis). The slowing down of all psychomotor activity, which is a caricature of the Metal constitution or of the hyposthenic diathesis, is accompanied by a lack of concentration, poor memory and impaired imagination. We see a slowness in movement, which is cautious and kept to a minimum. Digestive problems are constant: constipation (Yang Ming) and anorexia (Tai Yin). Amenorrhea is common, as is a deficiency of libido and sterility (see Endocrinology above and in Tai Yin). We find bradycardia, but the heart appears big and spread out in the x-rays. When we examine by auscultation, it seems muffled and far away, which might indicate pericardiac effusion, as is sometimes the case. In Chinese medicine this may be explained by an insufficient rong energy coming from zu tai yin[197] to the heart meridian. This is very different from the cardiac erethism, typical in cases of excess of Yang Ming, and the beating of the pulse which is visible beneath the skin in cases of excess of xu li.

A more serious dimension of this energetic imbalance is represented by the myxedema coma accompanied by extreme bradycardia, a drop in blood pressure and marked hypothermia. The intense adrenal and renal insufficiency is in proportion to the deficiency of Shao Yin energy. The insufficiency was initially energetic. Shao Yin is not the first to be affected, but rather Tai Yin, which fails to pass on enough energy. Biologically, we notice normochromic anemia, or even pseudo-Biermerian macrocytic anemia caused by a vitamin B12 deficiency. This corresponds to the disturbance of the Earth viscera, stomach and spleen (for the connection between the spleen and hematopoiesis, see Hematology in Tai Yin). The perfect clinical correlation observed among Yang Ming, Tai Yin and hyperthyroidism is maintained in treatment. Zou Lien, in *La nouvelle science de l'acupuncture et des moxas,* indicates the Yang Ming points, hegu (LI-4), quchi (LI-11) and, locally, tiantu (CV-22) for this condition. We suggest tonifying zusanli (ST-36), whose semiology in the *Da Cheng* includes "swollen skin and great sensitivity to cold,"[198] and sanyinjiao (SP-6), which is indicated in amenorrhea, as are hegu (LI-4) and quchi (LI-11), the latter noted for cases of "the four limbs frozen."[199] We understand why. The spleen is incapable of circulating fluids for lack of energy.

We may needle these points, but moxibustion is even better. A very effective part of this treatment is massage of the cervical and cervico-occipital regions, the trapezius, the back muscles down to the first dorsal vertebrae, the front and sides of the neck, the lower mandible and the clavicles. This should be done in a very lively manner with the Chinese roller, with almost no pressure at all on the skin. This is how I have obtained good results in treating thyroid deficiencies.

The main points to be used are: LI-4, LI-11, CV-22, ST-36, and SP-6, with moxibustion and massage of the cervical region.

There is a good correlation with the trace elements:

Dysthyroidism may also be found in the hyposthenic diathesis (Metal) and may take on the aspect of hypothyroidism. The association of manganese-copper and opotherapy and iodine is indicated.[200]

If there is evidence of an incapacity to adapt (Earth constitution), Menetrier recommends the prescription of zinc-copper, which is particularly indicated in the Tai Yin-spleen temperament. The pituitary deficit that it implies may even represent hypopituitarism (see Tai Yin). The physiological relationship between thyroid and parathyroid (calcitonin) is now proven; their disorders seem to vary in an inverse proportion. Patients who present hypothyroidism often present hyper-parathyroidism, with its common digestive symptomology: nausea, vomiting, anorexia with loss of weight, gastroduodenal ulcer and organic pancreas disorders (chronic calcifying pancreatitis). In the etiologies of secondary hyperparathy-roidism, we find various deficiencies, gastrectomy aftereffects, chronic pan-creatitis and diarrhea.[201] These temperaments are Tai Yin and Yang Ming. The opposite, hyperthyroidism and hypoparathyroidism — with tetany and spasmophi-lia — are found among Shao Yang and Jue Yin subjects, Jue Yin more particularly for tetanoid syndromes and spasmophilia.

Diabetes

This is a disease that affects Yang Ming and Tai Yin subjects. It is discussed in the chapter devoted to Tai Yin.

Neurological Pathology

Cerebrovascular Accidents

The neurological pathology of Yang Ming is dominated by cerebrovascular accidents, including cerebral hemorrhage as well as cerebral ischemia. These accidents occur among patients suffering from high blood pressure, from atheroma or from cardiac syndromes. This is not surprising if we recall the plethoric profile of Yang Ming in excess with heat in the stomach. This constitutes an arterial ter-rain (atheroma, cardiopathy, arteritis and cor pulmonale) that is frequently aggra-vated when associated with diabetes.

• Physiopathology

Among these patients, the cephalic region is very sensitive, as the energy of Yang Ming, according to tradition, rules over the upper part of the body.

> Energy is a whole, but when energy acts in the upper part of the body, it is Yang Ming that represents it.[202]

Excess and deficiency of energy or of blood are linked to vasomotricity, which itself is linked to the cold and heat (atmospheric temperature, but also perverse energy and its accumulation in certain regions of the organism).

> Qi Bo explained, "Energy and blood like the heat and hate the cold; their circulations stop when it is cold and circulate only when it is warm. This is why, when energy is enclosed within the Yang, there is a deficiency of blood, and when the blood is enclosed within the Yin, there is a deficiency of energy."

> Huang Di then asked, "You are talking about deficiency. May there also be excess?"

347

> Qi Bo replied, "All the great and small secondary channels lead to the meridians. If the blood and the energy concentrate in a certain part of the body, there is excess. If the excess dwells in the head, there is apoplexy, occasionally with sudden death. Should the energy resume its circulation, the patient will live; if not, it means death."[203]

The same energy imbalance, termed an "excess of Yang," can cause agitated madness (see Psychiatry):

> The energy of Yang Ming is easily agitated, whereas that of Tai Yang and of Shao Yang is not.[204]

Husson's version is particularly interesting:

> Yang Ming is normally animated with pulsations — at the points renying {ST-9} and qishe {ST-11}. The same is not true for Tai Yang and Shao Yang, whose points tianrong {SI-17} and tianyou {TB-16}[205] are "animated" only in serious illness. It stops immediately if we stop eating.[206]

Fasting, or at least a prolonged diet, is likely to diminish the excess heat that is about to surge upward as "the destructive wind," and lead to "furious madness" or apoplexy, depending on the case. However, as we have seen:

> If there is an excess of energy with heat in Shao Yang as well as in Tai Yang, there will be congestion of blood with symptoms of feng.[207]

This means transformation of blocked heat into jue, the wind that destroys.

Among the vascular disorders that this internal wind may lead to is the cerebrovascular accident. The same description is indicated for Yang Ming in the fourth paragraph of the same chapter of the *Su Wen*.[208] Thus, we may understand the term zhong feng, or bian feng, describing the cerebrovascular accident, and generally translated as "the wind that goes straight to its target,"[209] refers to the upsurge of blocked heat, jue, that is transformed into wind and rises to disturb the circulation of energy and blood in the upper part of the body causing excess. The wind is an internal wind, an internal movement of energy, as we find in cardiac and acute pulmonary accidents in a subject of predisposed temperament. These occur in subjects under the stress of external perverse heat (or food), which triggers or aggravates this internal movement. We may say that the perverse heat attacks the bowel directly. Summer is a likely time for this to happen, as indicated in the *Su Wen:*

> Yang energy grows during the summer; if it is disturbed, sight and hearing problems will appear. If Yang energy is exacerbated, it takes to the head and will cause coma or syncope, and affect the muscles and the limbs. If the perspiration is too strong, hemiplegia may occur.[210]

This explains why summer cases of hemiplegia, which are most often of "bowel" origin, are easier to cure, as reads an ancient Japanese text:

348

> Those of the summer are as easy to cure as those of the autumn are difficult.[211]

Autumn cases are more specifically organ hemiplegia, vascular accidents that follow a deep metabolic disorder or a visceral organic affection, and are hard to treat.

In the chapter devoted to Tai Yin and Yang Ming, Qi Bo blames the possibility of a direct attack by the feng specifically on Yang Ming:

> The perverse energy that attacks the Yang is generally the feng; that attacking the Yin is generally the humidity. The Yin begins in the foot and rises towards the head, then passes into the upper limb to terminate in the fingers; the Yang begins at the fingers, goes to the head and then descends to the feet. {See the meridian pathways.}

> This is why, in aggression by the feng, it is always the upper part of the body that is affected.[212] In aggression by humidity, it is always the lower part of the body that is affected.[213]

Here we understand that it is possible for perverse wind to penetrate into the meridians and thus affect the body.

In the chapter of the *Su Wen* devoted to all the affections caused by the wind, the following discrimination is made. Huang Di asked:

> The aggression of the wind may cause either a cold heat or an internal heat, or an internal cold or a li feng, or a hemiplegia or a wind. So many illnesses with different names. No doubt they affect all the viscera internally. I don't understand, and would like to know your theory.

Qi Bo answered:

> When the wind is retained within the skin, it may neither enter into the interior of the body nor exit out of the body. The wind is mobile and changing. If the cutaneous orifices open, there is cold with shivering. If the orifices close, it is heat with languor. In case of cold, the appetite is diminished. In case of heat, the flesh is consumed. When the patient trembles and cannot eat, this is a "cold heat." When the wind penetrates into the stomach, through Yang Ming, and rises through this channel, it affects the internal angle of the eye. In a fat person, it may not dissipate to the outside, and causes interior heat (re zong) with yellow eyes.[214] In a thin person, it dissipates and is eliminated, causing an internal cold (han zong) with tears.[215]

We see here that the same perverse energy will have different effects on a patient, depending on his physical constitution. Once again we have a confirmation of the importance of constitutions and temperaments in Chinese medicine. We may relate this text to one we have already quoted concerning the cor pulmonale:

> If the carotid is agitated, the patient presents a cough with dyspnea, the internal corner of the eye is a bit swollen, at the point jingming

349

{BL-1}, there is a disturbance of the equilibrium of the organic fluids.[216]

It is the combination of external heat and wind that presents the highest risk of vascular accidents.

When there is an attack of feng and of Yang, without pain but with paralysis of the four limbs, without disturbing the mind of the patient who can still speak normally, the affection is curable. If he loses his capacity to speak, it is incurable.[217]

When there is an attack of this perverse energy, the mechanism will be as follows:

If the perverse energy attacks only one half of the body, it penetrates into the territory where rong and wei energies circulate. These energies go away, and in place of rong qi and wei qi there is only perverse energy, and hemiplegia settles in.

If the perverse energy is not so strong, then only one half of the body is painful.[218]

Everything tends to indicate that Yang Ming is the most sensitive of the meridians, the first to become agitated and cause cerebrovascular accident. This is seen in the pulse, in the premonitory symptoms and in the etiology of ischemia in particular.

• **Clinical Signs**

In the edifying chapter of the *Su Wen,* "Relations between the Pulses and the Arteries," Qi Bo says:

If the pulse of Yang Ming is dominant, this is a sign of excess Yang energy. We must disperse the Yang {stomach} and tonify the Yin {spleen} by needling the shu points of the lower limbs.[219]

A deficiency of the spleen accompanies this Yang Ming excess. This imbalance causes headache, among the dominant symptoms, most often with a rise in blood pressure. Such a headache is organic and is described in the *Ling Shu* in the chapter, "Disturbance of the Circulation of Energy." This physiopathology may, however, correspond to a purely functional headache as well (see Headaches, Tai Yin).

The disturbances of the circulation of energy cause headaches, with swollen face, and the patient has the feeling that the energy is rising and that he has malaise in the heart. We must needle zu yang ming {stomach meridian} and zu tai yin {spleen meridian}.[220]

Another passage from the same text:

In migraines with loss of memory, without specific localization of the pain, we must first needle the points on the artery of the head, on both sides {on the stomach meridian}, then the points of zu tai yin.[221]

350

This cephalic point seems to correspond to touwei (ST-8), located on the superficial temporal artery,[222] and not to renying (ST-9) as Chamfrault supposed, which is located on the neck.

For the point touwei (ST-8), the *Da Cheng* gives a richer and more significant symptomology than for renying (ST-9).[223] This includes hemiplegia with facial paralysis as well as migraine:

> Violent headache like a hatchet blow because of the feng, pain in the eyes and in the head, unclear vision {amaurosis, hemianopia}.[224]

We find also for this point:

> Cerebral congestion, hemiplegia, facial paralysis, numbness of the face.[225]

Thus, touwei (ST-8) corresponds to the treatment of migraine which is a warning symptom of cerebrovascular accidents. In the same chapter of the *Ling Shu* devoted to energy disturbances, we find:

> In migraines really the result of a serious disturbance of energy, the whole brain is painful, the limbs are frozen up to the elbows and knees. This affection is fatal: there is an attack of perverse energy; the head is the dwelling of the supreme Yang, it must not be entirely attacked.

The *Da Cheng* mentions another premonitory sign or alarm signal for cerebrovascular accidents, the intermittent claudication common to arterial disorders:

> One, two, three or more months before the apoplexy, from time to time and suddenly, the leg and foot become numb and heavy, with pain and paralysis. After a while it goes away, only to return. This is a precursory sign of apoplexy. Hasten to stimulate zusanli {ST-36} with three moxas and xuanzhong {GB-39} with three moxas.[226]

We will now study the clinical forms and etiologies of cerebrovascular accidents.

• **Etiological Forms**

Three texts enable us to discriminate between these forms: Zu Lien's *General Treatise on Acupuncture*, the *Trung Y Hoc* from Hanoi and the *Da Cheng*. In Zu Lien's *General Treatise on Acupuncture*, we read:

> The symptoms of gravity of the apoplexy attack are the following: the patient presents trismus, his eyes are closed {coma with total loss of consciousness}. He has incontinence of urine and fecal matter, and is stertorous.[227]

> We must then differentiate between apoplexy caused by an affection of the organs and that caused by an affection of the bowels.[228]

> If we are faced with an affection of the bowels[229] the patient presents hemiplegia with facial paralysis, but he can still feel pain. As he has

not lost his sensitivity, he is not in a coma, he can speak normally, and his complexion, by way of comparison with the organ apoplexy, is unchanged — he sometimes complains of itching. The illness heals more easily than that form caused by an illness of the organs.[230]

This is the symptomology of easily regressing superficial or temporary affections that may be more serious with coma. They relate more particularly to ischemia or an embolism, which does not exclude the possibility of hemorrhage or cerebral infarction.

Even if these signs get worse, with little alteration of consciousness, the etiology is clearly in favor of ischemia, which is classically more frequent (due to affection of the bowels). There are three possibilities: an affection of Yang Ming, of Shao Yang or of Tai Yang. The *General Treatise on Acupuncture* itself says:

In the apoplexy of the bowels, the stomach {Yang Ming} and the gallbladder {Shao Yang} are most often at the origin of the attack.[231]

In decreasing order, we will examine Yang Ming, Shao Yang, Tai Yang.

For a stroke, or for another accident of Yang Ming origin, the symptomology is as follows:

If the stomach is affected, the patient can neither eat nor drink, he has copious phlegm that comes to the mouth and has a dark yellow facial complexion.[232]

We may add that in this case, the symptomology will correspond to the deficit of the carotid region, on the pathway of the meridian, with hemiplegia, aphasia if the dominating territory is affected, and dominating brachiofacial paralysis if the deficit involves the superficial sylvian artery.

For a cerebral accident of Shao Yang origin, the symptomology is as follows:

If the gallbladder is the cause of the problem, the patient's eyes are always closed and his face is dark green.[233]

We may add here that the symptomology will correspond to a deficit of the vertebrobasilar territory, with sudden onset, posterior headache, dizziness and vomiting in the case of Wallenberg's syndrome (bulbar); and cerebellar syndromes[234] or hemianopia if other territories (peduncular, posterior cerebral) are affected. Awareness deficits, present in thrombosis of the basilar trunk, with sleepiness and akinetic mutism are comparable to the Chinese description of "closed eyes." If the cerebral accident is of Tai Yang origin, the symptomology will be posterior, as in the Shao Yang case. The onset is particularly brutal and might accompany an epileptic fit.

All these "bowel" affections are described in the chapter, "Ting Feng" of the *Trung Y Hoc* from Hanoi. According to this text, such a pathology corresponds to the direct penetration of the wind into the bowel or into its meridian,[235] and, we might add, to the transformation of the heat into the "wind that destroys" as mentioned in the chapter devoted to jue in the *Su Wen*. The *Trung Y*

Hoc distinguished two clinical forms. The first is the result of obstruction of energy and corresponds to jue:

> This affection is caused by excess, with the following manifestations: mouth shut {trismus}, reddish face, hands closed, gasping breath, sliding and hard pulse.[236]

The second is caused by the escape of energy:

> This affection is the result of deficiency with the following manifestations: eyes closed, mouth open, hands open, arms loose,[237] whistling breath with flaring nostrils, involuntary loss of urine, abundant perspiration, weak and small pulse.[238]

The latter form corresponds to organ apoplexy, identified by limb paralysis, which distinguishes it from bowel apoplexy.

The medieval text, *Yi Xue Ru Men,* also makes a distinction between two forms of apoplexy, the one due to obstruction and the other to escape — the one Yang and the other Yin. It makes the following comment:

> In the Yang disorder, the body is warm, in the Yin disorder the body is cold.[239]

The *General Treatise on Acupuncture* states:

> If it is an affection of the organs, the patient is in a coma. If he drools, his throat is obstructed with abundant phlegm, causing his breathing to seem more like growling. He presents paralysis, total loss of his senses and aphasia.[240] The illness will be difficult to cure.[241]

This clinical form is a serious cerebrovascular accident with continual coma and deficits that are hard to regress.[242] It may be the result of an escape of stomach energy (deficiency) concomitant with, or more probably, secondary to an aggravating obstruction of the corresponding bowel.[243] It also may be the result of a complete desertion due to the direct affection of the organ. Its etiology may be the perverse wind of the cerebrovascular accidents, but not exclusively. The word feng, which means wind, refers to a brutal and internal movement of energy within the body. This covers all the etiologies likely to bring on a coma. In the etiologies of ting feng (eight feng), the *Trung Y Hoc* notes eight possible physiopathologies of the coma:

— *Direct aggression by heat.* For example, external perverse heat, as in fulminating viral hepatitis.

— *Aggression from deficiency of energy.* This corresponds to the escape of energy of organic origin. The Yin of the exhausted organ is no longer sufficient to balance the Yang, whose natural tendency is to rise, and that escapes upwards, causing the feng. This aggression corresponds to all severe organ exhaustion, whatever may be the etiology, even perverse.

— *Direct aggression by cold.* Under this affection the *Trung Y Hoc* includes coma in patients buried beneath the snow (avalanche) as well as perverse cold that has evolved for a long time within the organ.

353

— *Direct aggression from humidity.* This is the case of neurological complications of neuropathy caused by humidity (see Tai Yin).

— *Aggression by psychic factors.* In Shao Yang, "an excess of anger may be fatal," etc.

— *Aggression by food.* Plethora is an antagonizing condition among Yang Ming subjects.

— *Aggression by toxic or vicious energy.* This corresponds to epidemics.

— *Aggression by perverse fire energy.* This is Yang heat energy. Its penetration or upsurge, typical in the Yang Ming bowel, or in others, corresponds to the "blockage of energy" etiology, or jue, and to bowel hemiplegia. These eight etiologies of comas have been described in detail by Nguyen Van Nghi.[244]

In summary, we may say that all the perverse energies (fire, heat, cold, humidity), as well as the psychic energies, food and epidemics, may directly affect the bowels, or deeply deteriorate the energy of the organs, thus leading to coma. Apoplectic comas or cerebrovascular accidents (CVA) are found in two forms: bowel apoplexy and organ apoplexy. In general, the perverse energy that penetrates directly and gives rise to "the wind that goes straight to its target" wounds the bowel. This corresponds to jue, energy blockage, and to our Western definition of CVA. It may cause a coma of varying depth with spasticity. This is bowel apoplexy. Such accidents may also be caused by energy desertion, particularly the energy of the liver or the heart, whose disturbance may lead to a CVA that is theoretically more severe with deep and flaccid coma. This is organ apoplexy.

This desertion of an organ's energy also describes imbalances that lead to the total deterioration of a viscera and to a terminal coma. For example, this is the meningeal hemorrhage of pulmonary tuberculosis, or the coma of chronic respiratory insufficiency. For the heart, this is the hemiplegia associated with Rendu-Osler-Weber's disease, or a cerebral embolism secondary to mitral stenosis, whose primary disorder involves Tai Yang. For the spleen desertion it is meningeal hemorrhage in spirochetosis with jaundice, or the cerebral metastasis secondary to leukemia or Hodgkin's disease. The kidney, when deserted, produces a terminal uremic coma associated with renal insufficiency; the liver, when deserted, produces the hepatic coma associated with cirrhosis.

However, the desertion of energy may take on a violent aspect without causing a CVA, as in acute atrophy of the liver. This occurs in fulminant hepatitis or in the hypothermic coma of subjects who are buried alive (Tai Yin). The semiology of these organ comas is hardly mentioned in Zu Lien's treatise on acupuncture, although in the *Trung Y Hoc* we read:

> In comas, if the liver is to blame, prior to the coma the patient would have been very sensitive to the cold. He would not perspire and his complexion would be greenish.

> If the heart is to blame, prior to the coma, the patient would be anxious.[245] His perspiration would be abundant and his complexion red.

If the spleen is to blame, the patient will have a fever, abundant perspiration and his complexion yellow. {This may represent cancer of the pancreas as well as spirochetosis, etc.}.

If the lungs are at the origin of this attack, prior to coma the patient would be sensitive to the feng. He would perspire abundantly and have a white complexion.

If the kidneys are to blame for this problem, the patient's body will be cold, his perspiration abundant and his complexion blackish {uremic coma}.[246]

Clinical Forms

The clinical forms of CVA may be defined, as these were categorized in ancient Chinese according to sex, laterality and age. In Chapter 48 of the *Su Wen* we read:

The stomach pulse is deep and undulating, but raspy. Associated with a small, hard and resistant heart pulse, it is a sign of hemiplegia. For men it will be on the left side, for women on the right; if the patient can speak, the illness is curable in thirty days. However if he can no longer speak, if the hemiplegia affects the left side in a man, the affection may heal after three years, unless the patient is under 25,[247] in which case he will die within three years.[248]

According to this text we understand that, more often than not, hemiplegia strikes men on the left and women on the right, and that these are the cases with a better prognosis. The *Yi Xue Ru Men* defines laterality according to physiopathology:

All hemiplegia is called bian feng {lateral wind}. In left-sided hemiplegia, there is a deficiency of blood, and fire and phlegm are affluent; the mouth cannot speak, the limbs cannot be raised. This is a weakness of blood.[249]

Weakness of blood, according to the *Su Wen*, implies excess of energy, as we saw in the physiopathology of blood congestion and the feng symptoms of Tai Yang, Shao Yang and Yang Ming: "There is a lack of blood and an excess of energy." Here we find that the aphasia is linked to a deficit of the dominating hemisphere (the left) and corresponds to a Yang etiology. This relates to an energy blockage (jue). In right-sided hemiplegia:

There is a deficiency of energy; fire and phlegm are replete in the right side; if the deficiency is extreme, there is urinary incontinence, snoring {stertor}, hypersialosis.[250]

This etiology corresponds to the desertion of energy. Incontinence is the Chinese indication of Yin deficiency. The text mentions quadriplegia, which is the combination of the two sides. In short, among male patients, the left-sided affection is the least serious. It represents the bowel etiology, jue. The right-sided attack is more serious and represents the organ etiology (Yin deficiency). Among women, the opposite is true.

Treatment

It is out of the question to discuss all the etiological treatments of CVA, particularly those of the five organs, cold, humidity, heat and emotional energy. The Yang etiologies, on the other hand, are worth expanding. The obstruction of energy from an excess of Yang in the bowels, or from the penetration of wind and heat into the meridians, is the most common cause of those vascular disorders that give rise to hemiplegia. Yang Ming subjects are the most susceptible. Treatment covers three aspects: emergency treatment of the coma, treatment of the aftereffects and preventive treatment.

• Emergency Treatment

In situations requiring emergency treatment, hemiplegia occurs as the result of a violent, global movement of energy towards the upper part of the body. The mechanism involves wei qi, the fierce defensive energy that is capable of sudden movement. In Chapter 52 of the *Ling Shu*, Qi Bo explains:

> When the meridians of the lower limbs are deficient, the patient feels as if his legs are frozen. When they are in excess, he feels that they are warm.

> When the meridians in the upper part of the body are deficient, the patient is dizzy;[251] if they are in excess, he feels painful heat in the upper part of the body. If there is excess in the upper part, we must needle to prevent it from rising.

> If there is deficiency, in the upper or lower part, we must draw energy there to reestablish the balance.[252]

The warning signs of excess in the upper part of the body relate to an excess of energy in Yang Ming and the stomach:

> When the thorax is swollen, the face is puffy as are the lips, and there is difficulty in speaking: if these symptoms arrive suddenly, unexpectedly, the points of the stomach meridian must be treated.[253]

We must remember that according to the *Su Wen*, Yang Ming is indicated in order to disperse both energy and blood.[254] Zu Lien has this to say:

> When the patient's face is red and puffy, his head hurts, he complains of dizziness, his pulse is ample, strong, rapid, he is about to go into a coma. We must needle or apply moxas immediately to draw the blood to another region of the body. We needle zusanli {ST-36}, shangjuxu {ST-37}, xiajuxu {ST-39}, sanyinjiao {SP-6}, hegu {LI-4}, shousanli {LI-10}.[255]

This treatment strengthens the energy of the spleen. If there is an excess of stomach energy, there is a deficiency of the spleen. In "Heat Diseases" in the *Ling Shu*, we note:

> In hemiplegia, if the patient is in pain, but does not lose his head, the illness is only in the flesh. We have only to stimulate with a big

needle, tonifying the deficiencies and dispersing excesses to obtain healing.[256]

The points indicated are those of Yang Ming. According to the modern Shanghai authors, hegu (LI-4) disperses heat.[257] This is also true of zusanli (ST-36), as indicated by Qi Bo in the *Ling Shu:*

> In illness resulting from an excess of the meridian or from congestion of blood, we must treat the stomach and needle its he point.[258]

The combination of zusanli (ST-36), shangjuxu (ST-37) and xiajuxu (ST-39) is important and deserves comment. In Chapter 54 of the *Su Wen,* the "Nine Ways of Needling," Qi Bo mentions these points:

> Zusanli {ST-36}, chongyang {ST-42},[259] shangjuxu {ST-37} and xiajuxu {ST-39} are very important points.[260]

Apart from chongyang, the three points are mentioned along with qichong in the *Su Wen* chapter, "The Art of Needling Affections Due to Perverse Yang":

> To disperse the Yang in the stomach, we use qichong {ST-30}, zusanli {ST-36}, shangjuxu {ST-37} and xiajuxu {ST-39}.[261]

It is no wonder that these points are indicated for CVA and hemiplegia.[262] Other points to be needled are: taodao (GV-12), wangu (SI-4), fengchi (GB-20), jianjing (GB-21), jianwaishu (LI-14) and jianzhongshu (SI-15).[263] These points have a global symptomatic action dispersing heat and feng in all the Yang: Tai Yang (small intestine), Shao Yang (gallbladder) and Yang Ming (stomach). In treating CVA before onset, we will utilize these points: ST-36, ST-37, ST-39, ST-30, SP-6, LI-4, LI-10, SI-4, GB-20, GV-12, SI-14 and SI-15.

• Treatment of Coma

Different protocols are recommended by classical authors. In cases of deep coma, the *Yi Xue Ru Men* reveals a curious technique:

> To save patients stricken with cerebral congestion, pull out the hair of the sinciput, over the forehead, and apply three to five moxas to the earlobes.[264]

This point is tinggong (SI-19), and is mentioned in the "Five Ways to Needle" in the *Ling Shu:*

> The second way consists in needling the shu points of the bowels: when one is suddenly struck deaf, or with ocular distress, we should needle tinggong {SI-19} over the earlobe. This point should be needled at noon. When we needle, the patient must block his nose[265] and this way the needling is more efficient. This point is to be needled as soon as one of the facial orifices is obstructed.[266]
>
> To needle in this way is to "emancipate."[267]

This point is, in all probability, the knot point of Yang Ming. Moxa applied here enables us to disperse the excess that is concentrated in the knot of the meridian.

357

The root of Yang Ming is the point lidui {ST-45}. The concentration, the knot of its energy is located between the ears and the maxilla.[268]

This is the approximate location of tinggong (SI-19). In the symptomology of the knot and root of Yang Ming we read:

If the axis {Shao Yang} fails to function and if there is paralysis of movement, we must needle Yang Ming, be it deficient or in excess.[269]

The symptomology thus corresponds to the location. The *General Treatise on Acupuncture* established this protocol:

When the patient is in a coma, with trismus and phlegm that obstructs his throat, we must bleed the shixuan points[270] and the ting points of all the meridians with a triangular needle.

This point is held to be fundamental by all authors, ancient and modern,[271] and is the classic treatment of deep coma, together with traction of the scalp at the sinciput and moxa at tinggong (SI-19).

• Treatment of CVA Without Loss of Consciousness

In cases of CVA without a loss of consciousness, such painful acts as described above must be avoided. A less unpleasant treatment is indicated for hyperthermic states caused by heat in Yang Ming and may be applied here:

If the patient presents a high fever throughout the body with delirium and visions, we must needle zu yang ming {stomach meridian} located on the capillaries. If there is congestion of blood there, we must bleed. In addition, with the patient lying on his back, we pinch the carotid between thumb and forefinger at the point renying {ST-9} for a rather long time, then we massage along the pathway of the meridians up to the clavicle. This is the art of dispersing heat.[272]

We may also add to this treatment the points mentioned in the discussion of precoma treatment. The *General Treatise on Acupuncture* indicates a slightly different protocol in cases of aphasia:

In apoplexy with Yang symptoms, the patient presents paralysis and aphasia. Needle hegu {LI-4}, jianyu {LI-15}, shousanli {LI-10}, zusanli {ST-36} and baihui {GV-20}.[273]

Moxibustion on baihui (GV-20) is indicated by all authors. Zu Lien also indicates certain Shao Yang points: fengchi (GB-20), jianjing (GB-21), huantiao (GB-30), yanglingquan (GB-34), as well as a single Tai Yang point, weizhong (BL-54). He describes a special technique for cases of hemiplegia, consisting of needling both sides of the body, starting with the unaffected side, before treating the paralyzed side.[274] If moxa is used, according to the *Da Cheng,* these must be applied on the opposite side.[275] Use of the heavenly window points, whose physiology was discussed in the introduction, is also justified and recommended.

It is necessary to determine which of the three Yang meridians is affected, and to take into account that two meridians may be combined. Physiologically:

> Shao Yang acts as an intermediary, it is the axis.

> If the axis does not function, and if there is paralysis, we must needle Yang Ming, be it in excess or deficient, for if the axis ceases to function, the energy circulating within the body stagnates and perverse energy will occupy the space where the body's energy no longer flows.[276]

If the obstruction is unilateral, the feng will occupy that space, as we have seen in our discussion of general physiopathology. This will cause hemiparesis, or even hemiplegia. The text goes on:

> If Shao Yang, the axis, does not function, the patient's muscles and articulations are relaxed to such an extent that he may no longer stand up. We must needle Shao Yang, after noting whether it is in excess or deficient.[277]

This is the reasoning that calls for the joint needling of zusanli (ST-36) and xuanzhong (GB-39) in the preventive treatment of CVA (see below). It justifies treatment of the Yang Ming knot, tinggong (SI-19), with needle or moxa, as we have seen in the treatment of comas.

We may make several remarks about the choice of xuanzhong (GB-39). First, Shao Yang is the axis, or the "hinge" that links the other two Yang meridians. This convergence of the three meridians occurs at two points, one in the arm on shou shao yang (triple burner) at sanyangluo (TB-8), the other in the leg, on zu shao yang (gallbladder) and xuanzhong (GB-39). These two points are among the four luo points, along with sanyinjiao (SP-6) and jianshi (PC-5) for the Yin meridians. Sanyangluo means "luo of the three Yang" and its semiology is presented in the *Da Cheng*. This semiology is purely neurological:

> Patients are fond of going to bed and sleeping, they show signs of obnubilation, are hard of hearing, suddenly become mute and do not want to move their limbs.[278]

The semiology of xuanzhong (GB-39) is as follows:

> There is a sensation of energy that rises to the upper part of the body, cerebral abscess or tumor, madness, anxiety, always angry and in a bad mood, after a fit of apoplexy, patients are paraplegic; epilepsy, paralysis of the feet.[279]

We read also:

> Epistaxis, sore throat {see ORL}, sensation of dryness in the nose, pain in the heart when he coughs, malaise and fullness in the chest with madness.

It is understandable that the modern Shanghai authors make use of this point in treating CVA motor aftereffects.

359

The multiplicity of bowel etiologies calls for discriminating use of the heavenly window points. Our choice of points will depend on neurological semiology. This depends, as always, on the energy level of the meridian's sensorial territory. As a rule, these symptoms are identical to the functional signs associated with a less serious affection.

The *Ling Shu* indicates:

> We needle futu {LI-18} for aphasia and we needle and bleed the points located at the base of the tongue simultaneously.[280]

Another heavenly window point is renying (ST-9):

> We needle renying {ST-9}, for violent pain in the head, when there is a sensation of fullness in the chest with respiratory difficulty. All these symptoms indicate that the energy cannot rise."[281]

This symptomology shows an affection of Yang Ming. As far as Shao Yang is concerned, the text indicates:

> We needle tianyou {TB-16} for sudden deafness or loss of visual acuity.[282]

And for Tai Yang:

> We needle tianzhu {BL-10} in presence of spasms, violent contractions, dizziness, when the patient cannot stand, and the feet will no longer hold up the body.[283]

To summarize the main points to be treated in CVA without coma, or as a treatment complementary to that recommended for coma, we have: LI-4, LI-10, LI-15, ST-36, ST-37, ST-39, GV-20, GB-20, GB-21, GB-30, GB-34, BL-40, GB-39, LU-9, LI-18, TB-16 and BL-10.

• Treatment of Aphasia

The *Da Cheng* indicates that aphasia with hemiplegia is difficult to cure. The *Ling Shu* claims that the disease is incurable when quadriplegia and aphasia are associated:

> When there is an attack of feng and of Yang, without pain and with paralysis of the four limbs, although the patient's mind is not overly disturbed, as he may still speak normally, the illness is curable. However, if the patient has lost the use of speech, it is incurable.[284]

The protocol recommended by the *Da Cheng* is baihui (GV-20) and qianding (GV-21) (seven moxas) for aphasia. The Shanghai authors indicate yamen (GV-15), tongli (HT-5), zhaohai (KI-6) and shanglingquan (M-HN-21).[285] We must remember futu (LI-18).

• Treatment of Headache

When there is headache, as in the case of accompanying migraines with motor deficits, we must follow the advice of the *Ling Shu:*

For migraine, we must not needle the beishu organ points. The same is true when there is a congestion of blood in a certain part of the body: we needle and bleed the painful points, but we do not needle the shu organ points, as these are not organic disorders but only energy circulation disturbances.[286]

Touwei (ST-8) is a good point to needle here, as we have seen.

• Treatment of Organ Apoplexy Due to Energy Desertion

Yin CVA caused by the escape of energy are common and call for the use of moxibustion with the beishu organ points to combat the extreme insufficiency of the corresponding organ. In these cases, we are not dealing with energy circulation disturbances, but with organ deficits. A prime example is hemiplegia secondary to the embolism associated with cardiac disease. The classic text, *One Thousand Golden Prescriptions,* referenced by the *Da Cheng,* advises:

> During apoplexy, if the heart is contracted, burn 100 moxas at xinshu {BL-15}, the beishu point of the heart, to dissipate this contraction.[287]

In the Yin form of cardiovascular accident, the points we find indicated are those intended to uplift the original energy, yuan qi, to come to the aid of the deficient Yin, no matter which of the organs are concerned. These are guanyuan (CV-4), the gate of the vital essence; qihai (CV-6), the sea of energy; and shenque (CV-8), treated with moxibustion.[288] The last point, shenque (CV-8), means "deficiency of the spirit" and corresponds to the navel.

• Treatment of Hemiplegia Aftereffects

We will discuss only the Shanghai protocol, which is well codified: electrostimulation of needles situated at the points hegu (LI-4), quchi (LI-11), jianyu (LI-15) and waiguan (TB-5) on the arm. On the leg, huantiao (GB-30), fengshi (GB-31), yanglingquan (GB-34) and xuanzhong (GB-39) are used. We choose groups of points surrounding the deficient muscles and deliver a low frequency, high intensity electrical current that elicits contraction of the muscles. This technique may be used without risk, according to Shanghai, as long as the blood pressure is not over 200/120. When improvement is slow, we apply moxa to shenque (CV-8).[289] Even when there is CVA caused by jue, that is, energy blockage in bowel apoplexy, the aftereffects may include exhaustion of the corresponding organ. Moxa on shenque (CV-8) will reinforce the central energy and is an indispensable part of the treatment.[290]

The meridian Yang Ming itself may show signs of exhaustion, with a high-low dissociation, described in the *Ling Shu:*

> If the energy of Yang Ming is exhausted, the eyes and the mouth move involuntarily, the patient is delirious, becomes anxious, his complexion is yellow. When the meridians above and below are in excess, but the energy does not circulate, there is death.[291]

This symptomology seems to correspond to the advanced aging associated with cerebral arteriosclerosis and infarction. This exhaustion of Yang Ming is clearly

361

similar to the desertion of organ energy, confirming once again the value of shenque (CV-8). This is not in contradiction with, but rather supports the possibility of a more focused cerebral infarction causing hemiplegia, or at least functional impotence. As we said earlier about the root and knot, check to see if there is excess or deficiency before needling.

• Preventive Treatment of Bowel Apoplexy

This treatment may be administered to patients who are imminently exposed to CVA, such as the plethoric, red-faced sanguine subjects, or those who present intermittent claudication, as the passage from the *Da Cheng* quoted above suggests. In this text, we will recall, we were urged to "hurry to simulate zusanli {ST-36} and xuanzhong {GB-39} with three moxas." The same text goes on:

> The moxas make the energy of the shock[292] leave the body through blisters. If this happens as spring gives way to summer, or as summer gives way to autumn, apply moxas, until both limbs produce blisters: the result is remarkable.[293]

The following bath therapy is subsequently indicated:

> Then take a raw onion, mint, willow leaves and che wei,[294] boil them, and add to the bath.

> If we don't trust these methods, and if we drink and eat without measure, with sexual intemperance, there will be sudden apoplexy.[295]

The text then gives another preventive therapy:

> We may also apply moxas to seven points: both zusanli {ST-36}, both xuanzhong {GB-39}, both earlobe tinggong {SI-19} and baihui {GV-20}. Three moxas to each point.[296]

This is not a bilateral treatment, as it is indicated:

> Affection on the right, moxas on the left; affection on the left, moxas on the right.[297]

The Shanghai authors recommend specific treatment of arterial hypertension and particularly, zusanli (ST-36); quchi (LI-11), needled deeply, as far as shaohai (HT-3); and taichong (LV-3).[298] To this treatment, I add the points shangjuxu (ST-37) and xiajuxu (ST-39).

• Preventive Treatment of Organ Apoplexy

A severe organ deficiency with an insufficiency of yuan qi necessitates preventive treatment with moxa at guanyuan (CV-4), qihai (CV-6) and shenque (CV-8). These are the three basic points of the most severe organic states. To these traditional points, Shanghai physicians add shenshu (BL-23), mingmen (GV-4), the point of origin of the kidney meridian, and shanzhong (CV-17), sea of energy point, with moxibustion.[299]

• **Treatment Conclusions**

The oriental literature dealing with CVA, ancient as well as modern, is rich, perfectly codified and coherent in so far as both diagnosis and treatment are concerned. All the ancient texts, the *Ling Shu,* the *Da Cheng* and Zu Lien's *General Treatise on Acupuncture,* claim relatively positive, rapid and complete results, depending on the clinical form of the affection and the age of the patient. Ischemic accidents, embolic or hemorrhagic, were already identified as the most common forms. The importance of Yang Ming, and particularly of the stomach and its meridian, was well known as early as the creation of the *Su Wen* and the *Ling Shu.* No matter which meridian is in excess, it is through the balancing of Yang Ming that we may regularize the excess in the upper part of the body.

There is every reason to attempt a systematic, long term program of acupuncture treatment under medical supervision in a public hospital. Today we are able to treat this pathology only symptomatically or through surgery, when possible. Recent Chinese research has shown that there are neurological zones that correspond to specific spots on the scalp. When craniopuncture is applied for these syndromes, the results are remarkable.[300] Here, more than elsewhere, we must try to initiate a collaboration between Eastern and Western medical paradigms, such as has been practiced in the People's Republic of China for the past 20 years.

As far as the correlation with the trace elements is concerned, CVA is not responsive to this therapy, although the degenerative vascular syndrome, atheroma and arteriosclerosis represent the inexorable evolution of all the other diatheses to the manganese-cobalt (Fire) diathesis, Diathesis III, the diathesis of old age. Menetrier indicates that the biological signs of aging should preferably be recognized early,[301] to attempt their stabilization by the prescription of manganese-cobalt. It is understandable that Yang subjects are more prone to this risk and that the premonitory techniques are of the utmost interest.

Psychiatric Pathology

As might be expected, the mental pathology found among Yang Ming patients depends on whether the pathological mode of Yang Ming is one of excess or of deficiency. The most common and well known is the excess mode that leads to manic behavior.

Manic Behavior

All the emotional symptoms of an excess of Yang Ming are described in Chapter 30 of the *Su Wen:*

First, the patient dislikes the heat.

The patient does not recognize family and friends.

He wants to get undressed, run naked, climb up everywhere, sing like a madman, swear at his parents: all these signs indicate an excess of Yang Ming.[302]

This manic agitation is the psychiatric form of an excess of Yang Ming, that may, given the right conditions, cause a fit of apoplexy in another patient. This symptomology is also described in the 10th Chapter of the *Ling Shu,* which includes a discussion of the semiology of the primary stomach channel:

> If the disturbance is severe, symptoms of excitation appear, the patient starts running like a madman, he wants to climb up high, to sing, to get undressed.[303]

Clearly the ancients held madness to be a disturbance of the stomach meridian. More precisely, in the same chapter, we find a link with the great luo of the stomach:

> If the luo channel of the stomach is in excess, this means madness.[304]

The sort of madness included in the semiology of the luo point of the stomach, fenglong (ST-40), corresponds exactly to the symptoms described above. The pathway of the luo channel of the stomach is described as:

> Rising to the upper part of the body, where it branches to the neck and head,[305] and from there, links up with the energy of the other meridians.[306]

The manic fit is caused by an excess of energy in Yang Ming that surges upwards, taking the shunt provided by the secondary luo channel. In the chapter of the *Su Wen* dealing with cardiovascular emergencies caused by blockage and upsurge of energy within Yang Ming, the Emperor asked Qi Bo to describe the symptoms corresponding to imbalance in the meridians. Qi Bo replied:

> In disturbances of Yang Ming, there are emotional troubles; the patient wants to run, to shout, he feels a fullness in the abdomen, heat in the face with blushing, he has hallucinations and his mind wanders.[307]

In order to understand all these symptoms, we may suggest two complementary interpretations, one energetic and the other psychological. The energetic interpretation is given by Qi Bo in Chapter 30 of the *Su Wen.* The psychological interpretation is my own.

The energetic interpretation of the symptoms is based on analogical reasoning. Though simplistic in appearance, it is the Chinese mode of perception.

> Huang Di asked, "When Yang Ming is gravely disturbed, the patient throws off his clothes to run around naked. He climbs to high places and sings. Sometimes he may go for days without eating, he jumps over walls and climbs up on roofs. He manages to climb up to places he normally couldn't reach. Is it the illness that gives him this capacity?"
>
> Qi Bo replied, "The limbs are connected to all the Yang meridians. When there is overabundance within the Yang, the limbs are sturdy and are able to climb."
>
> Huang Di asked, "Why does the patient throw off his clothes to run around naked?"

364

Qi Bo replied, "The body is too full of heat, and it is to cool off that he throws off his clothes and goes around naked."

Huang Di asked, "And his nonsense, his cursing, his singing and disregard for those around him?"

Qi Bo replied, "When a patient talks nonsense, curses and will listen to no one, this is an overabundance of Yang, and he refuses to eat because he is wandering around without his senses."[308]

The psychological interpretation is clear. In its physiopathology the manic fit occurs commonly among subjects with an Earth constitution, more particularly among Yang Ming subjects. These are the sanguine subjects, people who are joyful, carefree, sometimes impulsive, who enjoy jokes, puns, word games, tricks (see Berger), who fail to heed social conventions and take advantage of all sensory pleasures at the table as well as in bed. The psychiatric symptoms described above are only an exaggeration of the normal Yang Ming behavior and are the expression of an excess of the stomach meridian. Abuse of food or drink, special climatic circumstances such as intense heat, and psychological conditions such as frustration, are likely to cause the blockage of energy (jue) and the brutal upsurge that are responsible for the manic fit. Psychiatrists find that the initial occurrence of these episodes comes around the age of thirty, among subjects of stout constitution, especially women. Heymans and Wiersma, Dutch psychologists, confirm our observations. Among psychiatric decompensations of sanguine subjects they mention the manic fit.[309]

This is obvious when we analyze the Western semiology associated with loss of the senses: affective outbursts, increase in muscular force, psychomotor agitation, the sensation of fatigue, which has not been accorded much importance, insomnia, nonsensical speech with strange word games. The loss of the senses is linked to a disturbance of the yi (thought, reflexion, shen of Earth). Thoughts flow endlessly, giving the impression of great intellectual wealth. The manic fit appears to be a running wild of the native tendency to enjoy word games and associations. There is a loosening of the inhibitions.

The manic is left prey to his instincts, alimentary and sexual, and engages in orgiastic behavior.[310]

The comparison extends to more general behavior. The manic fit is described as either an absence of hunger or, on the contrary, an accentuation of hunger and thirst that leads to excesses of food and drink. There is a loss of weight (spleen) and a slight rise in temperature (heat, comparable to the thermophobia of Yang Ming described above). There is also constipation, coated tongue and warm breath (heat).[311]

The digestive symptomology shows the involvement of the Earth and of its two viscera in this pathology. The increase of the secretions, with hypersialosis and unending perspiration, concerns the stomach as well as the spleen (see Tai Yin). As is indicated in the *Su Wen:*

When there is an excess of Yang Ming in the pulse, we must disperse the Yang {stomach} and tonify the Yin {spleen}.

365

This excess of zu yang ming, particularly in its secondary channel, is necessarily accompanied by a deficiency of the spleen. The most eloquent proof of this is found in the indications of the tonification point of the spleen meridian. For dadu (SP-2), the tonification point, we find the following symptoms of deficiency:

Lack of moral conscience (perceives his desires and not their consequences), lack of internal discipline, lack of emotional control.

Inability to fix attention or to concentrate on any given subject.

Lack of associations. . . failure to compare new facts to past knowledge, believes all he is told.

Euphoric, outgoing, selfish, tactless.

Superficial spirit, without personality, lack of introspection, lack of perspicacity.[312]

The symptomology of the dispersion point is just the opposite, as we shall shortly see.

The treatment of manic fits is obvious. We must tonify the spleen meridian, but above all and to start with, we must disperse the luo channel of the stomach, with fenglong (ST-40), which means "contains the excess"[313] and then needle taibai (SP-3), the yuan point of the meridian, to shunt the excess of Yang of the stomach luo channel into the spleen, through the transverse luo channel. Taibai (SP-3) is indicated in the *Da Cheng* for "Agitation, revolt of energy."[314] We reinforce this action by tonifying dadu (SP-2), in the direction of the meridian.

We may complement this action by dispersing chongyang (ST-42). This point, which means the "assault of Yang," includes the symptomology of the manic fit as well as the neurovascular symptomology. It is to Yang Ming what taichong (LV-3) is to Jue Yin. One is called the "assault of Yang," the other the "supreme assault." It is also useful to disperse baihui (GV-20) and to stimulate it for a good while by hand. This treatment may be combined with the dietary advice found in the *Su Wen:*

Huang Di asked, "How does the furious madness come about?"

Qi Bo replied, "It comes from the Yang. Anger is caused by a brutal repression of the Yang, which is prevented from overflowing; this is a blockage of Yang {Yang jue}. . .

Abstention from food stops it immediately. Food enters the Yin, and makes it become Yang. Avoidance of nourishment stops this. We must have the patient drink water containing iron,[315] to stop the qi diseases."[316]

The points to remember in treating the manic fit are: ST-40, ST-42, SP-2, SP-3, GV-20.

If we were to prescribe a single trace element, it would be zinc-nickel-cobalt, although Menetrier indicates this treatment only for functional disturbances of mood and imagination of lesser gravity but identical to those presented in the manic fit. There is, nonetheless, an obvious correlation between the two systems of reference.

Melancholia and Obsessional Neurosis

The mental deficiency caused by a deficiency in Yang Ming is less well known. The semiology of the primary stomach channel is defined in the *Ling Shu:*

> The patient is very sensitive to the cold.[317] He whines and yawns frequently. His complexion is blackish. He is misanthropic and hates fire. He does not like to hear the sound made when wood is struck; he likes to be alone.[318]

This semiology may correspond to the fit of melancholia that follows the manic fit in bipolar cases of cyclothymia. This is the manic-depressive syndrome.

There is a sudden inversion. Yang Ming (stomach) is suddenly deficient and Tai Yin (spleen) is in excess. This is still a luo pathology, with a Yin-Yang alternation between the two Earth viscera, stomach and spleen. In the monopolar manic forms, there is only the excess of stomach and the deficiency of spleen that comes and goes with relative abruptness. In the monopolar depressive forms, there is only the deficiency of Yang Ming and excess of Tai Yin that brings on what we call melancholia or obsessional neurosis. The excess of spleen tends to aggravate a secondary deficiency of kidney (Earth destroys Water) when the origin of the imbalance, or the temperament, initially implicates the spleen (Yang Ming or Tai Yin apathetic subjects). In the monopolar form, when the patient is Shao Yin (see Melancholia of Shao Yin), the origin may be a primitive deficiency of kidney (depressive state), which increases the excess of spleen and aggravates the symptoms. Knowledge of a subject's temperament allows us to determine the organ initially responsible and thus to conceive the most sophisticated treatment.

A deficiency of Yang Ming that does not give rise to melancholia may elicit obsessional behavior. This is a disturbance of the yi, which is very different from the euphoric manic behavior. On the contrary, there is obsession: rigid preoccupations that are stuck in the mind, compulsions, acts or sequences of acts, always the same, that the compulsive patient feels forced to execute to avoid unbearable anxiety. Classical psychiatric literature stresses that obsessional and compulsive behavior is elaborated over a superstructure of asthenia or psychasthenia that we may relate to anergy (Water), or on the contrary, of an asthenic or anal nature that we relate to hyposthenia (Metal). In asthenic or anal forms of obsessional neurosis, depression is an exaggeration of the incapacity to take action, with doubt, indecision and scruples. The temperament of these subjects is Yang Ming (deficient). Their already phlegmatic activity is inhibited and they become overly apathetic.[319] "Their complexion is blackish,"[320] and this is striking, their faces and whole bodies look grey or dirty.[321]

As the symptomology is indicative of a deterioration of the yi,[322] the neuralgic points of the imbalance are located within the Earth. There is a deficiency of Yang Ming (stomach) and an excess of spleen. That the ancient Chinese knew all this is demonstrated by the semiology of the dispersion point of the spleen, shangqiu (SP-5), as given in the *Da Cheng:*

> Pessimism, worry about the future, exaggeration of the importance of problems, absence of joy, great sorrow, obsessions, scruples, excessive religiousness,[323] excessive altruism (to the point of being masochistic), nightmares, lack of appetite due to lack of spleen.[324]

367

The treatment of monopolar or bipolar melancholia involves the dispersion of gongsun (SP-4), the luo point of the spleen, and the tonification of chongyang (ST-42), the yuan point, reinforced by shangqiu (SP-5). Chongyang (ST-42) is indicated in the *Da Cheng* for:

> Yawning, shivering from the cold, lack of appetite, jumps at unexpected noises, at the cracking of wood.[325]

The fear of cracking wood is an excellent sign of a deficiency of Yang Ming, as we have seen in the *Ling Shu,* above. Husson translates this as follows:

> Huang Di asked, "When Yang Ming is diseased, the subject fears people and fire. A ringing bell does not upset him, but the resonance of wood frightens and contracts the patient. Why?"

> Qi Bo replied: "Yang Ming is the channel of the stomach, Earth. The Earth fears Wood, and this is why the sound of wood frightens."[326]

Tonifying the kidneys will help appease the spleen (see Melancholia in Shao Yin). In pure obsessional states, in absence of cyclothymia, we must concentrate on treating the spleen and the stomach, and stimulate the corresponding shu-mu points. To treat manic depressive patients in an effort to stabilize their condition between onsets of pathological behavior, it would seem logical to needle zusanli (ST-36) and sanyinjiao (SP-6) again and again.

Dermatological Pathology

Facial Complexion

The examination of a Yang Ming subject's complexion enables us to differentiate excess (sanguine, red-faced) and the deficiency (phlegmatic or apathetic, blackish or dark face) of Yang Ming at a glance.[327] In practice, I find that the theoretical distinction between apathetic (Tai Yin) and the phlegmatic (Yang Ming) subjects is not at all absolute. The pathological inhibition of activity makes a difference.

How to best distinguish between apathetic Tai Yin and apathetic Yang Ming patients? By their complexion. The apathetic Tai Yin is most often pale, white, tall and/or thin and often has blue eyes. His personality is often schizoid. The Yang Ming apathetic subject is, on the other hand, dark-skinned and grey. The eyes are most often brown. His personality is rather compulsive. His skin is dry and often prematurely wrinkled. At the age of 35, the Yang Ming channel deteriorates, the face begins to wilt[328] and the hair begins falling out.[329] Husson points out that "Yang Ming is visible in the hair and face."[330] Elsewhere, we read, "When dryness triumphs, it causes dessication."[331] Just looking at Yang Ming patients (Yang Ming-dryness) enables us to observe that they wrinkle more and at a younger age than others. This is especially the case of Yang Ming-Metal subjects.

Cutaneous Disorders

Because of the Metal aspect of the large intestine, Yang Ming patients have sensitive skin. All the cutaneous pathology studied in the chapter devoted to Tai Yin[332] may be found among these subjects: acne, eczema, urticaria, psoriasis, problems with the fingernails, hair and teeth. Very frequently there is hereditary premature baldness, which is logical, judging from what we have read in the *Su Wen* concerning the deficit of Yang Ming. In practice, we find that Yang Ming patients suffer less often from these disorders than do their Tai Yin counterparts. As children they less often have eczema and as teenagers they do not suffer nearly as much from acne.

ORL Pathology — Stomatology

Yang Ming is very involved in the ORL sphere, given its pathways around the nose, the ears, the sinuses and the pharynx. Yang Ming subjects are therefore especially exposed. Anatomically, the narrow link between the maxillaries, the dental alveoli and the sinuses lies in the middle of the intersection between shou yang ming (large intestine meridian) and zu yang ming (stomach meridian).

Sinusitis

This is a typical Yang Ming disorder, so much so that in the presence of sinusitis coupled with several other typical factors, we may diagnose a patient as being Yang Ming with little further investigation. Sinusitis strikes Earth and Metal subjects alike. On closer investigation we find that Yang Ming-Earth patients who suffer from this disorder were generally of Metal constitution in their childhood or adolescence and have evolved a Metal-Earth equilibrium or an Earth temperament. Sinusitis is classically a Yang Ming affection, resulting from the penetration of perverse energy into either the stomach or large intestine meridians, because of a constitutional or acquired weakness of the lungs, or of the element Metal. More precisely, there is a penetration of the organ, either the lung, or of the bowel, the large intestine, or of both. These are the viscera that govern the nose, ears, sinuses and maxillaries.

The perverse energy involved may be heat or cold. The patient interrogation will enable us to determine whether the disorder was triggered by summer heat or by overheated rooms. If we notice congestion, or pronounced erythrosis in the cheeks, we may conclude that perverse heat was the cause. When heat stagnates in a certain part of the body, it may lead to a stagnation of the blood that is responsible for suppuration. This is confirmed by Qi Bo:

> If perverse Yang energy {heat} is concentrated in a certain part of the body, which suppurates, we must also disperse the Yang.[333]

Therefore, when there is an attack by perverse heat, the production of pus is considerable whether it is drained or retained in the infected cavities.

If perverse cold is the triggering factor of the affection, there will be an abnormal sensitivity to cold and cold will be an aggravating factor. We might suppose that cases of cold sinusitis would be less purulent. This is true in general, but is not absolutely the case. We must understand:

> The compression of perverse cold that has invaded the body may transform it into heat. An excess of Yin may be transformed into Yang.

This is particularly true of anergic patients (Shao Yin). They will be affected by the cold in proportion to the kidney deficiency.

Perverse heat will tend to attack the stomach meridian, which is sensitive to heat, as we have seen. Perverse cold will tend to attack the large intestine meridian ("the lungs dislike the cold," lungs-Metal-large intestine). However, this distinction is not important, as the whole of Yang Ming is affected. For example, in contagion of infected cysts, or of atypical granuloma of the second premolars or the first and second molars, this is the case. The floor of the maxillary sinus is close to the roots of the teeth (see Stomatology, below). From the large intestine meridian the perverse energy may spread to the frontal sinus through its ascending pathway, from yingxiang (LI-20) to jingming (BL-1). The pathway is anastomotic with the stomach meridian at chengqi (ST-1). From there it passes to zanzhu (BL-2). In the same way, the perverse energy in the stomach meridian may reach the cheek, the concentration point of Yang Ming, and penetrate into the maxillary sinus, or reach zanzhu (BL-2).

Treatment of sinusitis has remained unchanged from ancient to modern times. It calls for needling hegu (LI-4) and quchi (LI-11) on the large intestine meridian, and zusanli (ST-36) and neiting (ST-44) on the stomach meridian. Neiting (ST-44) is needled only in sinusitis of perverse heat origin, as it is the rong point, the cold point that combats the heat. Other points may be stimulated to reinforce the treatment. In the *Elements of Chinese Medicine,* we read:

> In all affections of the nose, needle the points hegu {LI-4} and taichong {LV-3}.[334]

The relationship between the liver and the nose explains the choice of taichong, especially in cases of sinusitis, where the beginning of the disorder was induced by rhinitis that became chronic. The allergic aspect is obvious from the start.

The chapter devoted to key points in the *General Treatise on Acupuncture* says:

> In cases of coryza with red face, headache and fever, we needle the two key points lieque {LU-7} and zhaohai {KI-6}, as well as the points tongli {HT-5}, quchi {LI-11} and xuanzhong {GB-39}.[335]

As is developed in further detail in the chapters devoted to Shao Yin and Tai Yin, the relationship between the kidneys and the lungs is fundamental. Zhaohai (KI-6) and lieque (LU-7) are the key points of yin qiao mai and ren mai. These are, as is written in the *Da Cheng,* "The two miscellaneous channels linked to the rhino-pharynx and the lungs."[336] Tongli (HT-5), the luo point of the heart meridian, is one of the paths leading to the face (sinus and eyes) that the perverse energy takes in Shao Yin. In the *Da Cheng,* tongli is indicated for:

Lack of energy, hot face, headache, sore throat, pain and congestion of blood in the eyes.[337]

Given the allergic aspect of these symptoms, xuanzhong (GB-39) may be a useful complement when a Wood constitution is mixed with Yang Ming. It is the equivalent of and acts in synergy with taichong (LV-3). Two other fundamental points are local points: yingxiang (LI-20), which acts against all nose affections, from rhinorrhea to sinusitis, and zanzhu (BL-2), the point of concentration of excess energy in the frontal sinus. This point must be needled and bled (with the triangular needle).

Acupuncture treatment of sinusitis is consistently effective; the results are fast and long lasting. Most acupuncturists attest to this. It enables patients to remain symptom-free for long periods between recurrences. Other treatments fail to do so. A series of 10 to 20 sessions (two to three per week), depending on the gravity of the case, should be undertaken at the onset of symptoms for maximum efficacy. I find that an average of one to four series with an interval of from three to six months, then one to two years, will remove this painful and handicapping affliction forever. The main points to be retained here are: KI-6, LU-7, LI-4, LI-11, ST-36, ST-44, HT-5, GB-39, LV-3, LI-20 and BL-2.

Trace element therapy enjoys an equivalent reputation if properly prescribed. Once again, the correlation with acupuncture is clear and precise. Menetrier says:

> In cases of sinusitis,[338] the hyposthenic profile is the most common,[339] associating physical, intellectual or emotional fatigue with intestinal problems, *i.e.,* left-sided colitis. The action of manganese-copper and of sulfur is often positive.[340]

This is the equivalent of needling the Yang Ming points. Menetrier adds that this action may be complemented in cases of allergic manifestation. This is exactly what we do with taichong (LV-3) and xuanzhong (GB-39). In cases with recurring infections, we identify the anergic profile and we must add copper-gold-silver. This corresponds to the kidney-adrenal deficiency described by Chinese medicine and its indication of the key points zhaohai (KI-6) and lieque (LU-7), along with tongli (HT-5, shou shao yin), to aid the lung and stimulate the defenses. In practice, we find that the association of acupuncture and trace element therapy is useful for a number of reasons. The results are fast and nearly total. We may reduce the number of acupuncture sessions prescribed, lengthen the interval between recurrences and increase the chances of a permanent cure. In acute cases,[341] phytotherapy can add a natural antibiotic action that is very effective. This enables us to avoid chemical antibiotics in almost all cases, a fact appreciated by these subjects who have such sensitive colons.

Chronic Rhinitis

These cases of rhinitis are quite different from the acute seasonal allergic rhinitis common among subjects of Wood constitution (see Shao Yang, Jue Yin). Such a case may, however, follow acute rhinitis. These are typically obstructive cases, with stuffed, dry nose. Most cases of Yang Ming rhinitis are characterized by rhinorrhea with a clear fluid that runs all the time. This signals an imbalance in Yang Ming caused by perverse cold energy. The physiopathology is exactly that of sinusitis caused by cold, except that here the cold is not compressed into Yang, does not transform into heat and remains chronic. The cold attacks the cavities defended by Yang Ming.

Treatment is approximately the same: hegu (LI-4), quchi (LI-11), yingxiang (LI-20), zusanli (ST-36), taichong (LV-3). The results are improved if we bring heat to these points with moxa or if we combine the jing (heat) points of the Yang Ming meridians: yangxi (LI-5) and jiexi (ST-41), using moxa as well. In trace element therapy for chronic rhinitis, Menetrier indicates manganese-copper and manganese, as well as sulfur, to treat the allergic aspect.

Tonsillitis, Sore Throat

Of all the energetic etiologies of sore throats, Yang Ming is commonly involved, especially in acute bacterial or viral infections among adults. Chapter 10 of the *Ling Shu,* dealing with the semiology of the meridians, tells us that disturbances in the heart, kidney (Shao Yin), small intestine (Tai Yang) and triple burner (Shao Yang) meridians may lead to sore throats, as may disturbances in the stomach and large intestine meridians. Here again we are shown the importance of determining the constitution and the temperament of a patient to determine precisely which meridian is likely to be imbalanced and thus to heed treatment.

In the semiology of the large intestine, we read:

The eyes are yellowish, the mouth is dry, there is epistaxis,[342] we may find a sore throat.[343]

For the semiology of the stomach, we find:

All disorders relating to blood disturbances must be treated through this meridian: epistaxis, sore throat, etc.[344]

There may also be a penetration of perverse energy in the longitudinal luo channel of the stomach:

If there is an imbalance of energy in this channel, the patient has a sore throat and becomes suddenly mute.[345]

Qi Bo states, in the chapter titled, "Various diseases":

In cases of tonsillitis that impedes speech, we must needle the points of the stomach meridian. If the patient can speak, we must needle the points of the large intestine meridian.[346]

Apart from perverse energy aggressions, a blockage of rong energy within the large intestine meridian may elicit the same symptom:

If there is blockage of the energy (jue) in the meridian shou yang ming with pain and swelling in the throat, we must needle the points of the large intestine meridian.[347]

We may conclude that this specific physiopathology corresponds to very bad sore throats, as the affection is one of blockage (jue).

Acupuncture treatment of Yang Ming tonsillitis focuses on the points hegu (LI-4), quchi (LI-11) and fenglong (ST-40).[348] The point hegu (LI-4) is the master point for this illness and may be needled no matter what the etiology. The classical indication of key points found in the *General Treatise on Acupuncture* leads us to add gongsun (SP-4) and neiguan (PC-6). If the throat seems obstructed, the key points of Tai Yang, houxi (SI-3) and shenmai (BL-62), may be added as well. If swallowing is impossible,[349] a sign of perverse heat in shou tai yang, the cold point qiangu (SI-2) is indicated.[350] The key points zhaohai (KI-6) and lieque (LU-7) must not be neglected, particularly if there is a history of repeated sore throats and an anergic terrain (weakness of zu shao yin).[351]

An excellent technique for treating sore throats among Yang Ming or Tai Yin patients with respiratory sensitivity is indicated for sore throats with white spots in the *General Treatise on Acupuncture*. We are advised to needle shaoshang (LU-11) and hegu (LI-4) contralaterally. Among Yang Ming subjects, we will primarily needle the points of the corresponding meridian.

There is a good correspondence with trace element therapy. Manganese-copper is indicated, combined with bismuth.

Tinnitus, Hearing Loss and Deafness

We must differentiate between auditory deficits of internal and external origin. Among those of external origin, we find acute or chronic labyrinthitis, post-traumatic complications, otitis complications, ototoxic drugs (antibiotics, among others), serious otitis (with aseptic inflammatory effusion), acute or chronic otitis. We may also include sudden deafness, either infectious (parotitis)[352] or vascular. In the latter case, which is a medical emergency, acupuncture is only an adjunctive therapy where vasodilator treatment is prescribed.

Auditory deficits among Yang Ming patients that are of internal origin include loss of cochlear perception as a result of degeneration (atherosclerosis), as well as central nervous system degeneration (vascular disorders). These are covered in the chapters dealing with Shao Yang and Tai Yang. We will discuss here only the etiologies of perception or transmission deficits that are likely to be influenced by acupuncture. Each of these involves Yang Ming.

Huang Di inquired about buzzing in the ears and Qi Bo had this to say:

> The ear is also a meeting point of the ancestral energies (zong qi).[353]
> When the stomach is deficient, the ancestral channel xu li is also deficient. The energy collapses to the lower part of the body and causes buzzing in the ears. We must tonify shaoshang {LU-11}.[354]

The ting point of the lung, shaoshang (LU-11) draws energy upwards when xu li fails to do so. Further on we read:

> When there is a deficiency of energy in the upper part of the body we hear a buzzing in the ears, we feel dizzy. In this case, we must also needle kunlun {BL-60}.[355]

Acupuncture is especially effective for serous and chronic cases of otitis, more so than in acute otitis. Their etiologies essentially consist of rhinopharyngitis among children and acute or chronic sinusitis. This is why rhinopharyngitis, sinusitis and serous or chronic otitis represent a single physiopathological entity in Chinese medicine where treatment focuses on the initial cause.

When the initial affection is otitis and if it becomes acute or chronic and recurring, we must track down the perverse energy that is responsible. This will be found within Yang Ming:

> If the perverse energy lodges in the secondary luo of the shou yang ming meridian {large intestine},[356] there may be an intermittent loss of hearing; the patient can hear and then he is deaf. We must needle shangyang {LI-1} and shaoshang {LU-11}. The patient will be able to hear at once.
>
> If there is no improvement, we must needle the point zhongchong {PC-9} on the opposite side.[357]

The last point relates to a vascular etiology, or more precisely, to a vasomotor etiology. This was not unknown to the Chinese (see Meniere's disease in Jue Yin):

> If the patient is permanently deaf, we must not needle these points, as the deafness is not due to perverse energy: it is an essential deafness {Shao Yang deafness, for example}. If the patient hears buzzing like the noise of the wind in the ears, we must needle the points mentioned above.[358]

These points, shaoshang (LU-11) and shangyang (LI-1), in association with kunlun (BL-60), are indicated for all cases of loss of hearing with or without dizziness of degenerative or vascular origin. Qi Bo makes a clear distinction between deafness caused by infection and deafness caused by degenerative or central nervous system factors. The main points to remember are: LU-11, LI-1, BL-60 and PC-9.

In acute or chronic serous otitis, manganese-copper is the basic trace element.

Epistaxis (Niu Xue)

A common medical emergency, epistaxis is a symptom that deserves special attention in the realm of ORL pathology. Most often the cause is local. However, in almost 10 percent of all cases, the problem is serious because of the abundance of bleeding, which necessitates rapid care, or because of the location of the bleeding. Epistaxis is, above all, an etiological problem. The causes are as multiple in Western medicine as in Chinese medicine, where there are several different physiopathologies. Before discussing the local causes, which are the most common, we will deal with the other etiologies. Among these, epistaxis may be the result of imbalances in Tai Yang, Jue Yin, Tai Yin, Shao Yin and Shao Yang. In the ORL sphere, a Yang Ming etiology is the most common.

• Tai Yang Epistaxis

Apart from epistaxis of local origin (ORL), in which Tai Yang may be active, we come across Tai Yang epistaxis in general affections. In the semiology of the primary channel of the bladder, the symptoms of excess, which may be isolated or compounded are:

374

Headache, pain at the top of the head {around the roots of the hair from GV-22 to GV-24}, torticollis, yellowish eyes with abundant tears, acute back pain, epistaxis.[359]

Tai Yang epistaxis may be caused by a more or less serious general infection. When there is blockage of the energy (jue) within Tai Yang, this is the case. The energy may surge upward as "the wind that destroys":

In imbalances in Tai Yang with coma, vomiting blood or frequent epistaxis, we must needle the points of the bladder meridian.[360]

Here, we are dealing with the cerebrovascular accidents among Tai Yang patients who suffer from high blood pressure or arteriosclerosis. Epistaxis is a way of escape for the excess heat of the blood within the head.

Tai Yang epistaxis may also be the first sign of aggression of perverse heat energy in this meridian, which produces other affections. This is the case in Rendu-Osler-Weber's disease, where epistaxis may endanger the life of the patient (see Cardiology in Tai Yang). Thus, the *General Treatise of Acupuncture* gives the key points of Tai Yang for epistaxis as houxi (SI-3) and shenmai (BL-62).[361] These are confirmed in the *Da Cheng,* which also gives the two rong-cold points of Tai Yang, qiangu (SI-2) and tonggu (BL-66).[362] In Chapter 26 of the *Ling Shu* there is a whole paragraph devoted to the treatment of continuous epistaxis with the points of Tai Yang:

Epistaxis that does not stop: if black blood flows abundantly, needle zu tai yang {bladder}; if the blood only trickles, needle shou tai yang {small intestine}. If we do not manage to stop the bleeding in spite of this treatment, we must needle houxi {SI-3}. If there is still no result, we must bleed the point weizhong {BL-40}.[363]

• Shao Yin and Jue Yin Epistaxis

"The liver produces the blood." We may therefore expect that functional disturbances of the liver will lead to coagulation problems and epistaxis. This is logical when we consider the cephalic and nasal pathways of the liver meridian. These cases include hemophiliac patients or those suffering from perverse heat aggressions, the best example of which is a case of epistaxis secondary to thrombocytopenic purpura or thrombocytopathic purpura. Here, the initial aggression is against Shao Yin [364] then passing to Jue Yin (liver). Qi Bo says,

When the perverse Yang {heat} passes from the kidneys to the liver, the patient is anxious and presents epistaxis.[365]

Because of the perverse heat the syndrome is probably infectious. This is confirmed in the description of the pulse of the liver:

If the pulse of the liver is ample, there is abscess, vomiting and frequent epistaxis.[366]

This is further confirmed in the chapter on "The Yang {Heat} Illnesses" in the *Ling Shu:*

375

In cases of fever with pain in the head, trembling of the lips and eyes and frequent epistaxis, we must needle the liver meridian.[367]

It is logical that ququan (LV-8), the cold and Water point of the liver meridian, is indicated here. This point ameliorates disturbances of the blood of the liver. The beishu points, ganshu (BL-18) and shenshu (BL-23), used classically to disperse heat, are also indicated.

Apart from serious organic pathology that may affect the liver (Jue Yin), epistaxis may be the result of a functional disturbance, either within the ORL sphere or in a disturbance of the endocrine aspect of zu jue yin. This is the case of catamenial epistaxis that most commonly occurs in the context of dysmenorrhea of ''dark liver'' origin. We also find cases of epistaxis with abundant bleeding during pregnancy because of the disturbance of the blood and the chong mai-ren mai equilibrium. These affect Jue Yin.[368] The main point to needle in these cases is ququan (LV-8).[369]

• **Tai Yin Epistaxis**

This problem signals the terminal stage of infectious pulmonary pathology. Perverse heat energy is responsible and has ravaged a weakened terrain:

If the patient coughs, with epistaxis, and if he cannot perspire, or if he perspires, he does not do so from the surface of the arms, this is a sign of approaching death.[370]

This is one of the nine cases of fever due to perverse heat in which acupuncture is contraindicated.

Epistaxis may also reveal a liver-lung conflict, as is mentioned in the chapter ''Shiver or Fever'' of the *Ling Shu:*

We needle tianfu {LU-3}[371] when the patient is suddenly thirsty. The lung and the liver fight each other, the patient has epistaxis and bleeds from the mouth.[372]

The perverse energy that has reached the liver tries to insult the lung. The lung defends itself, if it is in good condition, but the perverse energy tries to invade the lung through the terminal anastomosis of the liver meridian that passes its energy to the lung. Jue Yin is the end of Yin, the last meridian before the return to the lung. This battle causes the internal compression of the energy, creating intense heat that stagnates, causing epistaxis, hemoptysis and thirst.

The therapeutic solution is to needle tianfu (LU-3), the heavenly window point that, with tianchi (PC-1), regulates the energy and blocked blood.

• **Epistaxis in ORL**

Epistaxis may accompany infections or inflammations in the ORL sphere, such as chronic infection of the nasal fossa or of the sinuses (not to speak of nasopharyngeal fibroma or other benign or malignant tumors). The preponderant imbalance of Yang Ming that produces sinusitis, rhinitis or rhinopharyngitis is responsible for the concomitant epistaxis. This is particularly common among children. In Western medicine we say that epistaxis is secondary to the inflammation; in Chinese medicine, the bleeding is seen as the result of excess heat accumulated in Yang Ming. In Chapter 10 of the *Ling Shu*, which discusses the semiology of the primary channels, epistaxis is related as much to the large intestine meridian as to the stomach. Aggression of perverse heat energy against the longitudinal luo channel of the stomach may also cause epistaxis:

> If the perverse energy lodges in the secondary channel of the meridian zu yang ming, this may cause epistaxis, the sensation of cold in the upper teeth; in this case we must needle the points lidui {ST-45} and neiting {ST-44} on the side opposite the affection.[373]

Thus, if there is bleeding from a single nostril, which is most often the case, we must needle the stomach meridian on the foot of the opposite side. This is an excellent symptomatic treatment for epistaxis. Even recurring epistaxis concomitant to infectious or inflammatory pathology (sinusitis, rhinitis) will respond to this etiological treatment. The important thing is to not confuse this with Tai Yang or Jue Yin epistaxis.

Jue Yin epistaxis goes hand in hand with springtime rhinitis and may be associated with chronic nasal or sinus affections (see Sinusitis). It will respond to stimulation of taichong (LV-3). I find that epistaxis is not uncommon in the springtime. Qi Bo says:

> The perverse feng of the springtime causes headaches and pain in the neck. This is also the reason that patients present epistaxis in the spring.[374]

Here we have, in a nutshell, the difference between infectious and allergic rhinitis. In the former, it is mainly Yang Ming that is affected and the perverse energy is heat or cold. In the latter, Jue Yin (liver) is mainly affected and the wind, feng, is the perverse energy at work, the wind that blows in the spring. The functional energetic condition of the liver is decisive. We must never wound this condition, even by therapeutic means. Remember the advice of the ancient physician:

> When we practice acupuncture on the ting and rong points during the winter, there will certainly be no epistaxis in the springtime.[375]

These are the classic points to be needled during winter. If we do indeed treat these points at the appropriate time of the year, and if we do not weaken the kidney during the winter, it will harmoniously pass on its energy to the liver in the spring. There will be no hepatic insufficiency to cause epistaxis.

The point xuanzhong (GB-39) is indicated whenever Shao Yang or the gallbladder influence the course of infectious rhinitis or sinusitis. Qi Bo says, in the *Su Wen:*

> When the perverse Yang {heat} passes from the gallbladder to the brain, the patient has rhinorrhea with cloudy fluid, followed by epistaxis. In addition, the patient cannot open his eyes.[376]

One last physiopathology of epistaxis deserves mention. This is the deficiency of the luo channel of the bladder (zu tai yang). This channel in excess causes head cold symptoms: stuffed up nose, headaches, dorsalgia.[377] In cases of deficiency, the symptomology of the luo channel of the bladder is "epistaxis."[378] This deficiency of the luo channel of the bladder may also be associated with an imbalance of Yang Ming in acute or chronic affections of the cavum and the sinuses. Occasionally it is isolated, but only in subjects who are exclusively Tai Yang. The point to needle, for cases of either excess or deficiency, is jinggu (BL-64), the yuan point of the bladder meridian.[379] The *Da Cheng* indicates tongtian (BL-7) as well. This may be explained by the pathway of the meridian and the accompanying symptomology. The popular expression "head cold" ("brain cold" in French) is absolutely justified.

Essential Epistaxis

In a good many cases we are unable to explain the etiology of epistaxis in spite of repeated clinical and paraclinical examination performed by specialists. In Western medicine this is called essential epistaxis. In Chinese medicine, we may always find a cause that is related to an imbalance of energy within one or more meridians. Sometimes there is a link with the menstrual period, but not necessarily the accompanying dysmenorrhea. Rather, the epistaxis appears along with ammenorrhea, which orients our investigation towards the liver (Jue Yin). As we read in the *Da Cheng*, "Women whose periods do not come, often present epistaxis."[380] In other cases, the study of the patient's behavior, functional signs in other spheres, periodicity of the bleeding and the precise time of day that the bleeding occurs will generally help us to identify which of the meridians is to blame.

In conclusion, this symptom is more often than not benign. It can be easily dispatched by an acupuncturist who always has his needles handy. Circumstances do not always permit hemostasis with the classical materials, catheters, cotton pledgets, silk sutures and gauze needed to pack the nose and stop the bleeding. More importantly, the Chinese symptomology enables us to understand the etiology to an extent far greater than that of Western medicine.

Pathology in Stomatology

Pathology in the sphere of stomatology is essentially dominated by Yang Ming.

• Hyposialosis — Xerostomia

In the semiology of the large intestine meridian, we read, "It is the primary channel that regulates the production of saliva."[381] This physiology is also related to the spleen meridian (zu tai yin). Hypersialosis is directly related to the disturbances of the spleen (see Tai Yin). A dry mouth, on the other hand, often implicates shou yang ming.

> In cases where the large intestine meridian is affected, the mouth is dry.[382]

We may conclude, in this case, that we are dealing with perverse heat and needle the rong-cold point, erjian (LI-2).

• Gingivostomatitis

Gingivostomatitis of local origin (tartaric, odontic, prosthetic) due to unhealthy teeth, is related to the pathology of the teeth and signals an imbalance of Yang Ming. This is indicated in the *Ling Shu,* especially as it concerns the luo channel of the large intestine meridian:

> If the luo channel of shou yang ming is in excess, we find toothache,
> pain in the gums. If there is a deficiency, there is a sensation of cold
> in the gums and in the teeth.[383]

In a condition of excess, we needle the luo point of the meridian, pianli (LI-6). In one of deficiency, or if there is no symptomology indicating perverse heat (infection), we needle lieque (LU-7) and hegu (LI-4). Gingivostomatitis secondary to generalized affections, such as eruptive fever, infections, hemopathy, lead poisoning or drug intolerances, are linked to disturbances of Tai Yin, particularly to those involving the spleen and its meridian, zu tai yin (see Tai Yin).

• Toothache, Tooth Decay, Pyorrheal Abscess

Miller's theory on the etiology of tooth decay — as a result of the acidogenous catabolism of carbohydrates — was confirmed by the research done by Gustafson in 1958. The role of sugar, the flavor linked to the element Earth, is likely to affect the organs associated with that element, the mouth and the teeth. This may explain why Yang Ming subjects, because of constitutional weakness of the stomach and its meridian, are particularly vulnerable to tooth decay and to the whole range of infectious pathology involving the mouth. The formation of tooth decay requires, however, the intervention of some external factor, *i.e.,* bacteria and their enzymes. The action of these enzymes is twofold. They proteolyze and hydrolyze the organic substances of the enamel and dentine. This leeches calcium and thus demineralizes the tooth. This may simply be called perverse heat in Chinese medicine; perverse energy that invades Yang Ming and lodges in the maxillae along the buccal pathway of its meridians. Toothaches are included in the semiology of the primary stomach and large intestine channels described in the *Ling Shu*. They are consecutive to an aggression against the luo channels of the large intestine: "If there is excess, we find toothache."[394] They follow as well an agression against the luo of the stomach:

> If the energy lodges in the secondary channel of the meridian zu yang
> ming, it may cause the sensation of cold in the teeth of the maxilla;
> we must in this case needle the points lidui {ST-45} and neiting
> {ST-44} on the opposite side.[385]

This is the same mechanism that produces certain cases of epistaxis, as we have seen above, and the treatment is the same. The sensation of cold in the teeth is unrelated to the perverse energy at work, which is nonetheless perverse heat (see Sinusitis).

We may differentiate between an imbalance in shou yang ming (large intestine) and zu yang ming (stomach) by paying attention to the semiological and anatomical signs. In Chapter 26 of the *Ling Shu,* we read concerning toothache:

> In cases of pain in the teeth, if the patient can tolerate cold water, we needle zu yang ming. If he cannot tolerate cold water, we needle shou yang ming.[386]

The anatomical distinction is also to be found in the *Ling Shu:*

> When we have toothache, the upper teeth are linked to shou yang ming {large intestine} and the lower teeth to zu yang ming {stomach}. Apart from the pain in the teeth, the patient will certainly feel heat along the meridian pathway, on the right, on the left, above or below.[387]

This last semiological factor is interesting because it reveals not only the perverse energy — heat — at work, but also the meridian and its laterality.

In treating this pain, we must not forget to needle on the opposite side:

> In presence of toothache, we must needle the points of the large intestine meridian. If there is no result, we must needle the points of the meridians that lead to the teeth.[388]

Chamfrault has the following commentary on this passage:

> If the pain is above and if we needle below, this is a form of opposite-side treatment. If the pain is on the right side and if we needle on the left side, this is opposite-side treatment. If there is toothache and we needle the points of the large intestine meridian, this is normal. If we needle any other meridian, this is a form of opposite-side treatment.[389]

Qi Bo goes on to say:

> If the perverse energy passes from the large intestine meridian to the stomach meridian, there will be pain and a sensation of cold in the teeth and lips. Before treatment, we must observe the back of the hand. If there is a congested zone, we must bleed it, disperse it, and apart from this, needle the point neiting {ST-44}; also the ting point of the thumb, shaoshang {LU-11}; and the ting point of the index finger, shangyang {LI-1}.[390]

Another point that must be considered in the treatment of toothache is daying (ST-5), mentioned by Qi Bo:

> "Daying {ST-5} is the jing point where the energy from shou yang ming passes into zu yang ming. The energy passes through this point and penetrates deeply into the teeth of the mandible; if the patient is sensitive to the cold, we tonify the point, if not we disperse it.[391]

The physician Bian Que advises us as well:

Do not forget to needle this point in toothache with swelling in the cheeks.[392]

Daying is located on the mandible, a little below (one unit) the angle of the maxillaries, over the lower dental nerve.

Among other Yang Ming points useful for treating toothache are the rong (cold) points erjian (LI-2) and neiting (ST-44), the great points hegu (LI-4) and zusanli (ST-36) and the luo point of the large intestine, pianli (LI-6). In the *General Treatise on Acupuncture* we find several mentions of taixi (KI-3), the point that corrects the anergic factor in chronic infections (see Shao Yin). For tooth decay and the symptomatic treatment of toothache the main points to remember are: LI-1, LU-11, ST-45, ST-44, LI-2, LI-4, LI-6, ST-36, ST-5 and KI-3.

Trace element treatment of tooth decay and toothache has been discussed in many doctoral theses. Keep in mind the correction of the terrain and the necessity of prescribing manganese-copper and occasionally copper-gold-silver (anergia) — or more simply and necessarily, copper alone. Copper acts locally on infections (Earth). The catalytic action of fluoride has been widely demonstrated[393] and its prescription by intensive electrolysis in tooth decay is of capital importance, with amelioration of the terrain. The decalcification and the catalysis that causes lysis of the hard tissues of the teeth may be arrested by trace element fluoride.

There is one factor that is widely recognized to be at the root of a patient's predisposition to dental caries — the histological quality of the enamel. This quality is linked to the terrain:

> Patients who consume many carbohydrates, even if their dental hygiene is insufficient, will have fewer cavities than those who consume fewer carbohydrates, have meticulous dental hygiene practice, but whose enamel is of poor quality.[394]

As a consequence, subjects of Metal constitution are those who are most exposed to tooth decay: Yang Ming-Metal and Tai Yin-Metal. This is confirmed in practice. The Yang Ming-Earth sanguine subjects and the Tai Yin-Earth amorphous subjects are not excluded from this predisposition. Their terrains, too, must be corrected by manganese-cobalt and zinc-copper, or zinc-nickel-cobalt respectively. They are perhaps more sensitive to carbohydrates and to the enzymatic phenomena that affect the collagenases (flesh = collagen).

In sum, we may say that the temperament that is the most sensitive to ORL pathology is Yang Ming-Metal, more so than Yang Ming-Earth, and to a lesser degree, Tai Yin. In Chinese medicine, it is common that a single physiopathology corresponds to several diseases that are individually defined by Western medicine. We often find that patients suffering from one disorder of the ORL sphere suffer at the same time from colitis or respiratory disorders.

Ophthalmological Pathology

Two passages from the ancient Chinese texts deserve mention. First, the words of Qi Bo in Chapter 30 of the *Ling Shu:*

> When the wei energy, created by the stomach, is deficient, the eyesight is weakened.[395]

381

Elsewhere, we find an anatomical observation concerning the energization of the eyeball:

> The point xuanlu {GB-5} is the point where the energy of shou tai yang {small intestine} penetrates through the little capillaries into the meridian of the gallbladder.
>
> It is the energy of zu yang ming that passes to the nose and reaches the face. But through this point xuanlu {GB-5}, it reaches the face and the eyes. In consequence, in any disorder affecting the eyes we must needle this point, tonify it or disperse it, depending on if there is an excess or a deficiency.[396]

This point is the convergence of the three Yang. This must be remembered when we are confronted with ophthalmological disorders such as ocular complications of high blood pressure or of diabetes due to imbalance in Yang Ming.[397]

Infectious Pathology

Yang Ming, like Tai Yin, plays an active role in infectious pathology. It closes inward; Tai Yin opens outward. The two meridians together represent the energy level at which the Yang (perverse energy) and the Yin (body energy) fight to win or to defend the energetic territory.

> Tai Yin is Yin, Yang Ming is Yang. One of the two meridians may be in excess or be deficient. The perverse energy may attack one or the other; this is why the symptoms are different. The meridian Yang Ming corresponds to the Yang, to the energy of the heaven, it governs the outside of the body; the meridian Tai Yin corresponds to the Yin, to the energy of the Earth, it governs the inside of the body. If the perverse energy attacks the Yang meridian, it enters the six bowels. If it attacks the Yin meridian, it enters the five organs.[398]

This passage presents us with the occasion to note that the deficiency or excess of one or the other of these two meridians is noticeable in so far as its vulnerability to the perverse energy is concerned. Husson translates:

> They are alternately in excess and deficient, in opposition to and in conformity with, the seasons.[399]

This allows us to assume a susceptibility to one perverse energy or another, depending on the temperament. The terrain will then physiologically determine relative excess or deficiency of energy within the meridian and also its vulnerability — its ability to adapt to the seasons. This is true for Yang Ming and Tai Yin and, generally speaking, for all the meridians and temperaments. Symptomologically:

> When the perverse energy attacks the six bowels, the patient presents a fever, he cannot stay calmly in bed {agitation} and he may have dyspnea.[400]

A rise in body temperature is a consistent sign of attack against the six bowels that involves Yang Ming. In all cases of fever that are obviously caused by attack of perverse energy, we will expect to treat Yang Ming.

• **Fever and Antipyretic Treatment**

This is confirmed in Chapter 31 of the *Su Wen* that deals with the signs of progression of the perverse energy through the six meridians, in chronological order: Tai Yang, Yang Ming, Shao Yang, Tai Yin, Shao Yin, Jue Yin. When the perverse energy[401] reaches Yang Ming, fever appears:

> The second day, the Yang Ming meridians are affected, these meridians pass beside the nose and to the eyes, the patient presents a fever, with the sensation of pain in the eyes[402] and of dryness in the nose, he cannot sleep tranquilly, he is agitated.[403]

The chapter then discusses a possible amelioration where the perverse energy leaves the meridians in the order of its chronological penetration. The departure of the perverse energy from Yang Ming corresponds with the disappearance of the fever:

> On the eighth day the meridians of Yang Ming quiet down, the fever drops.[404]

A specific case, the aggression against Yang Ming and Tai Yin, is described:

> If the meridians of Yang Ming and Tai Yin are affected at the same time, on the second day, the patient presents fullness in the abdomen, anorexia, and delirium.[405]

Another case involves the intermittent fevers associated with malaria. In the symptomology of the primary channel of the stomach we read:

> All the disorders caused by disturbances of the blood must be treated through this meridian: madness, intermittent fevers {malaria} etc.[406]

We may also read in Chapter 26 of the *Ling Shu:*

> For intermittent fever, when the patient is not thirsty and has a fever every other day, we must needle the stomach meridian zu yang ming. On the contrary, if he is thirsty, with fever every day, we must needle the large intestine meridian shou yang ming.[407]

And in the *Su Wen:*

> The meridian Yang Ming in excess is a sign of energy and of a lack of blood. This will cause imbalance of the blood, with frequent fevers.[408]

For all these reasons, the antipyretic treatment depends on the points of Yang Ming.

The doctor Zang, in the *Treatise on Acupuncture and Moxibustion,* advises us to "needle quchi {LI-11} for fevers of long duration."[409] The choice of the modern authors for the symptomatic treatment of fevers is quchi (LI-11) and dazhui (GV-14).[410] We must remember that the *Ling Shu* does not recommend needling when there is high fever. These points alone, however, seem able to bring down the temperature. If we hesitate, we may always apply the sudorific treatment indicated in the *Ling Shu* (see Infectious Pathology in Tai Yin). For a high temperature, we may treat Yang Ming with massage. This enables us to avoid needling as much as possible. This advice is given by Qi Bo in the chapter "The Art of Needling":

> If the patient presents a high temperature throughout the body, with delirium and visions, we must needle the points of zu yang ming located over the capillaries. If there is a congestion of blood in this region, we must bleed them. Besides this, with the patient lying on his back, get behind his head and pinch the carotid between thumb and forefinger, renying {ST-9}, for a while, then massage along the pathway of the artery as far as the clavicle.[411] This is the art of dispersing heat.[412]

Yang Ming seems to be the primary meridian for fighting fever and heat. We may needle and bleed the capillaries and massage the heavenly window point, renying (ST-9).

The explanation of this antipyretic property of Yang Ming is energetic. Qi Bo explains:

> The meridian Yang Ming in excess indicates an excess of energy and a lack of blood.[413]

This applies to the three Yang. But for Shao Yang the resulting pathology is muscular,[414] while for Tai Yang it is osseous.[415] For Yang Ming types, the clinical consequences of excess of energy and lack of blood involve "imbalance of the blood, with frequent fevers."[416]

This indicates the importance of Yang Ming in the physiology of the blood, in short, in immunity. It is addressed, in a more general sense, to the element Earth and to the importance of the spleen in this pathology. This observation sheds light on the passage dealing with semiology in Chapter 10 of the *Ling Shu* concerning the stomach meridian:

> All the disorders caused by disturbances of the blood must be treated through this meridian — profuse sweating, epistaxis, intermittent fevers, affections of the lips {post infectious herpes}, sore throat.[417]

This shows that the Chinese understood perfectly the relationships between immunity, hematology, spleen and stomach (see Physiology in this chapter). These are examined in our discussion of malaria and the hematological diseases and their classical infectious complications in the chapter devoted to Tai Yin.

There are many reasons to choose the points of Yang Ming in treating patients for fever and infection. A sanguine subject is particularly exposed to these pathologies, because of his constitutional excess of Yang Ming.

Chronobiology of Yang Ming

Diurnal Rhythm

Shou yang ming's hour is mao: from 5 am to 7 am. Its animal is the dragon. Zu yang ming's hour is chen: from 7 am to 9 am. Its animal is the serpent.

Annual Rhythm

The rhythm of Yang Ming corresponds to the summer.[418] Its various disturbances are likely to be exacerbated during summer. Depending on their nature, the symptomology varies:

> Shivering with cold: Yang Ming carries the number seven {wu in the 12 terrestrial branches}. In May the Yin begins within the Yang at its full strength; shivering with cold is the result of the interference of Yin with Yang in its fullness.

> Swelling in the tibia region with inability to move the thigh: The decline of Yang commences and the Yin makes its first appearance. The struggle between these two is the cause of swelling in the tibia region with inability to move the thigh.

> Choking and ascites: The Yin again appears from below and brings about the xie {perverse energy} that comes to reside between the viscera where it causes ascites.

> Chest pain with lack of qi: a damp qi is in the viscera {spleen and stomach}. Water is Yin and if the yin is central it leads to dyspnea and a lack of qi. In severe cases of blockage of qi, there is aversion to people and to fire, convulsive fears {starts} caused by the noise of wood: this is a rivalry between the Yin and the Yang; the fire and water are incompatible.[419] There is desire for seclusion and confinement: rivalry of Yin and of Yang, exhaustion of Yang and ripening of Yin.

> Delirious fits, desire to perch in a high place, to undress and wander aimlessly: the struggle between the Yin and the Yang has removed to the exterior and causes the victim to cast off his clothing.

> Settling of the xie in the vascular branches triggering headache, epistaxis, swelling of the abdomen: The qi of Yang Ming flows upward in the plexus of Tai Yin.[420]

The preceding text shows that the rhythm of Yang Ming coincides with the end of summer (heat wave), the height of Yang. In another reference, referring to the two Earth viscera, the stomach and the spleen, we are informed that these viscera are not linked to any particular rhythm:

> The energies of the spleen and the stomach are not influenced by the four seasons; they are constantly in activity in all seasons.[421]

385

Terrestrial Duodecimal Rhythm

The fourth and tenth years correspond to Yang Ming.[422]

Monthly Rhythm

Shou yang ming corresponds to the second month of spring, Zu yang ming corresponds to the third month of spring.[423]

Rhythm of Yang Ming in the Lower Limb

The third and fourth months correspond to zu yang ming in the left and in the right.[424]

Rhythm of Yang Ming in the Upper Limb

In the upper limb the energy evolves in ten-day cycles: the fifth day represents shou yang ming on the left; the sixth day shou yang ming on the right.[425]

Synopsis of the Yang Ming Temperament

In summary, Yang Ming subjects are ambivalent and correspond to two different temperaments. The Yang Ming-Earth is the sanguine type described by Gaston Berger, stout and often in a good mood. The Yang Ming-Metal is Berger's phlegmatic type, distinguished and reserved, sometimes dark, ill-tempered and misanthropic. Except for some sanguine subjects, both are characterized by activity that is regular, consistent, efficient and discrete. Each individual may be more or less jovial or restrained, opportunistic or regular and may be distinguished for his judgement or his faithfulness.

In pathology, the biggest danger is that of vascular disorders that affect the arteries without functional or neurotonic antecedents (angina pectoris, infarction, arteriopathy, high blood pressure, stroke), particularly during the second half of their lives. The progressively plethoric and apoplectic complexion of certain sanguine Yang Ming patients, within whom arteriosclerosis is developing, signals long in advance the approaching vascular accident. Our surprise is great when it occurs among Yang Ming-Metal patients. Neither the complexion nor the behavior, the lifestyle nor the lack of anxiety allows us to predict vascular disorders. It is in these subjects that heart attacks surprise us the most. Gastric and intestinal pathology is characteristic of Yang Ming. It involves either hiatal hernia early in life or chronic disorders. These are the same chronic stomach pains, the same "indigestion," the same constipation presented by the patient's father or mother. This delicate digestive syndrome is recognizable from its association with certain typical symptoms — respiratory sensitivity during childhood, asthma, regular sinus trouble (with or without epistaxis), chronic rhinitis and numerous dental cavities. It is among these patients that we occasionally find hemorrhagic recto-colitis, when the temperament is associated with the anergic Shao Yin behavior.

Rheumatologically, Yang Ming patients suffer more often than others from epicondylitis, or from scapulo-humeral periarthritis, if not from rheumatoid arthritis or psoriatic rheumatism. They are also given to hypothyroidism and to diabetes. The latter aggravates the vascular risk. Psychiatrically, the manic fits that characterize an excess of Yang in Yang Ming have become rare. We more often witness fits of melancholia, depression or the obsessional neuroses that happen only to these patients. Yang Ming patients are often feverish, sometimes inexplicably so, with a shivering that has been likened to malaria. Malaria is a risk for these patients. Such are the characteristics of this double temperament and of its pathology.

Yang Ming is the meridian to treat when we wish to act upon the body's temperature and on arterial disorders, acute pulmonary edema, hematemesis and ascites. It contains much blood and much energy. It is easy to understand that the needling of hegu (LI-4), zusanli (ST-36) and even sanyinjiao (SP-6) is beneficial for these subjects. The perfect correlation observed between the behavior and pathology of Yang Ming patients and manganese-cobalt and manganese-copper justifies their prescription in the treatment of Yang Ming patients. Zinc-nickel-cobalt and zinc-copper may also be considered.

387

Notes

[1] See Hematology in Shao Yin.

[2] Pancreozymin and cholecystokinin are structurally very similar to gastrin and possess the same tetrapeptide terminal.

[3] *Su Wen* (8), Chapter 8, p. 46.

[4] *Su Wen* (28), Chapter 8, p. 95.

[5] Nguyen Van Nghi (66), p. 15.

[6] The posterior projection point of this zone is surely gaohuang (BL-38), as its name indicates: "envelope of the region between the heart and the diaphragm."

[7] Vander *et.al.* (114), pp. 378-379.

[8] Malmejac (42), p. 361.

[9] Vander *et.al.* (114).

[10] *Su Wen* (8), Chapter 8, p. 46.

[11] Nguyen Van Nghi (66), p. 15.

[12] *Ling Shu* (8), Chapter 18, p. 395.

[13] Some authors, based on certain translations of the *Nan Jing*, include the kidneys and the liver within the lower burner. This interpretation is not incompatible with the other one. The kidneys and the liver may be considered as sites of concentration and distribution of wei qi. For the moment, the different opinions are unclear.

[14] *Ling Shu* (8), Chapter 18, p. 395.

[15] *Ibid.*, Chapter 48, p. 475.

[16] This carotid point is just over the baroreceptors of the carotid artery.

[17] This comparison is not exclusive, as wei qi is also active in thalamic thermoregulation, and the stomach, which produces wei qi, is in harmony with the subject's mood, with the pancreas, and thus with the pituitary gland. (*Cf.* Earth constitution and corticothalamic adaptation disorders.)

[18] *Ling Shu* (8), Chapter 12, p. 382.

[19] *Su Wen* (8), Chapter 24, pp. 104-105.

[20] Shanghai quotes the *Ling Shu* on this, as Roustan points out: "Wei qi, which initially circulates superficially in the skin, flows first into the luo mai." The modern authors stress the importance attributed to wei qi in the *Su Wen* regarding the physiology of the acupuncture points: "Man possesses twelve great points {shu points on the meridians} and 354 small points, which are the places where wei energy lodges and where the perverse energy is located" Roustan (99), p. 26. See also wei qi, capillaries and blood in Dermatology in Jue Yin.

[21] *Su Wen* (28), Chapter 18, p. 121.

22 This corresponds to lieque (LU-7), jingqu (LU-8) and taiyuan (LU-9), the points on the lung meridian at which we palpate the pulse and determine the quality of the blood and energy of the different Chinese functions. The stomach's part of the energy is gathered by the lung at zhongwan (CV-12), xiawan (CV-10) and shangwan (CV-13), and transmitted through the anastomotic loop of the twelve primary channels.

23 The "one-meter pond" corresponds anatomically to the forearm, from the wrist to the inside elbow, particularly along the path of the large intestine meridian.

24 The translation, "one-meter pond," is actually incorrect, as the meter is not a Chinese measurement. It has become established through usage, however.

25 *Ling Shu* (8), Chapter 60, p. 504.

26 We find this among some chronic polyarthralgic patients, and in Dupuytren's contracture, where the skin of the hand and forearm is very dry and rough. These are feng-wei diseases (see Tai Yin).

27 *Ling Shu* (8), Chapter 74, pp. 534-535. See also Chamfrault (7), pp. 177-179.

28 *Su Wen* (8), Chapter 18, p. 74-78.

29 *Ibid.*, p. 78.

30 Nguyen Van Nghi (59), p. 301.

31 *Su Wen* (8), Chapter 18, pp. 74-78. The pulse of Yang Ming (and of Shao Yang and Tai Yang) is taken at three levels of the left wrist (thumb, bar and foot). See Introduction.

32 *Su Wen* (28), Chapter 21, p. 96.

33 As a whole, *i.e.* thumb, bar and foot together.

34 *Su Wen* (59), Chapter 7, p. 301.

35 *Ibid.*, p. 303.

36 *Ibid.*

37 "Qi hao allows us to judge the state of the Yin; ren ying allows us to judge the state of the Yang" *Ling Shu* (8), Chapter 19, p. 402.

38 It is also important to take the femoral pulse (qichong, ST-30) and the temporal pulse (touwei, ST-8).

39 *Ling Shu* (8), Chapter 10, p. 361.

40 *Ibid.*

41 Shanghai (106).

42 Roustan (99), p. 25.

[43] *Ling Shu* (8), Chapter 75, p. 541.

[44] *Ibid.*, Chapter 23, p. 442.

[45] The hollow of the chest refers to the intercostal spaces. *Cf.* Dinouart (16).

[46] *Ling Shu* (8), Chapter 26, p. 429.

[47] Chamfrault (8), p. 359.

[48] *Ling Shu* (8), Chapter 60, p. 504.

[49] The beishu or yu points of the back (BL-13, BL-15, BL-18, BL-20, BL-23).

[50] *Ling Shu* (8), Chapter 2, p. 315.

[51] *Ibid.*

[52] *Ibid.*, Chapter 60, pp. 503-504.

[53] Together, they make up the organ and bowel of Metal, which explains the characteristic hyposthenia among Metal subjects, which is blatant among apathetic patients and, to a lesser extent, among plegmatic ones.

[54] *Ling Shu* (8), Chapter 2, p. 315.

[55] *Ibid.*, Chapter 4, p. 328.

[56] It is not unusual to find this sign among children whose parents or grandparents present diabetes or vascular disorders.

[57] *Su Wen* (8), Chapter 62, p. 226.

[58] This may be aggravated by external perverse heat.

[59] Since the upper and lower burners are insufficient, the excess Yang (fire) will tend to rise.

[60] It is interesting to note the meaning of these terms.

[61] There is a direct link with cardiac rhythm.

[62] Nguyen Van Nghi (66), Chapter 18, p. 266.

[63] *Ling Shu* (8), Chapter 26, p. 429.

[64] Chamfrault (7), pp. 346-351.

[65] *Ibid.*

[66] Zusanli is the origin of a secondary channel that diffuses the energy downwards and terminates in the third toe. See Nguyen Van Nghi (67), p. 106.

[67] *Da Cheng* (8), p. 343.

[68] Chamfrault (8).

[69] Nonetheless, we find cardiac and respiratory dyspnea symptoms mentioned for the thoracic stomach meridian points qihu (ST-13), kufang (ST-14), wuyi (ST-15), yingchuang (ST-16), rugen (ST-18) and chengman (ST-20). It is worthwhile to apply pressure to these points before needling to determine those that are the most painful.

[70] *Ling Shu* (28) , Chapter 24, p. 422.

[71] From chongyang (ST-42), the meridian is connected to Tai Yin at yinbai (SP-1) by way of a small liaison channel, which is not the transverse luo channel.

[72] *Ling Shu* (8), Chapter 65, p. 514.

[73] See mechanism of cold compression in the discussion of sinusitis in ORL, this chapter.

[74] *Ling Shu* (8), Chapter 21, p. 406.

[75] This point is over the carotid artery, and caution must be exercised when needling it.

[76] *Ibid.*

[77] *Su Wen* (8), Chapter 49, p. 181.

[78] See Mai Van Dong (40), pp. 19-22.

[79] *Ling Shu* (8), Chapter 35, pp. 446-448.

[80] *Ibid.*

[81] *Su Wen* (8), Chapter 21, p. 96.

[82] *Su Wen* (28), Chapter 44, p. 167.

[83] Chong mai, every bit as much as zu yang ming, is an essential channel active in the distribution of energy within the body: Yang Ming distributes wei qi and rong qi, while chong mai distributes yuan qi and jing qi.

[84] At the point taixi (KI-3), at the posterior tibial artery.

[85] *Ling Shu* (8), Chapter 38, p. 453.

[86] As does the stomach meridian (see Physiology of Yang Ming).

[87] This is evocative of the celiac trunk and its branches; the arteries beside the umbilicus, integral with the ramifications of the stomach meridian, suggest the bilateral point tianshu (ST-25), "celestial pivot," encountered above.

[88] *Ling Shu* (8), Chapter 62, p. 507.

[89] If the excess of Yang energy is Shao Yang, the result may be the opposite: the feet are burning hot. This is certainly linked to a phlebitis type pathology.

[90] See jing qi and its relationships with cholesterol and the vascular system (a "curious bowel") in the constitution of arteriosclerosis (Shao Yang).

[91] *Ling Shu* (8), Chapter 75, p. 541.

[92] The adjective "warm" here applies to the needles, and not necessarily to the limbs. *Ling Shu* (8), Chapter 21, p. 407-408.

[93] Here, the *Su Wen* is quoted in *Ling Shu* (8), Chapter 21, pp. 407-408.

[94] *Ibid.*, Chapter 73, p. 533.

[95] For the physiology of xuanzhong (GB-39), see Cerebrovascular Pathology (Neurology).

[96] This is true if treatment is initiated immediately.

[97] *Su Wen* (8), Chapter 63, p. 231.

[98] *Su Wen* (28), Chapter 7, p. 91.

[99] *Su Wen* (59), p. 313.

[100] *Su Wen* (8),p. 44.

[101] The carotid pulse corresponds to renying (ST-9).

[102] Close to jingming (BL-1). Tai Yang is linked with the body fluids in the upper part of the body, which affects its meridian at the point jingming (see Tai Yang and Opthalmology in Jue Yin).

[103] *Su Wen* (8), Chapter 18, p. 77.

[104] *Su Wen* (28), p. 123.

[105] Husson translates, "If the stomach flows backwards, decubitus is intolerable," and, "this is a reflux within Yang Ming." This is a clear indication of a backward flow along the stomach meridian.

[106] Husson says, "Stasis of the water qi," (28), p. 174.

[107] *Su Wen* (8), Chapter 34, p.130-131.

[108] Up to this point, the tendency for excessive energy within a meridian to turn into upsurging wind has been associated especially with the liver and gallbladder meridians.

[109] *Ling Shu* (8), Chapter 34, pp. 444-445.

[110] Jue, which means blockage, is the equivalent of what Chamfrault and Nguyen Van Nghi termed *kut* in their studies of the disorder. In the chapter devoted to these jue, we find descriptions of most emergencies. Jue is the underlying mechanism responsible for all cardiovascular accidents.

[111] Husson translates this as a blockage of the energy of the lung (rather than the meridian), which makes more sense.

[112] *Su Wen* (8), Chapter 45, p. 171.

[113] *Ling Shu* (8), Chapter 34, pp. 444-445.

[114] Chamfrault (7), p. 346.

[115] Husson translates thus: ''In energy blockages of the stomach. . .''

[116] *Su Wen* (8), Chapter 45, pp. 170-171.

[117] *Ibid.*, Chapter 59, p. 498.

[118] For accumulation in the belly alone, see Ascites, below.

[119] See Fabre (18).

[120] Although burong (ST-19) seems ambivalent.

[121] We must therefore include the vomica associated with an abscess of the lung.

[122] Chamfrault (7), p. 339. Thoracic fullness may also be treated by the following points: ST-12, ST-13, ST-14, ST-15, ST-16, ST-18, ST-19 and ST-21. The *Da Cheng* is more descriptive and insists on kufang (ST-14) and chengman (ST-20) in cases of pulmonary disorders. In cases of cardiac disorders, on the other hand, only burong (ST-19) is indicated. Thus in cases of pulmonary disorders of cardiac origin (acute or chronic cor pulmonale), burong (ST-19) seems to be the preferable point.

[123] *Ibid.*, p. 335.

[124] *Su Wen* (8), Chapter 23, p. 102.

[125] Studied in detail in Requena (92).

[126] Diarrhea is studied below.

[127] *Ling Shu* (8), Chapter 29, p. 436.

[128] These subjects are indeed given to vomiting, because of their gastric vulnerability and also because of their sensitivity to the ''bitter'' flavor, the nemesis of all who have an excess of fire.

[129] *Su Wen* (8), Chapter 10, p. 52.

[130] *Ling Shu* (8), Chapter 59, p. 498.

[131] *Ibid.*, Chapter 28, pp. 432-433. See Gastritis in the chapter devoted to Shao Yin. See also Requena (79).

[132] This is the opposite, a deficiency of Yang Ming.

[133] *Su Wen* (8), Chapter 64, p. 238.

[134] This is because the heat of the stomach evaporates the liquids.

[135] *Ling Shu* (8), Chapter 10, p. 361.

[136] *Su Wen* (8), Chapter 17, p. 71.

[137] *Ibid.*, Chapter 60, p. 214.

[138] *Ling Shu* (8), Chapter 33, pp. 441-442.

[139] *Ibid.*, Chapter 80, p. 557.

[140] Requena (90).

[141] Symptoms described by the *Trung Y Hoc,* in Nguyen Van Nghi (65).

[142] The skin is related to the element Metal; a dull skin is a sign of an imbalance in the stomach. Indeed, Yang Ming subjects sometimes have a blackish complexion (see Psychiatry).

[143] *Ling Shu* (8), Chapter 46, p. 471.

[144] *Ibid.*

[145] *Cf.* Shao Yin.

[146] *Su Wen* (28), Chapter 17, p. 118.

[147] Nguyen Van Nghi (65).

[148] Chamfrault's translation of "degenerative stomach disease." Chamfrault (7), pp. 430 and 632.

[149] *Ibid.*

[150] See this semiology in the *Da Cheng* (Gastritis in Shao Yin).

[151] *Da Cheng* (7), pp. 343-448.

[152] Menetrier (46), p. 78.

[153] Requena (86).

[154] *Ling Shu* (8), Chapter 4, p. 330.

[155] The large intestine is a bowel.

[156] *Ling Shu* (8), Chapter 19, p. 399.

[157] *Ibid.*, p. 401.

[158] Probably bronchial and asthmatic. We must therefore be wary of the semiological definition, "feeling of energy which rises to the upper part of the body," which does not only correspond to the cardiovascular jue.

[159] Chamfrault (7), p. 626.

[160] *Ibid.*, p. 641. The *Ling Shu* goes on to discuss the excess of the small intestine, and describes the symptoms we have considered to be those of the renal colic attack. The *Ling Shu* is consistent in its treatment: qihai (CV-6) alongside xiajuxu (ST-39), with the dispersion of the lung meridian (see Tai Yang).

[161] This is tianshu (ST-25), which is the mu point of the stomach.

[162] *Ling Shu* (8), Chapter 26, p. 429.

[163] Vander *et.al.* (114), p. 379.

[164] *Su Wen* (8), Chapter 23, p. 102.

[165] *Ling Shu* (8), Chapter 29, p. 436. A specific form of epidemic cold (see our discussion of curious perverse energy in the Introduction) is responsible for cholera. There are two other forms of cholera: cholera from heat and aberrant cholera. See Nguyen Van Nghi (70), p. 671.

[166] *Ling Shu* (8), Chapter 34, pp. 444-445.

[167] *Ibid.*

[168] *Ling Shu* (28), Chapter 17, p. 116.

[169] This corresponds to xiawan (CV-10).

[170] The problems involved in translating the Chinese terms are such that "swelling of the belly" and "fullness of the chest" may mean distension and thoracic oppression, whereas they may also refer to ascites or pericarditis with dyspnea. This all depends on the clinical context. The former interpretation may also represent an earlier phase that evolves into the latter phase.

[171] Especially when it is concentrated at xiawan (CV-10).

[172] *Ling Shu* (8), Chapter 35, pp. 447-448.

[173] *Ibid.*

[174] *Ibid.*, Chapter 22, p. 413. This represents the third case of mental disorder whose origin is organic and falls outside the realm of psychiatric pathology, which is discussed in the chapter devoted to "madness," as translated by Chamfrault. The first case is the apoplectic coma (see Neurology in Yang Ming), the second is the uremic coma (see Nephrology in Shao Yin). We must, then, read "mental disturbance" or "alteration" where Chamfrault writes "madness."

[175] *Su Wen* (8), Chapter 28, p. 116.

[176] The usual point is zhongwan (CV-12).

[177] *Cf.* Nguyen J. and Reboul J.L., "Techniques speciales des aiguilles," Conference au troisieme seminaire d'acupuncture du G.E.R.A., Toulon, 1978.

[178] Chamfrault (7), p. 347.

[179] *Ling Shu* (8), Chapter 19, p. 402.

[180] G.E.R.A. translation of the Shanghai treatise, quoted by Nguyen (57), p. 122.

[181] See Cardiovascular Pathology, above.

[182] *Su Wen* (28), Chapter 7, p. 91.

[183] *Ibid.*

[184] Chamfrault (7), p. 314.

[185] *Ling Shu* (8), Chapter 19, p. 401.

[186] *Su Wen* (28), Chapter 41, p. 192.

[187] *Cf.* Rheumatology in Tai Yin.

[188] *Ling Shu* (8), Chapter 10, p. 360.

[189] *Ibid.*, Chapter 21, p. 409.

[190] *Ibid.*, Chapter 10, p. 361.

[191] *Ibid.*, Chapter 26, p. 426.

[192] Nguyen Van Nghi (67), p. 159, as well as the modern Shanghai charts.

[193] Nguyen Van Nghi (65), p. 311.

[194] *Da Cheng* (7), p. 352.

[195] *Ling Shu* (8), Chapter 10, pp. 360-361.

[196] *Ibid.*

[197] In the order of anastomosis of the meridians, zu tai yin precedes shou shao yin (heart).

[198] *Ling Shu* (8), pp. 351-352.

[199] *Ibid.*

[200] Menetrier (46), p. 91.

[201] The physiopathology of hyperparathyroidism is complex because Shao Yin is also involved (polyuro-polydipsic syndrome, calcic lithiasis, renal insufficiency, etiology of dialysis). The Shao Yin knot, lianquan (CV-23), seems more closely related to the parathyroid than to the thyroid.

[202] *Ling Shu* (8), Chapter 9, p. 353.

[203] *Su Wen* (8), Chapter 62, p. 224.

[204] *Ibid.*, Chapter 46, p. 173.

[205] All these points, with the exception of qishe (ST-11), are heavenly window points.

[206] *Su Wen* (28), p. 208.

[207] *Su Wen* (8), Chapter 64, pp. 237-238.

208 *Ibid.*

209 Translation of the *Trung Y Hoc,* quoted in Nguyen Van Nghi (67), p. 667.

210 *Su Wen* (8), Chapter 3, p. 24.

211 Soulie de Morant (107), p. 717.

212 Such is the case in apoplexy.

213 *Su Wen* (8), Chapter 29, p. 118.

214 See yellow eyes and semiology of the large intestine meridian in Chapter 10 of the *Ling Shu.* The physiological explanation is the evaporation of the body fluids because of the heat (see also Small Intestine, Tai Yang).

215 *Su Wen* (28), Chapter 42, p. 197.

216 *Su Wen* (8), Chapter 18, p. 77.

217 *Ling Shu* (8), Chapter 23, p. 414.

218 *Ibid.,* Chapter 75, p. 543.

219 *Su Wen* (8), Chapter 21, p. 96.

220 *Ling Shu* (8), Chapter 24, p. 420. "Glair creates heat; heat creates the wind," according to the *Zu Dan Xi,* a classical text mentioned by the modern authors of Shanghai (105). This implicates the deficiency of the spleen, related to the excess of glair, which is transformed into heat.

221 *Ibid.*

222 On the hairline, linqi (GB-15) is located directly over the pupil; benshen (GB-13) directly over the outer canthus of the eye. Touwei (ST-8) is also located on the hairline, outside of benshen, and as far from benshen as benshen is from linqi.

223 However, this point is mentioned in the *Ling Shu* in relation to vascular accidents (see below).

224 Chamfrault (7), p. 327. See also, Bossy and Maurel (3), p. 63.

225 *Ibid.*

226 *Da Cheng* (107), Chapter 11, p.718.

227 Translation of the Chinese term, "growling in the throat."

228 Chamfrault (7), pp. 776-782.

229 Tai Yang represents the bladder and small intestine, Shao Yang the gallbladder and Yang Ming the stomach and large intestine.

230 Chamfrault (7), pp. 776-777.

231 *Ibid.*

[232] *Ibid.*

[233] *Ibid.*

[234] All these symptoms represent the functional symptomology of Shao Yang apart from any organic disease and unrelated to vascular pathology, as we have already seen to be the case of Yang Ming headaches. Symptoms are occasionally common to functional and organic diseases where there is no necessary link between the two.

[235] Nguyen Van Nghi (67), pp. 667-668.

[236] *Ibid.*

[237] Deep coma with limpness does seem to correspond to Yin accidents.

[238] *Ibid.*

[239] Soulie de Morant (107), p. 718.

[240] Aphasia is a symptom of considerable gravity and is considered to represent an organic illness.

[241] Chamfrault (7), p. 776.

[242] We may compare this with the mention of incontinence of fecal matter and the departure of shen referred to in gastroenterology.

[243] For example, the desertion of the energy of the spleen that accompanies an excess of Yang Ming is responsible for the vascular accident. The desertion is secondary to a primary obstruction of the energy. This corresponds somewhat to the aggravation of a coma after a bowel accident. The Yin symptoms follow the Yang symptoms.

[244] Nguyen Van Nghi (67), pp. 285-290.

[245] This could represent the anxiety that precedes or accompanies embolisms, such as pulmonary embolism, whose warning signal was no mystery to the ancient Chinese, as we have seen in our discussion of pulmonary infarction.

[246] Zu Lien, quoted in Chamfrault (7), p. 777.

[247] If the patient is young, the most probable etiology is the rupture of an aneurism, whose prognosis is not a bright one.

[248] *Su Wen* (8), Chapter 48, pp. 179-180.

[249] Soulie de Morant (107), p. 718.

[250] *Ibid.* All these signs show that the corresponding organs have been abandoned by their shen, leading to incontinence, in a broad sense of the term, of the secretions that correspond to the territory of each organ (urine, bronchial mucus, saliva, etc.).

[251] Dizziness in the context of lipothymia, weakness and sometimes hypotension such as spasmophilia or Meniere's vertigo. See Jue Yin.

[252] *Ling Shu* (8), Chapter 52, pp. 487-488.

[253] *Ibid.*, Chapter 26, p. 426.

[254] *Su Wen* (8), Chapter 24, p. 105.

[255] The arm sanli, shousanli (LI-10), is a point on the arm that is the equivalent of the leg sanli, zusanli (ST-36). The former is located on shou yang ming, the latter on zu yang ming. It has considerable neurological action.

[256] *Ling Shu* (8), Chapter 23, p. 414.

[257] Hemiplegia, Shanghai (105).

[258] *Ling Shu* (8), Chapter 44, p. 468.

[259] See chongyang (ST-42) in the treatment of manic fits in the discussion of psychiatry.

[260] *Su Wen* (8), Chapter 52, p. 192.

[261] *Ibid.*, Chapter 32, p. 125.

[262] Shangjuxu (ST-37) means "great excess in the upper region." It is the special action he point for the large intestine (Yang Ming) on the stomach meridian (also Yang Ming). Xiajuxu (ST-39) means "great deficiency in the lower region." It is the special action he point of the small intestine (Tai Yang). We have seen how needling the three points disperses the gallbladder as well (see Functional Colonopathy). These three points thus represent all the Yang. This is certainly why shangjuxu (ST-37) and xiajuxu (ST-39) are the shu points of the du mai (see *Ling Shu,* Chapter 33).

[263] Chamfrault (7), p. 776.

[264] Soulie de Morant (107), p. 718.

[265] That is, if the treatment is undertaken on a subject who is not in a coma. Otherwise, block the nose manually if needles are to be used. If moxa is used, this is unnecessary.

[266] Blocking of the facial orifices is often recommended in the texts dealing with loss of consciousness and coma.

[267] *Ling Shu* (8), Chapter 75, pp. 538-539.

[268] *Ibid.*, Chapter 5, p. 334.

[269] *Ibid.*

[270] In the geometrical center of the palmar aspect of the distal phalange of the ten fingers.

[271] Shanghai (105).

[272] *Ling Shu* (8), Chapter 75, p. 542.

273 Chamfrault (7), p. 778.

274 *Ibid.* See also, Shanghai (105).

275 Soulie de Morant (107), p. 719.

276 *Ling Shu* (8), Chapter 5, pp. 334-335.

277 *Ibid.*

278 *Da Cheng* (7), pp. 518 and 565. Paresis of the four limbs may be neurological or psychiatric (hysteria).

279 *Ibid.*

280 *Ling Shu* (8), Chapter 21, p. 406. The points beneath the tongue are the points yuye on the right and jinjin on the left, also indicated for cases of aphonia (Nguyen Van Nghi, *Le mensuel de medecin acupuncteur,* No. 1, May 1973, p.37). See physiology of the points in the discussion of psychiatry of Tai Yang.

281 This paragraph was quoted from in our discussion of cor pulmonale. The semiology includes migraine and a risk of stroke. The energy that may only rise to the upper part of the body does so because of a blockage of the energy within xu li, which prevents the lung from performing its task of injecting energy into the general energy flow within the twelve meridians and creates a deficiency of energy in its cephalic channel. This is why the luo point, lieque (LU-7), is needled to resolve the imbalance, as well as in cases of cerebrovascular accidents. This is another way of acting upon the imbalance, *i.e.* downstream from the obstruction, to reinforce the organ's pumping action.

282 *Da Cheng* (7), pp. 518 and 565. See also ORL and ophthalmology in Shao Yang.

283 *Ibid.*

284 *Ling Shu* (8), Chapter 23, p. 414.

285 Shanglianquan (M-HN-21) is one unit above lianquan (CV-23).

286 *Ling Shu* (8), Chapter 24, p. 421.

287 Soulie de Morant (107), p. 718.

288 *Trung Y Hoc,* quoted by Nguyen Van Nghi (67), p. 668. See also Shanghai (105).

289 Shanghai (105). See also *Da Cheng* (107), p. 719.

290 *Ibid.*

291 *Ling Shu* (8), Chapter 9, p. 357.

292 Shock refers here not to the Western notion of collapse, but rather to the shock caused by a sudden transport of wind to the brain.

[293] *Da Cheng* (107), Chapter 11, p. 718.

[294] Che wei is the Chinese name for *Polypodium Lingua,* a type of fern whose stem and spicy tasting leaves are diuretic, according to Chamfrault (9), p. 219.

[295] *Da Cheng* (7), Chapter 11, p. 718.

[296] *Ibid.*

[297] *Ibid.*

[298] Shanghai (105).

[299] *Ibid.*

[300] See Roustan (98), Mai Van Dong and Nguyen Van Nghi (41), Cheng-Kong and Hsing-Tai Liu (12), pp. 41-43.

[301] *Cf.* Shao Yang.

[302] *Su Wen* (8), Chapter 30, p. 119.

[303] *Ling Shu* (8), Chapter 10, p. 361.

[304] *Ibid.,* pp. 375-376.

[305] And converges at baihui (GV-20), according to Nguyen Van Nghi (67), p. 163.

[306] *Ling Shu* (8), Chapter 10, pp. 375-376.

[307] *Su Wen* (8), Chapter 45, p. 619.

[308] *Su Wen* (28), Chapter 30, p. 163.

[309] *Encyclopedia Universalis* (113), pp. 767-769.

[310] Perlemuter and Cenac (70).

[311] *Ibid.*

[312] Soulie de Morant (107), p. 498.

[313] The semiology for this point is, ''Sees ghosts, laughs, sings, undresses, runs'' Chamfrault (7), p. 357.

[314] Soulie de Morant (107), p. 499.

[315] Chamfrault writes that the patient should drink water in which rusty nails have been boiled.

[316] *Su Wen* (28), Chapter 46, p. 208.

[317] *Cf.* Hyperthyroidism.

[318] *Ling Shu* (8), Chapter 10, p. 361.

[319] As they are both non-emotive, what distinguishes the phlegmatic type from the apathetic is that the former is active while the latter is inactive. Activity is inhibited as the pathology evolves, transforming the patient's behavior.

[320] *Ling Shu* (8), Chapter 10, p. 361.

[321] The blackish complexion of the kidney predominates in the face, especially below the eyes. The black complexion characteristic of Yang Ming is uniform, as if the subject were dirty.

[322] Especially when there is obsession. In melancholia, the thymic aspect may be a sign of Water as it may be of Earth. This complexion has given these subjects the name "atrabilious" (black bile), which they share with those who suffer from a kidney deficiency. See Shao Yin.

[323] Whose behavior is of course compulsive and exorcistic.

[324] Soulie de Morant (107), p. 501.

[325] *Ibid.*, p. 442.

[326] *Su Wen* (28), Chapter 30, p. 163.

[327] *Ling Shu* (8), Chapter 10, p. 360.

[328] Chamfrault translates, "to wrinkle."

[329] *Su Wen* (28), Chapter 1, p. 72.

[330] *Ibid.*

[331] *Su Wen* (8), Chapter 4, p. 32.

[332] See the chapter devoted to Dermatology of Tai Yin, in Vol. II of *Terrains and Pathology.*

[333] *Ling Shu* (8), Chapter 75, p. 540.

[334] Chamfrault (7), pp. 797-798.

[335] *Ibid.*

[336] Nguyen Van Nghi (62), p. 130.

[337] Chamfrault (7), p. 388.

[338] As well as in rhinopharyngitis and otitis, as we will see below.

[339] The allergic (Wood) or anergic (Water) behavior may dominate, but then the hyposthenia is always subjacent.

[340] Menetrier (46), p. 101.

[341] Apart from the special case of acute suppurating ethmoiditis found among children, which presents a risk of orbital suppurative accumulation.

[342] These symptoms are also present in imbalances of the small intestine meridian, which complicates the diagnosis based solely on the semiology of the meridians when we do not take temperament into account.

343 *Ling Shu* (8), Chapter 10, pp. 360-361.

344 *Ibid.*

345 *Ibid.*, p. 375. This may be confused with a pathology of the luo channel of the heart, as sore throat and aphonia are common to both.

346 *Ling Shu* (8), Chapter 26, p. 427.

347 *Su Wen* (8), Chapter 45, p. 171.

348 Points mentioned in the *General Treatise on Acupuncture,* Chamfrault (7), pp. 792-793.

349 *Ibid.*

350 *Ibid.* See ORL in Tai Yang.

351 *Cf.* Shao Yin.

352 Parotitis is rather a Tai Yin (spleen) affection (see Tai Yin).

353 The original energy of the body, not to be confused with the essential energy (jing) that is linked to the kidney, and that also causes deafness when it is deficient (see ORL in Shao Yin).

354 *Ling Shu* (8), Chapter 28, pp. 434-435.

355 This point on zu tai yang is linked with the occiput and the teroauricular region.

356 Concerning the symptomology of the luo of the large intestine, deafness corresponds to an excess of the luo. See *Ling Shu* (8), Chapter 10, p. 375.

357 *Su Wen* (8), Chapter 63, pp. 231-232.

358 *Ibid.*, p. 232.

359 *Ling Shu* (8), Chapter 10, p. 365.

360 *Su Wen* (8), Chapter 45, p. 170.

361 Chamfrault (7), pp. 801-802.

362 *Ibid.*, pp. 398-463.

363 *Ling Shu* (8), Chapter 26, p. 427.

364 Capillary microcirculation and diseases caused by perverse heat with purpura are Shao Yin imbalances, energetically similar to acute articular rheumatism (see Shao Yin).

365 *Su Wen* (8), Chapter 37, p. 144.

366 *Ling Shu* (8), Chapter 4, p. 326.

[367] *Ibid.*, Chapter 23, pp. 416-417.

[368] See Gynecology in Jue Yin.

[369] As might be expected, the semiology for ququan (LV-8) includes epistaxis. Chamfrault (7), p. 583.

[370] *Ling Shu* (8), Chapter 23, pp. 416-417.

[371] Tianfu is the heavenly window point on the lung meridian.

[372] *Ling Shu* (8), Chapter 21, pp. 406-407.

[373] *Su Wen* (8), Chapter 63, p. 232.

[374] *Ibid.*, Chapter 4, p. 27.

[375] *Ibid.*, Chapter 61, p. 218.

[376] *Ibid.*, Chapter 37, p. 145.

[377] *Ling Shu* (8), Chapter 10, p. 375.

[378] *Ibid.*

[379] The *Da Cheng* includes in the semiology of this point the symptom ''unceasing epistaxis'' Chamfrault (7), p. 461.

[380] Soulie de Morant (107), p. 854.

[381] *Ling Shu* (8), Chapter 10, p. 360.

[382] *Ibid.*

[383] *Ibid.*, p. 375.

[384] *Ibid.*, Chapter 10, pp. 361-375.

[385] *Su Wen* (8), Chapter 63, p. 232.

[386] *Ling Shu* (8), Chapter 26, p. 427.

[387] *Ibid.*, Chapter 74, p. 536.

[388] *Su Wen* (8), Chapter 63, pp. 234-235.

[389] *Ibid.*

[390] *Ibid.*

[391] *Ling Shu* (8), Chapter 21, p. 407.

[392] Chamfrault (8), p. 332.

[393] Legrand (37).

[394] Perlemuter and Cenac (70).

[395] *Ling Shu* (8), Chapter 30, p. 438.

[396] *Ibid.*, Chapter 21, p. 407.

[397] See also Presbyopia and zusanli (ST-36) in Jue Yin.

[398] *Su Wen* (8), Chapter 29, p. 117.

[399] *Su Wen* (28), Chapter 29, pp. 161-162.

[400] *Ibid.* Husson adds "dyspnea if the illness relapses." This is an allusion to cardiovascular and respiratory accidents.

[401] The perverse energy here is cold: "Fever occurs generally subsequent to exposure to cold," the first sentence of the chapter.

[402] See mention of xuanlu (GB-5) in Ophthalmology, above.

[403] *Su Wen* (8), Chapter 31, pp. 120-122.

[404] *Ibid.*

[405] Fullness in the abdomen and anorexia are Tai Yin symptoms. Delirium is, on the other hand, a Yang Ming symptom. There is an association of the two symptomologies.

[406] *Ling Shu* (8), Chapter 10, p. 361.

[407] *Ibid.*, Chapter 26, p. 427.

[408] *Su Wen* (8), Chapter 64, p. 237. We may relate the case of a typical sanguine subject, who was diabetic, arteritic, plethoric, talkative, jovial and given to excess, and who suffered periodically (summer and winter) from pseudopaludism. All paraclinical and radiological test were negative; moreover, the patient had no case history of malaria. However, only quinine brought him relief. This sort of case is not exceptional in clinical practice.

[409] Chamfrault (7), p. 314.

[410] The *Ling Shu* indicates also dazhu (BL-11), a point that is close to dazhui (GV-14), is one of the specific points of du mai. *Ling Shu* (8), Chapter 75, p. 539, and Chapter 33, p. 443.

[411] Thus, from renying (ST-9) to qishe (ST-11).

[412] *Ling Shu* (8), Chapter 75, p. 542. This is the same chapter in which the sudorification treatment is mentioned.

[413] *Su Wen* (8), Chapter 64, p. 237.

[414] "This will lead to muscular disorders and swelling in the sides," says Qi Bo (see Shao Yang).

[415] See Rheumatology in Tai Yang, Vol. II.

[416] *Su Wen* (8), Chapter 64, p. 237.

[417] *Ling Shu* (8), Chapter 10, p. 361.

[418] *Cf.* relationship with Fire and with manganese-cobalt.

[419] Here, Yang Ming is comparable to Fire (as we have said at the beginning of this chapter) and in opposition to Water.

[420] *Su Wen* (28), Chapter 49, p. 215. This passage says much regarding the morbid vulnerability of Yang Ming, as we have pointed out throughout this chapter.

[421] *Su Wen* (8), Chapter 29, p. 118. Husson translates this as follows: "The earth, which gives birth to the creatures, follows the model of the universe. She is above, below, at the head and the feet, and she cannot limit herself to a single season. (28), p. 162.

[422] *Ibid.* (8), Chapter 66, p. 250.

[423] *Su Wen* (28), Chapter 7, p. 91.

[424] *Ling Shu* (8), Chapter 41, pp. 459-460.

[425] *Ibid.*

Bibliography

(0) Barlow, J.B., *et.al.* "The Significance of Late Systolic Murmurs." *Am. Heart J.* 66 (1963).

(1) Bensky, D., and J. O'Connor, trans. *Acupuncture, a Comprehensive Text.* Chicago: Eastland Press, 1981.

(2) Berger, G. *Traite pratique d'analyse du caractere.* Paris: Presse Univ. de France, 1974.

(3) Bossy, J., and J.C. Maurel. *Monographie de reflexotherapie appliquee: acupuncture.* Paris: Ed. Masson, 1976.

(4) Caen, J. *Communication au colloque sur la regulation de la fecondite.* Paris: 1979.

(5) Caroli, J., and Y. Hecht. "Foie." *Encyclopedia Universalis.* Paris: 1976 ed. 7: 83-92.

(6) —. *Le foie et ses maladies.* Paris: Presse Univers. de France, 1967.

(7) Chamfrault, A. *Traite de medecine chinoise.* Vol. 1. Angouleme: Ed. Coquemard, 1964.

(8) —. Vol. 2. Angouleme: Ed. Coquemard, 1973.

(9) —. Vol. 3. Angouleme: Ed. Coquemard, 1959.

(10) Chamfrault, A., and Nguyen Van Nghi. *Traite de medecine chinoise.* Vol. 6. Angouleme: Imp. de la Charente, 1969.

(11) Chein, E.Y.M. "Acupuncture: Useful Adjunct in the Treatment of Carbon Monoxide Poisoning." *Amer. J. Acup.* 3.2 (1975): 154-156.

(12) Cheng-Kong, N.G., and Hsing-Tai Liu, M.D. "Experiences with Head Acupuncture in Cerebral Hemorrhage." *Amer. J. Acup.* 2.1 (1974).

(13) Criley, J.M., *et.al.* "Prolapse of the Mitral Valve: Clinical and Cineangiocardiographic Findings." *Br. Heart J.* 28 (1966): 448.

(14) Debeaux, J.O. *Essai sur la pharmacie et la matiere medicale des Chinois.* Paris, 1865.

(15) Dessertene, F., *et.al. Etude des souffles mesosystoliques de pointe, et leurs rapports avec le fonctionnement de l'appareil mitral.* Coeur, 1974. 5: 543-642.

(16) Dinouart, P. "Un aspect particulier de la pathologie viscerale." *Actes du Troisieme Seminaire d'Acupuncture.* Toulon: G.E.R.A., 1978. 62-70.

(17) D'Omezon, Y. "Comment concevoir aujourd'hui la spasmophilie de l'adulte." *Medit. Med* 156 (1978).

(18) Fabre, J. "Resultats d'une etude comparative de maladies asthmatiques traites par acupuncture specifique et placebo." *Actes du Quatrieme Seminaire d'Acupuncture.* Toulon: G.E.R.A., 1979.

(19) Faubert, A. *Traite didactique d'acupuncture traditionelle.* Paris: Ed. Tredaniel Guy, 1977.

(20) Filliozat, J. "La nature du Yoga dans sa tradition." Preface to *Etudes instrumentales des techniques du Yoga.* By T. Brosse. Paris: Ecole Francaise d'Extreme-Orient (Maisonneuve), 1963.

(21) Gourion, A. "A propos de la theorie du Triple Rechauffeur." *Mens. Med. Acup.* 51-56 (1978).

(22) Granet, M. *La pensee chinoise.* Paris: Ed. Albin Michel, 1974.

(23) Guiguet, L. "Etude critique des resultats obtenus par acupuncture pendant six mois dans une consultation hospitaliere." M.D. dissertation. Marseille, 1977ᵢ

(24) Hamburger, J., *et.al. Petite encyclopedie medicale.* Paris: Ed. Flammarion Medecine, 1972.

(25) Hanania, G. "Prolapsus valvaire mitral." *Act. en Card.* 32 (1978).

(26) Harrison, T.R. *Principes de medecine interne.* Paris: Ed. Flammarion Medicine-Sciences, 1975.

(27) Huard, P., and M. Wong. *La Medecine chinoise.* Paris: Presses Univ. de France, 1969.

(28) Husson, A., trans. *Huang Di Nei Jing Su Wen.* Paris: Ed. A.S.M.A.F., 1973.

(29) Ionescu-Tirgoviste, C., *et.al.* "The Hypoglycemic Mechanism of the Acupuncture Point Spleen-Pancreas 6." *Am. J. Acup.* 3.1 (1975): 18-33.

(30) Kappas, A. "Biologic Action of some Natural Steroids on the Liver." *N. Eng. J. Med.* 278 (1978).

(31) Kay, C.R. "Incidence des contraceptifs oraux." *Le Quotidien du Medecin* 1879 (1979).

(32) Kespi, J.M. "Diagnostic des diarrhees par les huit regles." *Actes du Quatrieme Seminaire d'Acupuncture.* Toulon: G.E.R.A., 1979.

(33) Laboratoire Labcatal. *Contribution a l'etude de la therapeutique fonctionelle.* Paris: Imp. Rivaton et Cie, 1972.

(34) Lamorte, J.R. "L'epaule douloureuse: approche occidentale et orientale des pathogenies et therapeutiques." M.D. dissertation. Marseille, 1977.

(35) Laugt, A. "L'electrobiophotographie: etude critique de la litterature mondiale, perspective d'avenir." M.D. dissertation. Grenoble, 1978.

(36) Lavier, J. *Histoire, doctrine et pratique de l'acupuncture chinoise.* Paris: Ed. Veyrier H., 1974.

(37) Legrand, S. "Role effecteur des cations metalliques sur les cinetiques enzymatiques parodontales." Third cycle doctoral thesis. *Scien. Odont.* (1976).

(38) Leung Kwok Po. "Maladie de shan." *Rev. Franc. d'Acup.* 11 (1977): 27-32.

(39) Lhermitte, F. *Pathologie medicale,* vol. 1. Paris: Ed. Flammarion, 1963.

(40) Mai Van Dong. "Etude etiopathogenique et therapeutique des hypertensions arterielles." *Mens. Med. Acup.* 9 (1974): 19-22.

(41) Mai Van Dong, Nguyen Van Nghi. "Applications therapeutiques de la craniopuncture." *Mens. Med. Acup.* 22 (1975): 61-66.

(42) Malmejac, J. *Elements de physiologie.* Paris: Ed. Flammarion, 1976.

(43) Maspero, H. *Le Taoisme et les religions chinoises.* Paris: Ed. Gallimard, 1971.

(44) Menetrier, J. *Introduction a la medecine fonctionelle.* Paris: Ed. Pacomhy, 1954.

(45) —. *Introduction a une psychophysiologie experimentale.* Paris: Ed. Le Francois, 1967.

(46) —. *La Medecine des fonctions.* Paris: Lib. Le Francois, 1974.

(47) —. *Les Diatheses: symptomes, diagnostic et therapeutique catalytique.* Paris: Ed. Le Francois, 1972.

(48) Meunier, C. *L'ametallose enzymatique.* Paris: Imp. Rivaton et Cie, 1976.

(49) Michel, D. ''Interet therapeutique de l'acupuncture dans la lutte contre l'intoxication tabagique.'' M.D. dissertation. Marseille, 1977.

(50) —. ''Traitement des gonarthroses.'' *Actes du Quatrieme Seminaire d'Acupuncture.* Toulon: G.E.R.A., 1979.

(51) Michel-Wolfromm, H. *Gynecologie psychosomatique.* Paris: Ed. Masson, 1964.

(52) Mussat, M. *Physique de l'acupuncture: hypotheses et approches experimentales.* Paris: Ed. Le Francois, 1974.

(53) —, trans. *Sou Nu King.* Paris: Ed. Seghers, 1978.

(54) Needham, J. *La science chinoise et l'Occident.* Paris: Ed. du Seuil, 1973.

(55) —. *Chemistry and Chemical Technology.* Vol. 3 of *Science and Civilization in China.* Cambridge: Cambridge Univ. Press, 1974.

(56) Nguyen, J., *et.al. La Rhinofaciopuncture.* Toulon: G.E.R.A., 1978.

(57) Nguyen-Recours, C. ''Acupuncture et gynecologie medicale: bases et interet therapeutique.'' M.D. dissertation. Marseille, 1978.

(58) Nguyen Van Nghi. ''Etats depressifs et medecine chinoise.'' *Mens. Med. Acup.* 1 (1973): 11-20.

(59) —, trans. *Hoang Ti Nei King Souenn,* vol. 1. Marseille: Imp. Sodecim, 1973.

(60) —. ''Les Icteres.'' *Nouv. Rev. Intern. d'Acup.* 20 (1971).

(61) —. ''Les Insomnies.'' *Nouv. Rev. Intern. d'Acup.* 25 (1972).

(62) —. ''Le Systeme des 'huit meridiens curieux'.'' *Mens. Med. Acup.* 44 (1979).

(63) —. ''Mo King, de Wang Chou Ho.'' *Mens. Med. Acup.* 31, 32, 34, 36, 37, 39 (1976-1977).

(64) —. ''Nan King, de Pienn Tsio.'' *Mens. Med. Acup.* 21-23, 25-30 (1975-1976).

(65) Nguyen Van Nghi, *et.al. Theorie et pratique de l'analgesie par acupuncture.* Marseille: Imp. Socedim, 1974.

(66) Nguyen Van Nghi, *et.al.*, trans. *Hoang Ti Nei King Souenn,* vol. 2. Marseille: Imp. Socedim, 1975.

(67) Nguyen Van Nghi, and E. Picou. *Pathogenie et pathologie energetiques en medecine chinoise.* Marseille: Don Bosco, 1971.

(68) Nguyen Viet Hong, P. "La pensee medicale chinoise." *Mens. Med. Acup.* 28, 30, 32-38 (1976-1977).

(69) Pasteur Vallery-Radot, *et.al. Pathologie medicale.* Paris: Ed. Med. Flammarion, 1963.

(70) Perlemuter, L., and A. Cenac. *Dictionnaire pratique de medecine clinique.* Paris: Ed. Masson, 1977.

(71) Pernice, C. "La Hanche douloureuse." *Actes du Quatrieme Seminaire d'Acupuncture.* Toulon: G.E.R.A., 1979.

(72) —. "L'Epiconcylite." *Actes du Deuxieme Seminaire d'Acupuncture.* Toulon: G.E.R.A., 1977. 127-130.

(73) —. "Les Dysmenorrhees." *Actes du Deuxieme Seminaire d'Acupuncture.* Toulon: G.E.R.A., 1977. 163-170.

(74) —. "Traitement des nevralgies cervicobrachiales par acupuncture." M.D. dissertation. Marseille, 1976.

(75) Picard, H. *Utilisation therapeutique des oligo-elements.* Paris: Ed. Maloine S.A., 1975.

(76) Rat, P. "Essai de traitement par acupuncture dans certaines affections hepatiques." M.D. dissertation. Marseille, 1977.

(77) Reid, J.V.O. "Mid-Systolic Clicks." *South Afr. Med.* 5.35 (1961): 353.

(78) Requena, Y. "Etude du trajet du meridien principal du poumon, ses branches et consequences en pathologie." *Mens. Med. Acup.* 59 (1979): 337-348.

(79) —. "Introduction a l'acupuncture en gastro-enterologie." M.D. dissertation. Marseille, 1974.

(80) —. "La Recto-colite hemorragique." *Actes du Quatrieme Seminaire d'Acupuncture.* Toulon: G.E.R.A., 1979.

(81) —. "Le Meridien de la vesicule biliaire: cours de premiere annee d'acupuncture." *Archives du G.E.R.A.* Marseille: Fac. Med., 1978.

(82) —. "Le Meridien de vessie: cours de premiere annee d'acupuncture." *Archives du G.E.R.A.* Marseille: Fac. Med., 1975.

(83) —. "Le Meridien du coeur: cours de premiere annee d'acupuncture." *Archives du G.E.R.A.* Marseille: C.E.D.A.T., 1979.

(84) —. "Le Meridien du foie: cours de premiere annee d'acupuncture." *Archives du G.E.R.A.* Marseille: Fac. Med., 1977.

410

(85) —. "Le Meridien des reins: cours de premiere annee d'acupuncture." *Archive du G.E.R.A.* Marseille: Fac. Med., 1975.

(86) —. "Les Colopathies fonctionelles en acupuncture." *Mens. Med. Acup.* 43 (1977): 97-108.

(87) —. "Les Neuropathies peripheriques." *Actes du Quatrieme Seminaire d'Acupuncture.* Toulon: G.E.R.A., 1979.

(88) —. "Observations et resultats a moyen terme sur le traitement anti-tabac par acupuncture (a propos de 100 cas)." *Medit. Med.* 5.118 (1977): 9-14.

(89) —. "Physiopathologie et traitement de la recto-colite ulcereuse en acupuncture." *Actes du Quatrieme Seminaire d'Acupuncture.* Toulon: G.E.R.A., 1979.

(90) —. "Traitement de l'ulcere de l'estomac par acupuncture." *Mens. Med. Acup.* 30 (1976): 389-396.

(91) —. "Traitement des conjonctivites par acupuncture." *Actes du Premier Seminaire d'Acupuncture.* Toulon: G.E.R.A., 1976. 41-46.

(92) Requena, Y., *et.al. L'Acupuncture en gasto-enterologie.* Toulon: G.E.R.A., 1977.

(93) —. "Theorie, pratique et resultats de la desintoxication tabagique par acupuncture." *Mens. Med. Acup.* 35 (1976): 193-202.

(94) Requena, Y., and Nguyen Van Nghi. "L'Acupuncture et les risques de transmission de l'hepatite virale." *Mens. Med. Acup.* 18 (1975): 295-297.

(95) Requena, Y., and P. Rat. "Traitement de l'hepatite virale par acupuncture." *Mens. Med. Acup.* 56 (1978): 219-229.

(96) Rideller, B., and H. Colognac. "'Un Souffle innocent' qui peut tuer: la maladie de Barlow." *Medit. Med.* 158 (1978): 41-50.

(97) Robert, L., *et.al. Enzymologie et immunologie dans l'atherosclerose.* Paris: Ed. Baillere, 1964.

(98) Roustan, C. "L'Acupuncture cerebrale." *Nouv. Rev. Int. d'Acup.* 30 (1973).

(99) —. *Bases fondamentales.* Vol. 1 of *Traite d'acupuncture.* Paris: Ed. Masson, 1978.

(100) Roy, J.C. "Approche theorique, clinique et experimentale de l'acupuncture." M.D. dissertation. Marseille, 1976.

(101) Rubin, M. *Manuel d'acupuncture fondamentale.* Mercure de France, 1974.

(102) Sal, J. *Les Oligo-elements catalyseurs en pratique journaliere.* Paris: Ed. Maloine, 1977.

(103) —. "Rapports entre acupuncture et therapeutique catalytique." *Nouv. Rev. Int. d'Acup.* 22 (1971).

(104) Schatz, J. "Precisions sur les energies hereditaires." *Mens. Med. Acup.* 39 (1977): 355-358.

411

(105) Shanghai Hospital Medical Group. *Traite d'acupuncture.* Trans. G.E.R.A. Toulon: Archives du G.E.R.A., 1975-1976.

(106) Shanghai Traditional Medical Research Institute. *Cahier d'explication pour les planches anatomiques.* Shanghai: Ed. du Peuple, 1975.

(107) Soulie de Morant, G. *L'Acuponcture chinoise.* Paris: Ed. Maloine S.A., 1972.

(108) Stoicescu *et.al.* "Contributions cliniques et experimentales concernant l'utilisation de l'acupuncture sur la mobilite du tube digestif." *Nouv. Rev. Int. Acup.* 5 (1967).

(109) Tomatis, A. *L'Oreille et la vie.* Paris: Ed. Robert Laffont, 1977.

(110) Tremollieres, J. *Nutrition et metabolisme.* Paris: Ed. Flammarion, 1971.

(111) Trinh, R. "A propos de quelques cas de lombalgies et lombosciatiques traitees par acupuncture." M.D. dissertation. Marseille, 1974.

(112) —. "Les nevralgies faciales." *Actes du Deuxieme Seminaire d'Acupuncture.* Toulon: G.E.R.A., 1977.

(113) "Typologies psychologiques." *Encyclopedia Universalis,* 1975 ed. 13: 767-770.

(114) Vander, A.J., *et.al. Physiologie humaine.* Montreal: Ed. MacGraw-Hill, 1977.

(115) Verdoux, B. "La Sphygmologie chinoise." M.D. dissertation. Montpellier, 1978.

(116) Vitiello, A. "Aspects theoriques et bilan des anesthesies par acupuncture realisees en France." M.D. dissertation. Marseille, 1973.

(117) Wilhelm, R., and E. Perrot. *Yi King le livre de transformations.* Paris: Librairie de Medicis, 1973.

412

Index

417

emphysema: 74, 344
encephalon: 233-234, 236, 312-313
endarteritis obliterans: 264
endemics: 261
endocarditis, bacterial: 192
endocrine: 84, 228, 243, 252, 376
endocrine disorders: 68, 70
endocrine obesity: 85
endocrine pathology: 157, 176, 228, 345
endocrinology: 190
endolabyrinthic: 276
endolabyrinthine fluids: 237
endometriosis: 219, 291
energy balance: 41
energy circulation: 16, 18, 38
energy circulation disturbances: 169
energy desertion: 361
energy excessive: 392
energy, internal: 339
energy, obstruction of: 356
energy points, CV-13, CV-12, CV-10: 341
energy-blood balance: 58, 333
enterocolitis: 73
enterogastrone: 310
enterohepatic cycle: 311
enuresis: 84, 253
envelope of heart: 255
envelope of menstrual blood and sperm: 216
envelope of uterus: 218, 255
enzymes: 36, 40, 379
eosinophilia: 259
epicondylitis: 387
epidemics: 354
epididymitis: 213
epigastralgia: 147
epigastric disorder: 336
epigastric pain: 77, 334
epilepsy: 58, 83, 120, 160-161, 230, 234, 238-239,
   248, 250-252, 254, 260, 281, 295, 359
epileptic attacks: 239, 352
epileptic organ etiologies: 238
epileptic psychosis: 248
epileptic seizures: 253
epileptic syndromes: 295
episcleritis: 269
epistaxis: 199, 222, 263, 359, 372, 374-379, 384-
   386, 404
equilibrium disorders: 239
equisetum arvense: 195
equisetum hiemale: 232
erection disorders: 224
erethism: 137-138, 191
erythema: 207
erythematous rash: 257
erythrosic complexion: 53
erythrosis in cheeks: 369
essential energy: 15, 22, 57, 194, 230, 266, 285

estradiol: 135, 292
estrogen: 195, 197, 292
estrone: 135
estroprogestative imbalance: 230
estroprogestins: 259
ethylic intoxication: 237
euphoria: 68, 240, 366
examination of the patient: 43
excess energy in shao yang: 348
excess, external: 238
excess, large intestine luo: 403
excess, lower body: 239
excess, lower limb meridians: 356
excitation: 158
exophthalmia: 157-158, 272
exophthalmic goiter, Grave's disease: 157
extrahepatic retention: 167
extra-uterine pregnancy: 223, 282
extroversion: 98
eye: 232, 239, 242, 349
eye affections: 232
eye, canthus bulging: 328
eye, ear nose and throat pathology: 168
eye of the knee: 345
eye problems: 239
eyes cannot open: 377
eyesight: 265
eyesight, and bleeding points: 173
eyesight weakened: 381

— F —
fa chen: 260
face puffy: 356
facial complexion: 51-52, 368
facial congestion: 146, 250
facial neuralgia: 19, 160, 170-171
facial paralysis: 139
facial tics: 160
fainting: 107, 158, 239-240
fall: 3
false pelvis: 215
family history: 70, 74, 86
fasciae: 5, 159
fasting: 348
fat intolerance: 218
fatigue, weakness, at end of day: 76
fear: 55, 106, 123, 225, 248, 302
fear of cold: 336
fear of wind and cold: 276
feeling of heat in the feet: 150
feet: 235, 242, 244-245
feet, paralysis: 359
fei qi: 206
femoral pulse: 389
feng: 167, 203, 206, 220, 260, 315, 348-350,
   355, 359-360
feng han: 206
feng jue: 225, 294

424

— *M* —